KU-004-086

OXFORD MEDICAL PUBLICATIONS

Oxford Handbook of
Cancer Nursing

KERRY GENERAL
HOSPITAL
HEALTHCARE LIBRARY
0667104216

Published and forthcoming Oxford Handbooks in Nursing

Oxford Handbook of Adult Nursing, 2e
Edited by Maria Flynn and Dave Mercer

Oxford Handbook of Cancer Nursing, 2e
Edited by Mike Tadman, Dave Roberts, and Mark Foulkes

Oxford Handbook of Cardiac Nursing, 2e
Edited by Kate Olson

Oxford Handbook of Children's and Young People's Nursing, 2e
Edited by Edward Alan Glasper, Gillian McEwing, and Jim Richardson

Oxford Handbook of Clinical Skills for Children's and Young People's Nursing
Edited by Paula Dawson, Louise Cook, Laura-Jane Holliday, and Helen Reddy

Oxford Handbook of Clinical Skills in Adult Nursing
Edited by Jacqueline Randle, Frank Coffey, and Martyn Bradbury

Oxford Handbook of Critical Care Nursing, 2e
Edited by Heather Baid, Fiona Creed, and Jessica Hargreaves

Oxford Handbook of Dental Nursing
Edited by Elizabeth Boon, Rebecca Parr, Dayananda Samarawickrama, and Kevin Seymour

Oxford Handbook of Diabetes Nursing
Edited by Lorraine Avery and Sue Beckwith

Oxford Handbook of Emergency Nursing, 2e
Edited by Robert Crouch, Alan Charters, Mary Dawood, and Paula Bennett

Oxford Handbook of Gastrointestinal Nursing
Edited by Christine Norton, Julia Williams, Claire Taylor, Annmarie Nunwa, and Kathy Whayman

Oxford Handbook of Learning and Intellectual Disability Nursing, 2e
Edited by Owen Barr and Bob Gates

Oxford Handbook of Mental Health Nursing, 2e
Edited by Patrick Callaghan and Catherine Gamble

Oxford Handbook of Midwifery, 3e
Edited by Janet Medforth, Linda Ball, Angela Walker, Sue Battersby, and Sarah Stables

Oxford Handbook of Musculoskeletal Nursing
Edited by Susan M. Oliver

Oxford Handbook of Neuroscience Nursing
Edited by Sue Woodward and Catheryne Waterhouse

Oxford Handbook of Nursing Older People
Edited by Beverley Tabernacle, Marie Barnes, and Annette Jinks

Oxford Handbook of Orthopaedic and Trauma Nursing
Rebecca Jester, Julie Santy, and Jean Rogers

Oxford Handbook of Perioperative Practice
Edited by Suzanne Hughes and Andy Mardell

Oxford Handbook of Prescribing for Nurses and Allied Health Professionals, 2e
Edited by Sue Beckwith and Penny Franklin

Oxford Handbook of Primary Care and Community Nursing, 2e
Edited by Vari Drennan and Claire Goodman

Oxford Handbook of Renal Nursing
Edited by Althea Mahon, Karen Jenkins, and Lisa Burnapp

Oxford Handbook of Respiratory Nursing
Edited by Terry Robinson and Jane E. Scullion

Oxford Handbook of Surgical Nursing
Edited by Alison Smith, Maria Kisiel, and Mark Radford

Oxford Handbook of Women's Health Nursing
Edited by Sunanda Gupta, Debra Holloway, and Ali Kubba

Oxford Handbook of
Cancer Nursing

Second edition

Edited by

Mike Tadman
Senior Specialist Nurse, Neuroendocrine Tumours,
Oxford University Hospitals NHS Trust, Oxford, UK

Dave Roberts
Senior Lecturer in Cancer and Palliative Care,
Oxford Brookes University, Oxford, UK

Mark Foulkes
Nurse Consultant and Macmillan Lead Cancer Nurse,
Royal Berkshire NHS Foundation Trust, Reading, UK

HSE South Kerry General Hospital
Library

KH05064

OXFORD
UNIVERSITY PRESS

OXFORD
UNIVERSITY PRESS

Great Clarendon Street, Oxford, OX2 6DP,
United Kingdom

Oxford University Press is a department of the University of Oxford.
It furthers the University's objective of excellence in research, scholarship,
and education by publishing worldwide. Oxford is a registered trade mark of
Oxford University Press in the UK and in certain other countries

© Oxford University Press 2019

The moral rights of the authors have been asserted

First Edition published in 2007
Second Edition published in 2019

Impression: 1

All rights reserved. No part of this publication may be reproduced, stored in
a retrieval system, or transmitted, in any form or by any means, without the
prior permission in writing of Oxford University Press, or as expressly permitted
by law, by licence or under terms agreed with the appropriate reprographics
rights organization. Enquiries concerning reproduction outside the scope of the
above should be sent to the Rights Department, Oxford University Press, at the
address above

You must not circulate this work in any other form
and you must impose this same condition on any acquirer

Published in the United States of America by Oxford University Press
198 Madison Avenue, New York, NY 10016, United States of America

British Library Cataloguing in Publication Data
Data available

Library of Congress Control Number: 2018964269

ISBN 978-0-19-870110-1

Printed and bound in China by
C&C Offset Printing Co., Ltd.

Oxford University Press makes no representation, express or implied, that the
drug dosages in this book are correct. Readers must therefore always check
the product information and clinical procedures with the most up-to-date
published product information and data sheets provided by the manufacturers
and the most recent codes of conduct and safety regulations. The authors and
the publishers do not accept responsibility or legal liability for any errors in the
text or for the misuse or misapplication of material in this work. Except where
otherwise stated, drug dosages and recommendations are for the non-pregnant
adult who is not breast-feeding

Links to third party websites are provided by Oxford in good faith and
for information only. Oxford disclaims any responsibility for the materials
contained in any third party website referenced in this work.

Preface

The editors of this book come from different nursing backgrounds but have had a primary focus on people with cancer for many years. Likewise, the contributors have been chosen for their wealth of experience and unique practice perspectives. The aim of this book is to support the development of cancer nursing practice. It does this by providing a concise reference book, as well as a handbook that is detailed and accessible to the nurse in a range of practice situations. It is aimed primarily at the nurse, or indeed other professional, who encounters people with cancer, whether in a specialist cancer role or a more general one.

Cancer treatments are changing constantly, in response to new developments, and we have aimed to represent the most recent developments in the science of cancer. To balance this, we have also tried to keep pace with the human experience of cancer, the psychosocial aspects of care, and the survivorship experience.

We have aimed to focus on the essential elements of knowledge the nurse needs to practise safely and effectively, by providing up-to-date, practice-focused, and evidence-based information. To make this accessible, we have included tables, boxes, and bullet points that emphasize key points. There are also summaries of the main implications for nursing care. As knowledge can date quickly, we have also included essential elements of the theory and principles of practice that can be adapted to the many day-to-day challenges of nursing. We hope that the concise nature of the book does not frustrate the reader, and we signpost additional reading and resources for nurses who want to take their knowledge one step further.

Of course, nursing practice is about more than just knowledge. Practice is also an art and an exercise of moral judgement and compassion. These are based on personal values and experience and are learnt through the practice of nursing and through interaction with colleagues and patients and their families. To facilitate this process, we have provided reflection points that stimulate thought, discussion, and reflection and the ongoing development of nursing skills.

We hope that this is a book that the nurse can keep to hand in practice, or at home for reference, and is friendly, supportive, and helpful.

Acknowledgements

It is not possible to acknowledge all of the people who have contributed over the years to the development of this second edition of the *Oxford Handbook of Cancer Nursing*. This includes all of the colleagues, patients, their families, and loved ones who have contributed to the wealth of practice experience on which this book is based. We owe you a deep debt of thanks.

We would also like to thank the contributors who have generously given their time to writing sections of this book, the contributors to the first edition, some of whose work has filtered through to this second edition, and the external reviewers, who have helped to shape this book with their constructive criticism and suggestions for improvements. The editors would like to thank Dr Madhumita Bhattacharyya for her contributions to the manuscript and expert review.

More specifically, we would like to thank the following.

Dave Roberts. I would like to thank all my former colleagues at the Oxford Cancer Centre and my current and former colleagues at Oxford Brookes University. This includes Mary Boulton, Eila Watson, Yolanda Eraso, and Verna Lavender, in particular, as working alongside them and sharing ideas have helped to shape my own vision of cancer care. On a personal note, I would like to thank my family and friends for their support, particularly Farzaneh, James, Mary, and Nia.

Mark Foulkes. I am very grateful for the support, help, and advice provided by my partner Catherine Bailey, whilst editing this new version of the book. I would also like to thank all my colleagues and friends at the Berkshire Cancer Centre (BCC) in Reading for their hard work and commitment on behalf of our patients. I am particularly keen to thank the members, past and present, of the Acute Oncology Service at the BCC for putting up with me and teaching me something new every day, particularly Dr Pompa Bhattacharyya, Dr Elias Pintus, Dr Esme Hill, Alice Andrews, and Mary Hill.

Mike Tadman. I would like to thank my colleagues at work who have guided my writing across a number of diverse topics, sharing ideas and challenging me constructively on many occasions. My family and friends have been unstinting in their support, particularly Nic, who keeps everything running smoothly whilst I worked on this, and without whose love and support, I could not have completed this project. Finally to my wonderful boys Morgan and Finlay, who put up graciously with my absence.

Acknowledgements

Dedications

Mark Foulkes.
This is dedicated to all those affected by cancer and those who care for them.

Dave Roberts.
I dedicate this book to the memory of my parents Irene Roberts and Griffith Davies Roberts.

Mike Tadman.
This is dedicated to all those people I've met affected by cancer, who every day teach me to be the best nurse that I can possibly be.

Dedications

Contents

Section 6 Management of Major Cancers

Section 7 Symptom management

Section 8 Oncological emergencies

Contributors

Heidi Allen

Chapter 34: Skin cancer

Macmillan Advanced Nurse
Practitioner for Skin Cancers,
Oxford University Hospitals
NHS Trust, Oxford, UK

Richard Brown

Chapter 16: Radiotherapy

Clinical Oncology Consultant,
Royal Berkshire Hospital,
Reading, UK

John Curtin

Chapter 46: Pain management

Consultant in Palliative Medicine,
Isle of Wight NHS Trust,
Mountbatten Hospice, Newport,
Isle of Wight, UK

Gail Eva

*Chapter 6: The social ex-
perience of cancer and
Chapter 10: Rehabilitation of the
cancer patient*

Senior Lecturer, Occupational
Therapy, Oxford Brookes
University, UK

Toby Eyre

*Chapter 18: High-dose therapy
(autologous transplant);
Chapter 19: Allogeneic
haematopoietic stem
cell transplantation;
Chapter 30: Haematological
cancers; Chapter 37: Bone
marrow suppression; and
Chapter 38: Blood product support*

Haematology Specialist Registrar,
Oxford Deanery, Oxford, UK

Paula Horne

Chapter 16: Radiotherapy

Radiotherapy Service Manager,
Royal Berkshire Hospital,
Reading, UK

Susi Lund

*Chapter 12: Palliative care and
Chapter 47: Symptom management at the end of life*

Nurse Consultant of End-of-
Life Care and Clinical Lead for
Hospital Palliative Care, Royal
Berkshire NHS Foundation
Trust, Reading, UK

Anne Margrethe Phillips

*Chapter 27: Upper gastrointestinal
cancers*

Upper Gastrointestinal
Advanced Nurse Practitioner,
Oxford University Hospitals
NHS Trust, Churchill Hospital,
Oxford, UK

Karen Sherbourne

*Chapter 35: Teenage and young
adult cancer*

Advanced Nurse Practitioner
and Nursing Lead for
Teenagers & Young Adults with
Cancer, Oxford University
Hospitals, Churchill Hospital,
Oxford, UK

Bridget Taylor

Chapter 50: Sexuality and cancer

Advanced Nurse Practitioner,
Community Palliative Care,
Sobell House Hospice,
Oxford, UK

Abbreviations

5FU	5-fluorouracil
ABVD	doxorubicin, bleomycin, vinblastine, dacarbazine
ACEI	angiotensin-converting enzyme inhibitor
ACS	American Cancer Society
ADH	antidiuretic hormone
AFP	alpha-fetoprotein
AHP	allied health professional
AHTR	acute haemolytic transfusion reaction
AI	aromatase inhibitor
AIDS	acquired immune deficiency syndrome
AIHA	autoimmune haemolytic anaemia
ALK	anaplastic lymphoma kinase
ALL	acute lymphoblastic leukaemia
AML	acute myeloid leukaemia
AND	Allow Natural Death
ANP	advanced nurse practitioner
ANV	anticipatory nausea and vomiting
APTT	activated partial thromboplastin time
ARDS	acute respiratory distress syndrome
ART	antiretroviral therapy
ASAP	atypical small acinar proliferation
ATRA	all-trans-retinoic-acid
AVP	arginine vasopressin
BCC	basal cell carcinoma
BCG	bacille Calmette–Guérin
BCSH	British Committee for Standards in Haematology
BEACOPP	bleomycin, etoposide, cytarabine, cyclophosphamide, procarbazine and prednisolone
BEAM	carmustine, etoposide, cytarabine, and melphalan
BEP	bleomycin, etoposide, cisplatin
BMI	body mass index
BNCT	boron neutron capture therapy
BPI	Brief Pain Inventory
CA-125	cancer antigen 125
CAM	complementary and alternative medicine; Confusion Assessment Method
CARES	Cancer Rehabilitation Evaluation System

CBT	cognitive behavioural therapy
CCG	Clinical Commissioning Group
CCM	Cancer Care Monitor
CDK	cyclin-dependent kinase
CDT	complex decongestive therapy
CEA	carcinoembryonic antigen
CHART	continuous hyperfractionated radiotherapy
CHM	complete hydatidiform mole
CHNC	Complementary and Natural Healthcare Council
CHOP-R	cyclophosphamide, doxorubicin, vincristine, and prednisolone plus rituximab
CIN	cervical intraepithelial neoplasia
CINV	chemotherapy-induced nausea and vomiting
CLL	chronic lymphocytic leukaemia
cm	centimetre
CML	chronic myeloid leukaemia
CMV	cytomegalovirus
CNS	clinical nurse specialist; central nervous system
COPD	chronic obstructive pulmonary disease
COSHH	Control of Substances Hazardous to Health
CPR	cardiopulmonary resuscitation
CRA	Clinical Research Associate
CRF	cancer-related fatigue
CRP	C-reactive protein
CSF	cerebrospinal fluid
CT	computed tomography
CTD	cyclophosphamide, thalidomide, and dexamethasone
CTZ	chemoreceptor trigger zone
CUP	cancer of unknown primary
CVAD	central venous access device
CVC	central venous catheter
CVP	central venous pressure
CXR	chest X-ray
DCIS	ductal carcinoma *in situ*
DIC	disseminated intravascular coagulation
DIEP	deep inferior epigastric perforator
dL	decilitre
DLI	donor lymphocyte infusion
DMSO	dimethylsulfoxide
DNA	deoxyribonucleic acid
DNACPR	Do Not Attempt Cardiopulmonary Resuscitation

DNAR	Do Not Attempt Resuscitation
DTC	differentiated thyroid cancer
DVT	deep vein thrombosis
EAPC	European Association for Palliative Care
EBMT	European Group for Blood and Marrow Transplantation
EBRT	external beam radiotherapy
EBV	Epstein–Barr virus
ECG	electrocardiogram
ECM	extracellular matrix
ECOG	Eastern Cooperative Oncology Group
EGF	epidermal growth factor
EGFR	epidermal growth factor receptor
EGFR-TK	epidermal growth factor receptor tyrosine kinase
EMP	extramedullary plasmacytoma
EMR	endoscopic mucosal resection
EONS	European Oncology Nursing Society
EPA	eicosapentaenoic acid
EPIC	European Pain in Cancer
EPO	erythropoietin
EPR	extrapyramidal reaction
EPS	erythropoiesis-stimulating protein
ER	(o)estrogen receptor
ERCP	endoscopic retrograde cholangiopancreatography
ESMO	European Society of Medical Oncology
ESR	erythrocyte sedimentation rate
EUS	endocospic ultrasound
FAB	French–American–British (classification)
FACT	Functional Assessment of Cancer Therapy
FAP	familial adenomatous polyposis
FBC	full blood count
FDG PET	fluorodeoxyglucose positron emission tomography
FFP	fresh frozen plasma
FISH	fluorescence in situ hybridization
FIT	faecal immunochemical test
FNA	fine-needle aspiration
FOBT	faecal occult blood test
FSH	follicle-stimulating hormone
FTC	follicular thyroid cancer
g	gram
G-CSF	granulocyte colony-stimulating factor
GCT	germ cell tumour

GFR	glomerular filtration rate
GHRH	gonadotrophin hormone-releasing hormone
GI	gastrointestinal
GIST	gastrointestinal stromal tumour
GM-CSF	granulocyte-macrophage colony-stimulating factor
GOJ	gastro-oesophageal junction
GORD	gastro-oesophageal reflux disease
GP	general practitioner
GU	genitourinary
GvHD	graft-versus-host disease
GvM	graft-versus-malignancy
Gy	gray
HADS	Hospital Anxiety and Depression Scale
Hb	haemoglobin
H&N	head and neck
HCC	hepatocellular carcinoma
HCG	human chorionic gonadotrophin
HDR	high-dose rate
HDT	high-dose therapy
HEPA	high-efficiency particulate air
HER-2	human epidermal growth factor receptor 2
HFS	hand and foot syndrome
HGPIN	high-grade prostatic intra-epithelial neoplasia
5-HIAA	5-hydroxyindoleacetic acid
HIV	human immunodeficiency virus
HLA	human leucocyte antigen
HNA	holistic needs assessment
HNPCC	hereditary non-polyposis colorectal cancer
HPV	human papillomavirus
HRT	hormone replacement therapy
HSCT	haematopoietic stem cell transplant
IASP	International Association for the Study of Pain
IBS	irritable bowel syndrome
ICHGCP	International Conference of Harmonisation Tripartite Guidelines for Good Clinical Practice
ICP	intracranial pressure
ICU	intensive care unit
IM	intramuscular
IMRT	intensity-modulated radiotherapy
INR	international normalized ratio
IOG	Improving Outcomes Guidance

IPS	interstitial pneumonia syndrome
IRMER	Ionising Radiation (Medical Exposure) Regulations
IT	intrathecal
ITP	immune-related thrombocytopenia
IV	intravenous
IVU	intravenous urography
J	joule
kcal	kilocalorie
kg	kilogram
KS	Kaposi's sarcoma
L	litre
LBC	liquid-based cytology
LCIS	lobular carcinoma *in situ*
LD	latissimus dorsi
LDH	lactate dehydrogenase
LFT	liver function test
LGBT	lesbian, gay, bisexual, or transgender
LH	luteinizing hormone
LHRH	luteinizing hormone-releasing hormone
LLETZ	large loop excision of the transformation zone
LMWH	low-molecular-weight heparin
LVEF	left ventricular ejection fraction
MA	megestrol acetate
MASCC	Multinational Association of Supportive Cancer Care
MBCT	mindfulness-based cognitive therapy
MBD	metastatic bone disease
MBP	methotrexate, bleomycin, and cisplatin
MBSR	mindfulness-based stress reduction
MDT	multidisciplinary team
MEN	multiple endocrine neoplasia
MHRA	Medicines and Health Care Products Regulatory Authority
MIBG	metaiodobenzylguanidine
mL	millilitre
MLD	manual lymphatic drainage
mm	millimetre
mmol	millimole
MMSE	Mini-Mental State Examination
MPA	medroxyprogesterone acetate
MPM	malignant pleural mesothelioma
MRCP	magnetic resonance cholangiopancreatography
MRI	magnetic resonance imaging

MSCC	metastatic spinal cord compression
MTC	medullary thyroid cancer
MTOR	mammalian target of rapamycin
MUD	matched unrelated donor
MUGA	multigated acquisition (scanning)
MUP	malignancy of unknown origin
MUSE	medicated urethral system for erections
MUST	Malnutrition Universal Screening Tool
NCAG	National Cancer Advisory Group
NCEPOD	National Confidential Enquiry into Patient Outcomes and Death
NCSI	National Cancer Survivorship Initiative
NET	neuroendocrine tumour
ng	nanogram
NG	nasogastric
NHL	non-Hodgkin lymphoma
NHLBI	National Heart, Lung, and Blood Institute
NHS	National Health Service (UK)
NICE	National Institute for Health and Care Excellence
NK	natural killer
NLPHL	nodular lymphocyte-predominant Hodgkin lymphoma
NM	nuclear medicine
NMC	Nursing and Midwifery Council
NPI	Nottingham prognostic index
NPSA	National Patient Safety Agency
NRES	National Research Ethics Service
NRS	Numerical Rating Scale
NRT	nicotine replacement therapy
NSAID	non-steroidal anti-inflammatory drug
NSCLC	non-small cell lung cancer
NSGCT	non-seminomatous germ cell tumour
O_2	oxygen
OM	oral mucositis
OOHS	Out of Hours Study
Pap	Papanicolaou
PBSC	peripheral blood stem cell
PCNSL	primary central nervous system lymphoma
PD-1	programmed cell death protein 1
PD-L1	programmed death-ligand 1
PDT	photodynamic therapy
PE	pulmonary embolus

PEG	percutaneous endoscopic gastrotomy
PET	positron emission tomography
PG-SGA	Patient-Generated—Subjective Global Assessment
PHM	partial hydatidiform mole
PICC	peripherally inserted central catheter
PJP	*Pneumocystis jiroveci* pneumonia
PLB	pursed lip breathing
PMR	progressive muscle relaxation
PPI	proton pump inhibitor
PR	progesterone receptor
PRN	*pro re nata* (as required)
PROM	Patient-Reported Outcome Measure
PSA	prostate-specific antigen
PSTT	placental-site trophoblastic tumour
PT	prothrombin time
PTC	papillary thyroid carcinoma; principal treatment centre
PTH	parathyroid hormone
PTHrP	parathyroid hormone-related protein
PTSD	post-traumatic stress disorder
PUVA	psoralen ultraviolet A
QALY	quality-adjusted life year
QoL	quality of life
RANKL	receptor activator of nuclear factor-kappa B ligand
Rb	retinoblastoma
RCC	renal cell carcinoma
RFA	radiofrequency ablation
RGF	Research Governance Framework
RhD	rhesus D
RIC	reduced-intensity conditioning
RIDDOR	Reporting Injuries, Diseases, and Dangerous Occurrences Regulations
RIG	radiologically inserted gastrostomy
RMI	Risk of Malignancy Index
RNA	ribonucleic acid
RNIV	radiotherapy-induced nausea and vomiting
RSV	respiratory syncytial virus
SABR	stereotactic ablative radiotherapy
SACT	systemic anti-cancer therapy
SALT	speech and language therapist
SaO$_2$	oxygen saturation
SBP	solitary bone plasmacytoma

SC	subcutaneous
SCC	squamous cell carcinoma
SCLC	small cell lung cancer
SGAP	superior gluteal artery perforator
SIADH	syndrome of inappropriate antidiuretic hormone
SIGN	Scottish Intercollegiate Guidelines Network
SIRT	selective internal radiotherapy treatment
SNRI	serotonin-noradrenaline reuptake inhibitor
SPARC	Sheffield Profile for Assessment and Referral to Care
SPECT	CT single-photon emission computed tomography
SPF	sun protection factor
SSRI	selective serotonin reuptake inhibitor
STI	sexually transmitted infection
STZ	streptozotocin
SUSAR	suspected unexpected serious adverse reaction
SVCO	superior vena cava obstruction
TACE	trans-arterial chemo-embolization
TCC	transitional cell carcinoma
TENS	transcutaneous electrical nerve stimulation
TK	tyrosine kinase
TKI	tyrosine kinase inhibitor
TLS	tumour lysis syndrome
TME	total mesorectal excision
TNF	tumour necrosis factor
TNM	tumour node metastasis
TRALI	transfusion-related acute lung injury
TRAM	transverse rectus abdominis muscle
TRUS	transrectal ultrasound
TSG	tumour suppressor gene
TSH	thyroid-stimulating hormone
TURBT	transurethral resection of bladder tumour
TURP	transurethral resection of the prostate
TYA	teenage and young adult
U	unit
UICC	Union for International Cancer Control
UK	United Kingdom
UKFOCSS	UK Familial Ovarian Screening Study
UKONS	United Kingdom Oncology Nursing Society
URT	upper respiratory tract
US	ultrasound
USA	United States

UTI	urinary tract infection
UV	ultraviolet
VAD	venous access device
VAS	visual analogue scale
VATS	video-assisted thoracoscopic surgery
VC	vomiting centre
vCJD	variant Creutzfeldt–Jakob disease
VEGF	vascular endothelial growth factor
VOD	veno-occlusive disease
VRS	verbal rating scale
VTE	venous thromboembolism
VUD	voluntary unrelated donor
WHO	World Health Organization

Section 1

Introduction

Chapter 1

Introduction

Scientific advances

Oncology and cancer nursing are both rapidly developing specialties. Major breakthroughs in science within the last two decades exert a major influence on practice in a number of different ways.

Continued advances in our understanding of cancer biology at a cellular level have enabled the development of a range of new biological treatments. At the time of writing, it seems that every month brings the development of new drug treatments, targeting specific changes in cancer cells. These offer hope and choice to many individuals with cancer. Their development also creates new challenges for practitioners, supporting patients with difficult treatment choices and complex symptom management. New chemotherapy drugs lead to new combinations of treatment for many cancers, with an ↑ use of concurrent chemotherapy and radiation and the addition of new agents to standard chemotherapy regimes.

Technological advances continue to enable quicker and more targeted radiotherapy planning and treatment. This has led to more intensive treatment regimes in a number of cancer sites.

These changes have occurred in the context of extended life expectancy, leading to increasing rates of cancer. More people are now living with cancer in the community. Over the last 5 years, there has been greater focus from within cancer nursing, and beyond, on addressing the needs of these individuals. Improved access to information has led to higher patient expectations about treatment choices and support. In the United Kingdom (UK), there has also been public criticism of poor cancer survival rates, compared to other developed world countries, which successive governments have sought to address.

Future scientific breakthroughs will ensure that these remain exciting and hopeful times for all those working within the cancer nursing specialty. However, the pressure of expensive new drug treatments, an ageing population, and ↑ patient expectations have created their own difficulties for health services at a time when financial resources are limited across the whole health economy.

Policy initiatives

England

The *NHS Cancer Plan* (2000)[1] set out the government strategy to tackle cancer, linking prevention, diagnosis, treatment, care, and research. This overall strategy was delivered through the 34 Cancer Networks in England and Wales and focused on reducing waiting times for cancer treatments, investing in cancer and palliative care services, and increasing the numbers of specialist cancer nurses. Specific quality standards of care were outlined in the *Manual of Cancer Service*[2] (2004), which were assessed through a process of peer review.

In 2007, the *Cancer Reform Strategy* was published, which further developed the themes from the *NHS Cancer Plan* and aimed to build on the progress made. The main headings within the strategy were:
- Preventing cancers
- Earlier diagnosis
- Ensuring better treatment
- Living with and beyond cancer
- Reducing cancer inequalities
- Delivering care in the most appropriate setting (i.e. closer to patients' homes where possible).

In 2011, following a change in government, the *Cancer Reform Strategy* was superseded by *Improving Outcomes: A Strategy for Cancer*. This document signposted a way forward for cancer services for the next 5 years, with key themes being:
- An ↑ emphasis on outcomes, rather than targets, with good data collection
- Improved information for patients, which will empower them to make choices
- Improved access to new cancer drugs via continued support of the cancer drugs fund
- A move away from acute hospital trusts being the providers of cancer care, with some elements of care being community-based or delivered by non-National Health Service (NHS) providers.

In 2015, an Independent Cancer Taskforce, chaired by the Chief Executive of Cancer Research UK, formulated and published a new strategic document *Achieving World-Class Cancer Outcomes: A Strategy for England 2015–2020*. From this document, the main priorities were:
- A renewed commitment to cancer prevention and achieving earlier diagnoses
- Establishing patient experience as being as important an indicator as safety and clinical effectiveness
- Improving support for people living with and beyond cancer
- Investment in technology and high-quality services
- Modernizing the commissioning of cancer services.

Criticisms of this document have included that, although the government commissioned the strategic review, the outcomes are not owned by it, or any particular department or organization, and that the financial investment required to transform the priorities into reality will therefore not be forthcoming.

Cancer Policy Wales

In 2016, the Welsh government published *The Cancer Delivery Plan for Wales*, which provides a plan for cancer services in Wales until 2020. This document builds on previous iterations to promote healthy lifestyles and improve early detection of cancer via ↑ public education and awareness of early cancer symptoms linked to improved access to screening. There was continued commitment to improving performance against cancer access targets, underpinned by more extensive and efficient collection of data around cancer treatment and outcomes. Access to cancer research was given a high priority, with key actions promoting higher numbers of cancer studies to be undertaken in Wales, alongside improved partnership working to try and improve the speed with which research findings are adopted in the public domain.

Cancer Policy Scotland

In 2016, the Scottish government published a wide-ranging update of its cancer strategy entitled *Beating Cancer: Ambition and Action*. Within the document, there is emphasis on outlining Scotland's particular challenges with regard to cancer, with inequalities nationally and an increasing number of patients with a cancer diagnosis—the latter being due to an ageing population and an ↑ number of patients living with cancer. The document also committed considerable funds to improving the infrastructure of cancer services in Scotland and establishing a robust cancer intelligence system.

The main focus in the document is in attempting to address the large inequalities in access to cancer and survival. These differences are most notable with areas of high social deprivation being linked to higher cancer incidence and poorer outcomes, in contrast to areas with low levels of deprivation.

Beating Cancer: Ambition and Action and other useful cancer publications can be found at the Scottish government website (⌘ http://www.scotland. gov.uk/Publications/Recent)

References

1 Department of Health (2000). *The NHS Cancer Plan: A Plan for Investment, a Plan for Reform.* London: Department of Health.
2 Department of Health (2004). *Manual for Cancer Services.* London: Department of Health.

Clinical implications

The clinical implications of recent advances and policy initiatives have been many:

- An increase in survival rates in some major cancers
- An increasing number of individuals being actively treated, including older patients and those with lower performance status, who are more susceptible to major side effects
- The development of targeted biological and immunological agents which have revolutionized systemic therapies
- Increasingly specialized cancer treatment and support
- The continued development of cancer multidisciplinary teams (MDTs) into major decision-making forums within UK cancer care
- An increasing move from inpatient care to ambulatory care, which has had major consequences for resources in outpatient and primary care
- The recent emphasis on delivering cancer care in a range of settings outside of large acute hospitals
- The cost of cancer treatments having major implications on resources in an economic climate with reduced financial resources, particularly within the public sector
- The development of acute oncology services catering for those patients presenting as emergencies with cancer-related problems
- The growth of non-medical prescribing, particularly in chemotherapy prescription.

These changes offer nurses many opportunities to develop new knowledge, skills, and career opportunities, e.g. running nurse-led clinics and prescribing medications, including subsequent doses of chemotherapy. However, as nurses take on a range of different tasks and roles, the blurring of professional boundaries, particularly with junior doctors, is also a potential area for conflict.

New treatments add another layer of complexity to decisions that patients and health-care professionals must face. It can be difficult managing patients' expectations of new treatments, which may, in reality, offer only limited advantages. Many of these new agents also create new challenges in patient management and side effect profiles, with which the cancer nurse must be familiar. Nurses have a major role to play in providing informational and psychological support for these patients.

The move to more outpatient treatment may improve the quality of life (QoL) for many patients and their families. However, patients now have less time to be fully assessed, informed, and supported by health professionals. Acute oncology services have been developed in order to rapidly assess patients with oncological problems when they are admitted as emergencies.

Cancer nurses will be expected to find ever more flexible and efficient ways of working within current resource levels, whilst specialist nurses may face increasing caseloads of patients to support. Other demands include the need for continuing professional and educational development, at a time when study leave is also under pressure. Cancer care and cancer nursing will continue to be an area of constant change and development in the near future. Though some of the developments can be predicted, and therefore planned for, e.g. the continuing increase in cancer prevalence, others are less certain. For instance, it would have been difficult to predict the great moves forward in 'personalizing' cancer care in the last 5 years where genetic profiling of patients linked to possible targeted therapies has become a reality. This has led to improved treatment, but also other challenges such as affordability of these treatments and international discrepancies in the availability of these treatments.

Specialist nursing roles

Clinical nurse specialists

One of the most significant developments in cancer nursing has been the continued development of specialist nurse posts. Many of these are site-specific clinical nurse specialists, nurses who have responsibility for the care of a particular cancer site. The clinical nurse specialist's (also sometimes known as advanced nurse practitioners, or ANPs) role allows patients and their families to receive a comprehensive and holistic approach to care from a single professional, who will often remain their 'key worker' throughout their cancer journey. The role of the 'key worker' has been formalized within national guidance for most cancer sites. With their in-depth knowledge of individual patients, clinical nurse specialists are well placed to facilitate continuity of care within MDTs and across the boundaries of primary, secondary, and tertiary care.

Clinical nurse specialists require a high level of specialist skills and knowledge. This includes expertise in the care of a specific cancer site and also broader communication, consultation, educational, managerial, and research skills. These enable them to effectively support patients and their families, and also to support non-specialist staff in working directly with cancer patients. Clinical nurse specialists often play a key role in developing and improving patient services. Examples include developing and improving patient pathways, reducing delays in diagnostic clinics, and providing patient- and family-centred follow-up. However, many nurse specialists have ever more complex roles, with continuously increasing caseloads, as new treatment options are developed. They will face increasing demands on their time.

Nurse-led clinics

Another important recent development has been the increasing number of nurse-led clinics. These often provide follow-up for patients after treatment and offer specific therapeutic interventions for groups of people with cancer or with specific cancer-related symptoms and problems. Examples include breathlessness clinics, relaxation, massage, and psychological support services, and oral chemotherapy support clinics. There is a growing evidence base for the effectiveness of many of these clinics, in terms of safety and job satisfaction, and for their popularity with patients.

Other nursing roles

As policy continues to demand a flexible workforce to meet the changing needs of the population, new nursing roles continue to develop. Nurse practitioners carry out a number of highly specialized investigative and treatment procedures within cancer care, e.g. nurse-led cystoscopy, intravesical chemotherapy, and proctoscopy services. Another area of extended practice for specialist cancer nurses is that of non-medical prescribing. There are increasing numbers of cancer nurses who are trained to assess patients on chemotherapy and prescribe subsequent cycles within their own nurse-led clinics. Nurse consultants, alongside consultants from allied health professions (AHPs), contribute a higher level of expertise, leadership, and practice development.

The role of the patient in cancer care

One of the most radical shifts in our understanding of cancer care in recent years has been the enhanced profile of the patient. This is, in part, due to the actions of patients themselves, making their voices heard in a variety of ways, including writing their own accounts in newspaper articles, autobiographical accounts, or blogs. Subjective patient experience is now also supported by a significant body of research. The accounts that have emerged are illuminating for the professional, and they also help patients and carers to feel less isolated by putting their experiences into a broader social context.

There are also a number of ways in which we, as professionals, have begun to rethink patients' and carers' place in the health-care system. Cancer is best understood as a chronic disease, one that people may live with for many years. Patients therefore need help to manage their own lives, as well as deal with the process of treatment and whatever outcome it has for them. Resources need to be targeted on supporting patients and their families and carers, as well as on treating the cancer. No one is better placed to identify the needs of people with cancer than the patients themselves, especially with the improvements that have taken place in accessing information about cancer and treatment options.

There are other political trends that support the centrality of patient experience. Consumerist ideas have now been active within the British health-care system for over a decade, and these ascribe rights to the user or consumer of services. For any improvements to be made to cancer services, the voice of the patient must be heard, recognized, and responded to. There are a number of ways in which this is taking place, but the most high-profile and influential of these are the national cancer patient surveys in England. The results of these surveys are used to assess the performance of individual providers of cancer care, and these providers are expected to improve their services in response to patients' views as identified within the surveys. In addition to these national schemes, user groups are frequently involved in, or consulted on, decisions about the allocation of resources. Services now aim to work in partnership with service users who are frequently asked to attend meetings next to health professionals. However, people with cancer do not always wait to be asked for their view. Debates over the availability of new cancer drugs have shown just how powerful the patient voice has become.

Various labels are used to represent the recipient of cancer services, e.g. 'service user' and 'consumer'. These terms have a role in redefining our views of people with cancer, but the term 'patient' remains popular with the public and professionals alike and is the term used mostly in this book.

The multidisciplinary team

The MDT is established as a feature of the effective management of cancer within the UK's NHS. It usually involves a number of medical, nursing, and AHP specialists and focuses on a specific cancer site. The size of the population served will depend on the incidence of the cancer. Increasingly, specialist cancer surgery [e.g. that for head and neck (H&N) and urological cancers] is centred in specialist hospitals, with many smaller hospitals referring their patients to them. 'Specialist' MDTs have been developed to discuss these patients, and these meetings can often involve clinicians from several hospitals coming together, frequently using video-conferencing. Regular meetings ensure that information is pooled, expertise shared, and the complexities of the patient's needs dealt with. This creates a managed care pathway for patients with a particular cancer. Once a treatment plan has been discussed and decided at the MDT meeting, this plan is then discussed and agreed with the patient.

Within each MDT, each patient should have a key worker who provides a clear point of contact and manages the continuity of their care. This person will often be the site-specific CNS, who is well placed to fulfil this particular role. Within specialist MDTs, the key worker may be the CNS from a referring hospital, depending on where the patient is being treated.

The contribution made by CNS to decision-making in the MDT is very important. The nurse's input into the MDT can enable a more patient-centred approach to be maintained, with a focus on the needs of the patient and their family. The key worker may also be a 'constant' in the care of a patient, as they move between surgery and oncology, or even in some treatment within other centres. This makes them ideally placed to represent the patient across a range of professional boundaries.

National guidelines aimed at cancer services, e.g. *Improving Outcomes Guidance* issued by the National Institute for Health and Care Excellence (NICE), highlight the importance of effective MDT work and recommend the overall make-up of different MDTs for specific cancers.

National Institute for Health and Care Excellence

NICE is an independent organization, which provides national guidance for the NHS. It does this through:

- Public health guidance: guidance on the promotion of health and prevention of ill health
- Health technology appraisals: these offer guidance on the use of new and existing medicines, treatments, and procedures for cancer within the NHS
- Cancer service guidance: these offer advice on appropriate treatment and care of people with cancer within the NHS.

Cancer networks throughout England and Wales are expected to take NICE guidance fully into account when planning services and treatments for individuals with cancer. In Scotland, specific clinical guidelines are issued by the Scottish Intercollegiate Guidelines Network (SIGN), which considers the implications of NICE guidelines for Scotland.

With the high cost of many new cancer treatments, the role of NICE will become increasingly important in ensuring equitable access to treatment throughout the UK.

NICE and this handbook

The suggested approaches to treatment laid out in ➔ Section 6 (Management of Major Cancers) and ➔ Section 7 (Symptom Management) in this handbook are based on the most up-to-date national guidance at the time of writing.

However, treatment guidelines are changing frequently in the light of new research, particularly via NICE service guidance and health technology appraisals.

Note: It is important that you check the latest guidance via the NICE website at: ℘ https://www.nice.org.uk. You can also check for local guidelines from your Clinical Network. Practice in individual centres may vary and may change, as new guidelines are updated and published. In England, chemotherapy guidelines may be increasingly centralized by NHS England (℘ http://www.england.nhs.uk/).

For the latest Scottish guidance, please go to the SIGN website at: ℘ https://www.sign.ac.uk

Websites

Department of Health and Social Care website. Available at: ℘ https://www.gov.uk/government/organisations/department-of-health-and-social-care

National Institute for Health and Care Excellence website. Available at: ℘ https://www.nice.org.uk

Scottish Government website. Available at: ℘ http://www.scotland.gov.uk

Welsh Government website. Available at: ℘ http://gov.wales/docs

Further reading

Cancer Research UK (2015). Achieving World-Class Cancer Outcomes: A Strategy for England 2015–2020. Available at: ℘ http://www.cancerresearchuk.org/sites/default/files/achieving_ world-class_cancer_outcomes_-_a_strategy_for_england_2015-2020.pdf

Department of Health (2000). The NHS Cancer Plan: A Plan for Investment, a Plan for Reform. London: Department of Health.

Department of Health (2004). Manual For Cancer Services. London: Department of Health.

Department of Health (2007). The Cancer Reform Strategy. London: Department of Health.

Department of Health (2011). Improving Outcomes: A Strategy for Cancer. London: Department of Health.

Llywodraeth Cymru (2016). The Cancer Delivery Plan for Wales 2016 to 2020. Cardiff: Welsh Government.

The Scottish Government (2008). Better Cancer Care: An Action Plan. Edinburgh: Scottish Government.

Section 2

The Cancer Problem

Cancer epidemiology

The cancer problem

Around 17 million people worldwide were diagnosed with cancer in 2018., and 8.2 million die from the disease (latest statistics for year 2012). This equates to around 12% of annual deaths worldwide. The most common cancers worldwide are lung, ♀ breast, bowel, and prostate cancers. These four account for around 4 in 10 of all cancers diagnosed worldwide (see Fig. 2.1).

Lung cancer now accounts for 11% of all cancers worldwide, and its incidence is predicted to increase in the next 20 years in areas of the world where smoking prevalence has risen such as Eastern Africa, Central America, and South East Asia.

The most common cancers diagnosed worldwide have changed little over the last 40 years, though lung cancer now accounts for more of the total due to ↑ tobacco usage. Prostate cancer now accounts for a greater proportion of the total, probably partly due to ↑ use of prostate-specific antigen (PSA) testing.

There are wide regional variations in the most common cancers. In Europe, breast, bowel, and lung cancers account for 50% of cancer incidence. This reflects an ageing population and lifestyle factors such as high-fat diets and levels of smoking. In Eastern Africa, Kaposi's sarcoma (KS) and cervical cancer account for 27% of the cancer incidence, reflecting the prevalence of acquired immune deficiency syndrome (AIDS) and high rates of sexually transmitted infections.

Survival rates vary from region to region. In resource-poor countries, there may be limited access to screening programmes, diagnostic procedures, and many of the drug treatments that may improve survival rates. The

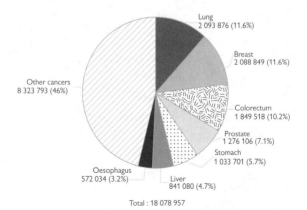

Total : 18 078 957

Fig. 2.1 Estimated number of new cases in 2018, worldwide, all cancers, both sexes, all ages.

Worldwide cancer statistics can be viewed at the Global Cancer observatory, http://gco.iarc.fr/

stigma associated with cancer and the burden of the cost of treatment may delay diagnosis and treatment.

The World Health Organization (WHO) is encouraging a public health approach to reduce the causes and consequences of cancer, focusing on:

- Developing and strengthening national cancer control programmes
- Early detection of cervical and breast cancers
- Developing guidelines on disease management.
- Support for low-cost approaches to respond to global needs for pain relief and palliative care.

The regional differences in incidence rates highlight the need for specifically targeted public health measures in each world region.

UK situation

Incidence

This is the number of new cancer cases arising in a specified period of time, normally over a period of 1 year. In 2015* over 360,000 people were diagnosed with cancer in the UK. The biggest risk factor for cancer is increasing age. Fifty-three per cent of cancers are diagnosed in those aged 50–74, with 36% of cancer being diagnosed in those aged 75 and over. The ageing population in the UK means that the incidence of cancer will continue to increase in the near future (see Fig. 2.2).

Although there are >200 different types of cancer, just four types— breast, lung, bowel, and prostate cancers—account for 53% of cancers diagnosed each year in the UK (see Fig. 2.3). Breast cancer is the most common cancer in the UK, despite being rare in men.

Common cancers by age

Children to young adults (0–24 years)

The most common cancers vary by age considerably. In children aged 0– 14 years, leukaemia and brain tumours account for over 50% of cancer incidence. Amongst teenage and young adults ♂, germ cell tumours and lymphomas are the most common. It is important to remember that cancer in children and teenagers is extremely uncommon, accounting for around 1% of cancer incidence.

Adults (25–49 years)

Ten per cent of UK cancer cases occur in this age group. Cases in women are nearly twice those of men, due to the high rate of breast cancer in this age group (accounting for 45% of ♀ cancers in this age group).

Adults (50 years and over)

In this age group, the most common cancers are breast, prostate, lung, and bowel.

UK males

Prostate cancer is now the most commonly diagnosed cancer in ♂ in the UK, with almost 47,000 cases diagnosed in 2014, accounting for 26% of all ♂ cancer cases.

The 'age-standardized' incidence of prostate cancer has ↑ threefold since the 1970s. This takes into account the different age structure of the population over time. The increase is mainly due to ↑ rates of transurethral resection of the prostate (TURP) and PSA screening. Lung cancer incidence dropped by over 45% during the same period, relating to a decrease in smoking amongst ♂. Bowel cancer is the third most common, and these three cancers account for over 50% of ♂ cancer incidence.

---

* The UK cancer registries do not release cancer statistics right up to the current year. There is normally a 4-year time lag with incidence statistics and a 2-year time lag with mortality statistics.

P/O NO:
ACCESSION NO: KHO5064
SHELFMARK: 610.730698

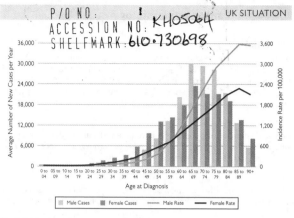

Fig. 2.2 Number of new cases and age-specific incidence rates by sex, including all neoplasms (but excluding non-melanoma skin cancer) (UK, 2002).

Statistics used courtesy of Cancer Research UK.

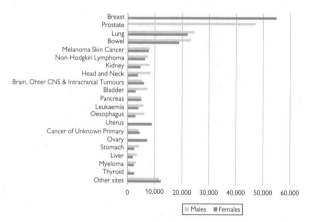

Fig. 2.3 The 20 most common cancers in the UK (incidence, 2002)*.

Statistics used courtesy of Cancer Research UK.

* Non-melanoma skin cancer is omitted from the Cancer Research UK statistics shown here. It is a very common condition, but virtually always curable. Registration is known to be incomplete, and up to 100,000 cases may be diagnosed in the UK each year. There is a delay of around 18 months compiling and completing cancer incidence registry statistics, and a slightly shorter delay in compiling the mortality statistics. This accounts for the time lag in the publication and statistics used within the book.

UK females

A little fewer than 55,000 women were diagnosed with breast cancer in 2015, accounting for 31% of ♀ cancers. The next most common cancers are lung cancer (12%), followed by bowel cancer (11% of cases). Rates of lung cancer have ↑ in women by 13% over the past 10 years as a result of high levels of smoking amongst women in the late 1960s and early 1970s.

Prevalence

This is the number of people who have received a diagnosis of cancer and who are alive at any given time. This reflects both the incidence of cancer and its associated survival pattern.

Risk

An individual's risk of developing cancer depends on many factors, including their smoking behaviour, diet, and genetic inheritance. It is estimated that, in the UK, around half of all cancers could be prevented through changes to lifestyle such as stopping smoking, limiting alcohol intake, eating healthily, and protection from sun exposure (see ➲ Aetiology, pp. 27–9).

UK mortality

Cancer is the cause of 28% of all deaths in the UK. In 2015, around 164,000 individuals were registered as having died from cancer. Over one-fifth of all cancer deaths are from lung cancer (21%). The next three most common cancers are bowel, breast, and prostate cancers. Forty-five per cent of all UK cancer deaths can be attributed to these four cancers (see Fig. 2.4).

The difference between incidence and survival statistics for particular diseases reflects the wide variation in 5- and 10-year survival statistics for each disease, with some cancers often being very successfully treated and others having a very poor overall prognosis (see ➡ Survival, p. 26).

Trends over time

The overall rate of mortality from all cancers has fallen by 9% in the last 10 years, despite an increase in incidence, though there are large variations in this trend between different cancers (see Figs. 2.5 and 2.6). Mortality has fallen in the four most common cancers in men and women, except for a small increase in women's lung cancer mortality. The main reasons for the decrease in mortality are:

• Primary prevention of cancer, e.g. a reduction in smoking
• Earlier detection through screening programmes
• Better treatment, e.g. new drugs to treat breast cancer.

Despite the fall in lung cancer mortality, it is still, by far, the most common cause of death from cancer in men in the UK, causing a quarter of all ♂ cancer deaths. Over 80% of lung cancer deaths are linked to tobacco smoking.

Mortality by age

Mortality rates increase with age for most cancers. More than half of cancer deaths occur in people aged 75 and over.

Children to young adults (0–24 years)

Cancer deaths are still very uncommon in this age group, accounting for <1% of all cancer deaths. Cancer is the most common single cause of mortality in children aged 0–14 years, accounting for 13% of deaths. In teenagers/young adults, it accounts for only 9% of mortality, with all accidents and suicide accounting for 50% of deaths in this age group.

Adults (25–49 years)

In this age group, cancer accounts for 18% of all deaths. It is the only age group in which ♀ cancer deaths exceeds ♂ cancer deaths, mainly due to the relatively high rates of death from ♀ breast cancer. This group still accounts for <5% of all cancer deaths

Adults (50 years and over)

This age group accounts for over 95% of all cancer deaths in the UK, with the most common cancers—lung and breast—accounting for the majority of deaths in this age group.

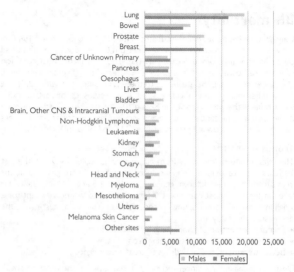

Fig. 2.4 The 20 most common causes of death from cancer (UK, 2004).
Statistics used courtesy of Cancer Research UK.

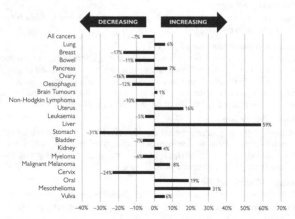

Fig. 2.5 Percentage change in European age-standardized mortality rates of major cancers by sex (UK 1995–2004).
Statistics used courtesy of Cancer Research UK.

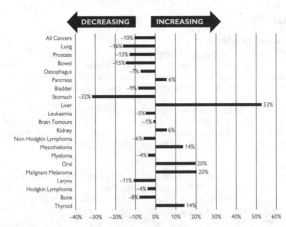

Fig. 2.6 Five-year age-standardized relative survival (%) in adults diagnosed in 1996–1999 in England and Wales, by sex and site.

Statistics used courtesy of Cancer Research UK.

Survival

Site and gender

Cancer survival has improved for most cancers in the last 20 years. In 2011, 49% of men survived cancer for 5 years or more. Survival for women is slightly higher at 59%. However, survival rates between different cancers vary dramatically and are very dependent on the stage of disease at diagnosis.

The variation in survival between disease sites is highlighted by testicular and pancreatic cancers. The UK 10-year survival rate for testicular cancer is around 98%, whereas for pancreatic cancer, it is around 1%. For most types of cancer, women have a small survival advantage over men.

Age

Survival decreases with increasing age for most cancers. This may be due to less aggressive treatment in the elderly, later diagnosis, and several cancers being more chemotherapy-sensitive in younger patients. Exceptions to this rule are breast and prostate cancers, which tend to be more aggressive diseases in the youngest age group. Screening in breast cancer may also increase survival in the screening age group, though some of this may be accounted for by lead time bias (see ➲ Evaluating screening programmes, p. 47).

Deprivation

There is lower survival in a range of cancers in more deprived groups, including prostate, colorectal, and breast cancers. The reasons for this could include:

• Later diagnosis, e.g. difference in access to PSA testing
• Treatment delays, poorer access, and lower compliance
• Worse general health and a higher prevalence of smoking.

In recent years, though gaps in deprivation have narrowed in some cancers, e.g. breast, lung in ♂, and prostate, in other cancers, the deprivation gap has grown, e.g. oesophageal and colorectal cancers in women. Though differences due to deprivation are small in percentage terms, the large overall number of diagnosed cancers in the UK means that deprivation could account for several thousands of avoidable cancer deaths each year.

Aetiology

The study of the causes of cancer is complex and fraught with difficulty. Epidemiological studies look at whole populations and try to correlate risk factors with specific cancers. Problems occur due to the complexity of factors such as diet and various chemicals. Confounding variables are a problem. For example, is it obesity, a high-fat diet, or a lack of activity which plays a role in bowel cancer, or is it all three to differing degrees?

Key factors in cancer causation

Host factors

- Age: cancer is primarily a disease of older age, with two-thirds of cancer being diagnosed in those over 65 years of age. This can be explained by increasing exposure to carcinogens, the fact that cancer development requires multiple genetic mutations (see ➔ Cancer biology, Introduction, p. 32), and the reduced effectiveness of the immune system in older people.
- Genetics: most cancers occur due to exposure to carcinogens that cause genetic mutations plus random damage to human deoxyribonucleic acid (DNA) that occurs during cell division during our lifetime. Around 5% of cancers may be caused by the inheritance of cancer-related genetic mutations (see Table 2.1). Hereditary cancers tend to occur at an earlier age, and people with an altered cancer gene can have a greater risk of developing other cancers. More cancer-related genes are being discovered each year, as research into the cellular causes of cancer continues.

Carcinogen

A carcinogen is any substance or agent that promotes cancer development. Carcinogens generally cause genetic mutations, i.e. they damage DNA in cells, therefore interfering with normal biological processes.

Table 2.1 Some inherited cancer genes and their related cancers

Implicated gene	Related cancer (and syndrome)
BRCA1, BRCA2	Breast and ovarian cancer
WT1, WT2	Wilms' tumour
Rb1	Retinoblastoma
APC	Adenomatous polyposis coli; bowel cancer
MLH1, MSH2	Hereditary non-polyposis coli, bowel cancer
RET	Thyroid cancer
p53	Li-Fraumeni syndrome; multiple types of cancer
XPA	Xeroderma pigmentosum, skin cancer

Environmental factors

Exposure to a range of **environmental** carcinogens increases the risk of developing cancer. This is supported by changes in cancer incidence found in migration studies and varying rates of cancer in different socio-economic groups.

Note: 'Environmental' refers to the physical environment in which we live, as well as lifestyle factors such as diet and smoking habits.

There are thousands of known carcinogens, but epidemiological studies suggest that radiation, pollution, and occupational exposure account for <10% of known cancer risk. More than 40% of all cancers in the UK are linked to tobacco, alcohol, diet, being overweight, inactivity, infection, radiation, occupation, post-menopausal hormones, or breastfeeding for <6 months.[1]

- Tobacco: this is, by far, the single most important risk factor for cancer worldwide, implicated not only in lung cancer, but also in H&N, oesophageal, and stomach cancers. The number of cigarettes smoked and the number of years that a person has smoked are risk factors. Smoking cessation programmes should have a major role to play in reducing the risk of cancer.
- Alcohol: the main effect of alcohol is its combined effect with tobacco smoking in H&N cancers and cancers of the oesophagus. Alcohol by itself is implicated in liver cancer and may contribute to some cancers of the breast and bowel.
- Diet: according to a range of epidemiological studies, diet may be the most important cancer risk factor. However, it is difficult to measure a person's diet over time, and we need to know what people ate in the past to explore links to cancer. High intake of red meat, especially processed meat, has been implicated in increasing the risk of bowel cancer. Diets high in fruit and vegetables may have a protective effect against a number of cancers, including stomach, oesophageal, and larynx cancers, though the evidence is limited. Similarly, high-fibre diets may offer some protection against bowel cancer. High levels of salt have been linked in several studies to stomach cancer. Contamination of food by aflatoxins (toxins produced by *Aspergillus* fungi) increases the risk of liver cancer.
- Being physically inactive is linked to excess cases of breast, colon, and uterine cancers. Breast cancer accounted for the largest number of linked cases highlighted in the recent review by Parkin *et al*.[1]
- Infections: these account for between 10% and 20% of worldwide cancer incidence, although in many developing regions of the world, this figure is far higher. A range of viruses are implicated in cancer incidence. Human papillomavirus (HPV) may account for over 90% of cervical cancers, and hepatitis B and C are linked to 80% of liver cancer. The AIDS epidemic [human immunodeficiency virus (HIV) infection] has seen a huge increase in KS and lymphomas. Other important infections relating to cancer incidence are Epstein–Barr virus (EBV) (lymphoma) and the bacterium *Helicobactor pylori*, which is an important risk factor for stomach cancer.

- Sun exposure: there is strong evidence that reducing exposure to ultraviolet (UV) radiation (sun exposure) reduces the incidence of melanoma. The most important risk factors are intensity and age of exposure (high risk from childhood exposure). Skin type plays a part, with fair and red-headed people at highest risk.
- It is estimated that over 40% of cancer cases each year in the UK are linked to common lifestyle factors. Targeting common behaviours could have a major impact on incidence (see Table 2.2).

Nearly 100% of cervical cancers could be prevented, due to the link with HPV infection. Nearly 90% of mesothelioma and lung and oral cancers could be prevented, and over 80% of melanoma cases due to links with UV radiation exposure.

Table 2.2 Common behaviours to target for cancer prevention

Behaviour	Preventable cases	Cancer incidence (%)
Smoke-free	64,500	19
Healthy weight	18,100	5
Eat more fruit and vegetables	15,100	5
Drink less alcohol	12,800	4
Sun-smart	11,500	3

Further reading

Cancer Research UK website. Available at: http://www.cancerresearchuk.org/cancer-info/cancerstats/ (excellent resource for UK cancer statistical information).

Pecorino L. *Molecular Biology of Cancer: Mechanisms, Targets, and Therapeutics*, 3rd ed. Oxford: Oxford University Press; 2012.

Weinberg RA. *The Biology of Cancer*, 2nd ed. New York, NY: Garland Science; 2013.

References

1 Parkin DM, Boyd L, Walker LC. The fraction of cancer attributable to lifestyle and environmental factors in the UK in 2010. *Br J Cancer* 2011;**105** Suppl 2:S77–81.

Cancer biology

Introduction to cancer biology

Knowledge of cancer biology has leapt forward in the last 20 years. This has improved the understanding of the disease process of cancer and has opened up the opportunity for targeted treatments and methods of screening.

Cancer is not one disease, but many, although there are some striking similarities in how all cancers develop. Cancer is a monoclonal disease, i.e. all the cells in a tumour come from only one ancestral cell. The transformation of a normal cell into its malignant counterpart is an accumulative, multistage process of gene mutation. As each mutation occurs, the cell's DNA becomes less stable. The genes involved control cell growth, cell division, genetic stability, cell mortality, and the ability of cells to migrate and develop blood supply.

It may take many years for multiple mutations of a single cell to occur. This explains the increasing risk of cancer, as we get older.

Cell cycle

The sequence of stages through which a cell passes between one division and another is known as the cell cycle (see Fig. 3.1). Loss of cell cycle control is a critical characteristic that all cancers share. Chemotherapy drugs target different phases of the cell cycle; some are cell cycle-dependent, whilst others are cycle-independent (➜ see Effects of cytotoxic drugs on the cell cycle, p. 207).

Therefore, a working knowledge of the cell cycle is important in order to understand treatment.

At any one stage, most cells in the human body are not dividing and are in an inactive phase called G_0. Growth factors can stimulate cells to move into the cell cycle and divide. For example, when the skin is cut, growth factors released by platelets at the site of injury stimulate skin cells to divide and close the wound.

The four stages of the cell cycle are: gap phases G_1 and G_2 where the cell builds up the energy required for division (see Fig. 3.1), S (synthesis) phase where replication of DNA occurs, and M (mitosis) phase where double-stranded DNA splits and two identical daughter cells are created.

A set of proteins (cyclins), and their associated enzymes called cyclin-dependent kinases (CDKs), control the cell cycle. The concentrations of these rise and fall during cell division. As the cell moves through the cycle, a series of controlling checkpoints have to be passed. These check the integrity of the DNA and ensure safe and accurate cell division.

Genes that code for proteins that regulate the cell cycle are known as oncogenes and tumour suppressor genes (➜ see Oncogenes and tumour suppressor genes, pp. 35–6). Damage to these genes can knock out the controlling aspect of cell division, driving division forward. This allows cells to ignore checkpoints and damaged DNA to be replicated, leading to out-of-control cell replication. Cancer can therefore be seen as a disease of the cell cycle.

Key genes that regulate the cell cycle include *p53* and *Retinoblastoma (Rb)*, which are implicated in a large number of different cancers when they become dysfunctional via mutation.

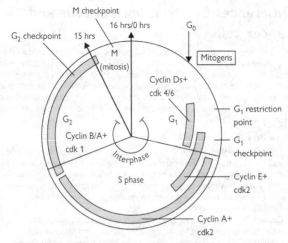

Fig. 3.1 The cell cycle and its checkpoints.

Reproduced from Pecorino L (2012) *Molecular biology of cancer: mechanisms, targets, and therapeutics* with permission from Oxford University Press.

Differences between normal cells and cancer cells

Normal cells reproduce in a controlled manner and will only divide when instructed to by other cells in their vicinity. This 'community' control means that cells cannot divide if there is not enough space or when nutrients are inadequate. There is a balance between the number of immature cells that can divide and the number of mature cells that are fully differentiated and lose the ability to divide. Normal cells are not able to migrate from their location in the body.

How do cancer cells differ?

- **Lack of control:** the key difference is that cancer cells are uncontrolled and do not obey the signals and rules of their own tissue and other cells in their vicinity. They are able to grow despite low levels of nutrients and growth factors required by normal cells. The cancer cell is rather like a renegade, behaving with complete independence from, and indifference to, its normal surroundings.
- **Growth inhibition:** cancer cells can grow when there is no room or when they are not attached to the same tissue. They lack contact inhibition (which will prevent normal cells from growing when there is no room) and anchorage dependence (the need to be attached to other cells of the same tissue, known as 'cell–cell adhesion').
- **Differentiation:** this is the process by which young, immature (unspecialized) cells take on individual characteristics and reach their mature (specialized) form and function. Cancer cells do not fully differentiate and therefore maintain the ability to divide. This lack of differentiation also means that cancer cells do not function as effectively as the normal cell counterparts of their original tissue. The lack of proper differentiation varies amongst cancer cells. The least differentiated cancers tend to be more aggressive and more likely to metastasize.
- **Metastatic spread:** cancer cells can develop the ability to invade other tissue space and grow at other sites. This is the most dangerous aspect of cancer and is the reason for a majority of cancer deaths (➔ see Metastasis (spread of secondary tumour), pp. 38–9).
- **Angiogenesis:** once a tumour reaches a size of around 1–2cm^3, its oxygen supply and nutrients are insufficient for further growth, unless it can establish its own blood supply. Cancer cells do this by sending out angiogenic factors, which stimulate new capillaries to grow towards the tumour from nearby blood vessels. The new blood vessels not only provide oxygen and nutrients for the tumour, but also create a route for metastatic colonization. Angiogenesis is not unique to cancer cells. However, in cancer, the process lacks effective controls.
- **Cell surface changes:** numerous changes take place on the surface of cancer cells. These lead to changes in behaviour, including a lack of proper cell–cell adhesion, promotion of metastasis, and ↑ response to growth factors.

Oncogenes and tumour suppressor genes

Of the estimated 20,000 human genes, there are now over 100 known oncogenes and tumour suppressor genes (TSGs). Each has a role in regulating growth. These genes code for a series of molecules, which transmit growth signals from the extracellular environment into the cell and onto the nucleus, known as a signal transduction cascade/pathway (see Table 3.1).

Oncogenes

These are genes that drive cell division (akin to an accelerator). These genes produce proteins that include growth factors, growth factor receptors, signal transducers, and nuclear transcription factors. When mutated, they can produce the wrong protein or too much protein, which can drive cell division inappropriately. Many of these molecules are now used as targets of more recent cancer drug therapies, such as trastuzumab which targets the ErbB2 receptor, or tyrosine kinase inhibitors (TKIs) (e.g. sunitinib, erlotinib) which target enzymes responsible for activating the signalling pathways within cells.

Tumour suppressor genes

These provide the negative feedback (or brakes) required in cell division. They can block growth signals at any point in the overall chain, from the surface to the nucleus. When mutated, their function is lost and cell division cannot be stopped.

Table 3.1 Common TSGs and oncogenes

TSG	Cancers linked with gene damage
APC (adenomatous polyposis coli)	Familial adenomatous and non-inherited colorectal cancers
BRCA1, BRCA2 (breast cancer 1 and 2)	Inherited breast cancers, ovarian cancers
DCC (deleted in colon cancer)	Colorectal cancers
p53	Over 50% of human cancers, including bladder, breast, colorectal, oesophageal, liver, and lung
Rb (Retinoblastoma)	Retinoblastoma, sarcomas; bladder, breast, oesophageal, prostate, and lung cancers
Oncogenes	
abl/bcr	Chronic myeloid and acute lymphoblastic leukaemias
HER2/neu	Breast and cervical
ras	Many cancers, including pancreas (90%), colon (50%), lung (30%), and thyroid (50%)
myc	Lymphoma, leukaemia, lung cancer
Src	Breast, colon, small cell lung cancer

Other key mechanisms

Other aspects of cell growth control are important in cancer development.

- **Apoptosis (programmed cell death):** cells normally have a protective mechanism to stop damaged DNA being replicated. If a cell is found to have damaged DNA, either the DNA is repaired or the cell self-destructs. Key genes in this process include *bcl-2* genes and also *p53*, known as the guardian of the genome, which is mutated in over 50% of cancers. If this gene is not functioning properly, then the accumulation of errors in DNA is speeded up, leading to a greater risk of developing cancer.

- **Immortal growth:** most cells can only divide a finite number of times. After each division, the tips of their chromosomes (telomeres) shorten. When these get too short, the chromosomes unravel and cannot divide. Some cancer cells can produce telomerase, an enzyme that maintains the length of these tips during division, therefore extending the number of potential divisions indefinitely.

- **Tumour heterogeneity:** as cancer develops, the inherent genetic instability leads to different cell populations within a single tumour. This can cause difficulty in treating tumours, as some cell populations within a tumour may be resistant to cytotoxic drugs and radiotherapy. This lack of uniformity makes it difficult to eradicate all cells in a tumour with systemic treatments.

Tumour growth

In normal tissue, homeostasis is maintained by the balance of cell replication, apoptosis (cell death), and differentiation. Fully differentiated cells tend to lose the ability to divide. Within a cancerous tumour, there is an imbalance. Tumour cells are not fully differentiated and maintain the ability to divide. The apoptosis functionality is not fully established, and due to telomerase (➔ see Apoptosis, p. 36), many cells can go on dividing indefinitely.

Note: it is this imbalance that causes tumour development.

Cancer growth is normally described in terms of 'doubling time' or the time taken for the number of cells in a tumour to double. This may vary from hours to many months. It varies across cancer types; for example, Burkitt's lymphoma, testicular cancer, and small cell cancers can have rapid doubling times, whereas many common cancers, such as colon and breast cancers, may have doubling times of many months.

From initial cancer development, 30 doublings will produce a tumour of about 1cm in diameter (~ a billion cells).

▶ Slower-growing tumours may therefore be many years old before being discovered.

Several mechanisms impact on the rate of tumour doubling time:
- **Average cell cycle time**: this is usually 1–5 days.
- **Growth fraction**: this is the fraction of cells within a tumour that are actively dividing at any one time. It is often well under 50%.
- **Cell loss**: the main reason that volume doubling times are so much longer than the average cell cycle time is the high percentage of cell loss in tumours. This is mainly due to cell death, through necrosis and apoptosis, but also includes loss due to metastatic spread.

Implications for treatment

Dividing cells are more sensitive to cytotoxic chemotherapy and radiotherapy than non-dividing cells. Tumours with a high growth fraction are therefore more susceptible to these treatments than those with a low growth fraction (➔ see Radiotherapy, Principles and uses, pp. 194–5).

Metastasis (spread of secondary tumour)

Metastatic spread is one of the unique characteristics of malignant disease and is the main reason for treatment failure and the eventual death of cancer patients. ~60% of cancer patients with solid tumours have metastatic disease at diagnosis, although only around half of these will be clinically detectable at that time. Not all cells within a tumour will have the ability to metastasize. This ability will develop in some cell populations if there are further mutations in their DNA.

Routes of spread

Blood and lymph circulation accounts for two-thirds of metastatic spread. Other methods of spread include direct extension along tissues, seeding in cavities such as the peritoneum, and spread via the central nervous system (CNS).

Where do cells metastasize to and why?

Most metastatic spread can be explained by anatomical closeness (e.g. ovarian cancer extending along the Fallopian tubes) and also by blood circulation. Cancer cells will get trapped in the first capillary bed they encounter, often in the lungs as part of the general circulation, e.g. in breast cancer, or in the liver via the portal blood system, e.g. in colon cancer. Cancer may metastasize to areas such as bone because of changes to cancer cell surface molecules allowing them to interact favourably with tissue or growth factors in specific new sites (see Table 3.2).

The metastatic cascade

Metastatic spread is known to be a complex process, requiring each of the following steps.

- **Angiogenesis (neovascularization):** development by a cancer of its own blood supply. The degree of vascularization of a tumour correlates poorly with survival, as it offers a perfect route for metastatic spread.
- **Intravasation:** changes in surface molecules (cell adhesion molecules) allow cancer cells to detach from the primary tumour and the extracellular matrix (ECM). They then invade the ECM by secreting digesting enzymes (proteases) and producing motility factors that assist their movement. By gaining access to local blood vessels, they can enter the circulation and be transported around the body.

Table 3.2 Areas where cancers metastasize

Common sites of metastatic spread	Cancers that commonly spread to these sites
Lung	Breast, colon, bladder, kidney
Liver	Colon, pancreas, lung, breast, stomach
Brain	Lung, breast, melanoma
Bone	Breast, lung, prostate

Note: this ability to invade tissue is similar to certain white blood cells, but in the case of cancer spread, it is completely unregulated.

- **Circulation and arrest:** during circulation, both mechanical turbulence and immune surveillance will destroy most cancer cells, probably >99.9%. However, some will survive and become trapped in small capillaries of a distant organ or tissue.
- **Extravasation:** the process of intravasation is then carried out in reverse and the cell establishes itself in the new tissue.
- **Growth:** further division and establishment of new blood supply are needed to enable the new tumour to develop and grow.

Note: after many years of remission, patients may get a sudden cancer relapse with metastatic cancer. This is thought to be due to dormant micrometastases—metastatic deposits which remain stable due to a lack of angiogenesis for many years, before further genetic changes enable them to grow again.

Treatment Implications of Metastatic Spread

The ability to control or prevent metastatic spread would be a major breakthrough in the management of cancer. Cell adhesion molecules, enzymes that cause ECM breakdown, and angiogenesis are amongst targets for new cancer treatments (➲ see Introduction to targeted and biological therapies, p. 227).

Immunology

The links between the immune system and cancer have been long established through a range of different evidence:

- Immune suppression has been shown to directly cause several cancers:
  - HIV and KS or non-Hodgkin lymphoma (NHL)
  - Long-term immunosuppressive therapy and lymphoma
- The presence of immune system cells in tumour biopsies
- Spontaneous regression of some primary tumours
- Effective use of immunotherapy, e.g. bacille Calmette–Guérin (BCG) to destroy tumours
- Graft versus leukaemia effect in allogeneic transplant (➔ see Graft-versus-malignancy, p. 258).

Recent improvements in the understanding of cancer biology and immunology have led to ↑ development and use of biological therapies, e.g. cytokines (➔ see Cytokines, pp. 231–3).

Understanding the basics of the immune system helps in our understanding of both cancer biology and cancer treatments.

Immune system

The immune system exists to defend the body against infections, e.g. bacteria, viruses, fungi, and parasite invasions, as well as malignant transformation. It consists of the following parts:

- Organs: bone marrow, thymus, spleen, lymph, nodes, Peyer's patches
- Cells: leucocytes—both myeloid and lymphoid
- Complement and cytokines: proteins which have a role in enhancing the immune response.

The immune system consists of two complementary components that closely interact during the immune response.

Innate immunity

This is also known as 'natural' or 'non-specific' immunity. It includes:

- Physical and chemical barriers such as skin, mucosa, mucus secretions, lysozyme, and cilia.
- Inflammatory response: phagocytes, neutrophils, monocytes, and macrophages which directly attack and destroy pathogens and release cytokines which stimulate further immune response (acquired immunity).
- Other cells, such as natural killer (NK) cells, that can directly kill virally infected cells and some tumour cells.
- Complement proteins which enhance the immune response.

Acquired immunity

This is lymphocyte-controlled and is a specific response to certain antigens. It has memory, allowing it to respond rapidly, in huge numbers, on a later exposure to the same antigen. It consists of:

- T-lymphocytes, of which the two main types are:
  - Helper T-cells: recognize foreign antigens and produce cytokines, e.g. interleukin/interferon and tumour necrosis factor (TNF). They also have a role in developing antibody response
  - Cytotoxic T-cells: directly lyse target cells

- B-lymphocytes: they produce antibodies in response to certain antigens and present antigens to T-cells, further stimulating the immune response.

The immune response

On encountering a pathogen, e.g. bacterial infection, phagocytes would immediately attack the bacteria, aided by complement. This leads to a release of cytokines, e.g. interleukins and TNF. This stimulates further macrophage and NK cell activation. Through phagocytosis, the antigen is degraded and presented to the acquired immunity system. A T- and B-cell response occurs, including direct pathogen destruction by cytotoxic T-cells, further cytokine release, and antibody production, leading to an enhanced immune response and cell destruction.

On destruction of the antigen, the immune system returns to its preactivated state but now has memory T- and B-cells for that antigen, to enable a more rapid and stronger future immune response.

Influences on the immune system

A number of factors impact on the overall functioning of the immune system:

- **Age**: as we age, there is a declining immune response, including reduced T-cell functioning
- **Stress**: though it is hard to clearly define, there is increasing evidence that long-term chronic stress has an immunosuppressive effect
- **Exercise**: moderate exercise has a generally positive effect; however, excessive exercise can reduce immune function
- **Diet**: nutrient deficiency, excess alcohol, and smoking all lower the immune response.

Immunology and cancer

Several cancers have antigen presentation different from normal tissue, e.g. CA-125 and ovarian cancer, carcinoembryonic antigen (CEA) and colorectal cancer (➔ see Tumour markers, p. 179).

These antigen changes can stimulate an immune response, activating NK cells, macrophages, and other cytokines. The ability of the immune system to destroy cancer cells is known as tumour surveillance. It is believed that such surveillance can explain spontaneous tumour regression and that the immune system is successfully destroying potential cancer cells throughout our lifetime.

However, tumour antigen presentation may only vary slightly from normal tissue and may not be sufficient to stimulate an effective immune response. Therefore, tumours continue to grow. Tumours may also 'downregulate' tumour antigens and other immune system molecules, such as human leucocyte antigens, making them more difficult for the immune system to target (➔ see Box 19.1 Human leucocyte antigen matching, p. 259).

Tumour classification

Tumour

A swelling or a mass of tissue that may be benign or malignant.

Benign tumours

Benign tumours cannot spread by invasion or metastasis; therefore, they only grow locally. Because benign tumours do not metastasize or destroy normal tissue, they are less likely to be life-threatening; an exception is benign brain tumours. Certain benign tumours, such as adenomatous polyps in the colon, can transform into malignant tumours.

Malignant tumours

Malignant tumours are tumours that are able to spread by invasion and metastasis.

Cancer

By definition, the term 'cancer' applies only to malignant tumours.

Main cancer types

There are hundreds of different cancers, due to the many tissue types and points of origin for cancer within the human body. They can be loosely classified into five main types: carcinoma, sarcoma, myeloma, leukaemia, and lymphoma, as well as mixed cell cancers.

Carcinomas are cancers of epithelial tissue and account for 80–90% of all cancer cases. Epithelial tissue lines the internal and external surfaces of the body and is found throughout the body. Carcinomas are divided into two major subtypes:
- **Adenocarcinoma**, which develops in an organ or gland, and
- **Squamous cell carcinoma (SCC)**, which develops in the squamous epithelium in many parts of the body.

Most carcinomas affect organs or glands capable of secretion, e.g. the four most common cancers in the UK—breast, lung, colon, and prostate.
- **Sarcomas** originate in supportive and connective tissues such as bones, tendons, cartilage, muscle, and fat.
- **Myeloma** is cancer that originates in plasma cells of the bone marrow.
- **Leukaemias** (blood cancers) are cancers of the bone marrow. They are further divided into myeloid and lymphoid types, based on the specific blood cell line from which they originate.
- **Lymphomas** are cancers of the glands or nodes of the lymphatic system. They may also occur in specific organs such as the stomach, breast, or brain. Divided into Hodgkin disease and NHL.
- **Mixed types:** some cancers arise from different aspects of the same tissue, e.g. adenosquamous carcinoma. Other cancers arise from the original germ cell layers of tissue and do not have any relationship to their tissue of origin, e.g. teratocarcinomas.

Further reading

Pecorino L. *Molecular Biology of Cancer: Mechanisms, Targets, and Therapeutics*, 3rd ed. Oxford: Oxford University Press; 2012.
Weinberg R. *The Biology of Cancer*. New York, NY: Garland Science; 2013.

Chapter 4

Cancer prevention and screening

Cancer prevention

Though the actual cause of an individual's specific cancer is often not known, many of the common forms of cancer have causative factors related to lifestyle such as smoking, sunbathing, and poor diet. They are therefore potentially preventable.

Estimates are that over half of all cancers could be preventable, so prevention, rather than attempts at cure, may have a greater impact on the rates of death from cancer.

Government targets

In 1999, the UK government set a target of reducing cancer deaths in people under 75 years by at least a fifth by 2010.[1] By 2010, this target had been virtually met, with a reduction of 19.3%.[2]

Inequalities in cancer health also need tackling. Rates of certain cancers are higher in deprived areas. For example, smoking rates remain extremely high amongst those living in poverty. Targeted policies aim not only to reduce cancer rates, but also to reduce the gap in cancer incidence and mortality between different groups in society. Once again, by 2010, there had been a reduction in the difference in cancer mortality between the most deprived and unhealthy sections of the UK and the population in general.[2] In 2011, the government published *Improving Outcomes: A Strategy for Cancer*, which laid out the aspiration that the UK should have cancer outcomes, to compare with the best in the world.[3] The focus on achieving further improvements was on prevention and earlier diagnosis.

Key areas of UK government policy on cancer prevention
- Smoking
- Poor diet
- Obesity
- Lack of exercise
- Alcohol

This is in line with the European Code Against Cancer (see Box 4.1), which, in 2014, entered into its fourth revision.

Approaches to cancer prevention

Generally classified as four levels:
- **Primary prevention**: strategies that reduce individuals' exposure to carcinogens. These can be medical interventions, such as immunization against HPV and hepatitis B, reducing the risk of cervical and liver cancer, respectively. However, most strategies are behavioural, involving health education, lifestyle, and environmental modification.
- **Secondary prevention**: this covers screening (➔ see Cancer screening, p. 47) and early detection measures. Early detection measures include individual and public education about common warning signs of cancer and, in the UK, referral guidelines for suspected cancer.[4]
- **Tertiary prevention and prevention of suffering**: these include avoiding complications from treatment, rehabilitation, and avoiding recurrence. It is often hard to separate from other aspects of treatment and nursing care.

Box 4.1 European Code Against Cancer

1 Do not smoke. Do not use any form of tobacco.
2 Make your home smoke-free. Support smoke-free policies in your workplace.
3 Take action to be a healthy body weight.
4 Be physically active in everyday life. Limit the time you spend sitting.
5 Have a healthy diet:
   • Eat plenty of whole grains, pulses, vegetables, and fruits.
   • Limit high-calorie foods (foods high in sugar or fat), and avoid sugary drinks.
   • Avoid processed meat; limit red meat and foods high in salt.
6 If you drink alcohol of any type, limit your intake. Not drinking alcohol is better for cancer prevention.
7 Avoid too much sun, especially for children. Use sun protection. Do not use sunbeds.
8 In the workplace, protect yourself against cancer-causing substances by following health and safety instructions.
9 Find out if you are exposed to radiation from naturally high radon levels in your home. Take action to reduce high radon levels.
10 For women:
   • Breastfeeding reduces a mother's cancer risk. If you can, breastfeed your baby.
   • Hormone replacement therapy (HRT) increases the risk of certain cancers. Limit the use of HRT.
11 Ensure your children take part in vaccination programmes for:
   • Hepatitis B (for newborns).
   • HPV (for girls).
12 Take part in organized cancer screening programmes for:
   • Bowel cancer (men and women).
   • Breast cancer (women).
   • Cervical cancer (women).

Extracted from Schüz J et al (2015) European Code against Cancer 4th Edition: 12 ways to reduce your cancer risk, *Cancer Epidemiology* **39**(1) S1–S10 with permission from Elsevier. These recommendations are the result of a project coordinated by the International Agency for Research on Cancer and co-financed by the European Commission.

Effective approaches

Evidence on cancer prevention suggests that it is most effective when political interventions are combined with individual interventions, e.g. the banning of smoking in public places throughout the UK, combined with well-resourced smoking cessation services.

A combination of different approaches is required. These should include:
• Properly resourced health promotion services
• Skilled professionals who receive training
• Using the media
• Targeting services in schools and the community
• Financial support for those living in poverty.

All health professionals should consider their own role in cancer prevention. For example, nurses may have many opportunities to assess an individual's cancer risk factors, advise smokers on smoking cessation clinics and drug therapy, or give dietary and exercise advice.

References

1 The Kings' Fund (2010). Have Targets Improved NHS Performance? Available at: ℜ http://www.kingsfund.org.uk/projects/general-election-2010/key-election-questions/performance-targets

2 Department of Health. *The NHS Cancer Plan: A Plan for Investment, a Plan for Reform.* London: Department of Health; 2000.

3 Department of Health (2011). *Improving Outcomes: A Strategy for Cancer.* Available at: ℜ https://assets.publishing.service.gov.uk/government/uploads/system/uploads/attachment_data/file/213785/dh_123394.pdf

4 National Institute for Health and Care Excellence (2005). *Referral Guidelines for Suspected Cancer.* Clinical guideline [CG27]. Available at: ℜ https://www.nice.org.uk/guidance/cg27

Cancer screening

Cancer screening involves testing a population of asymptomatic individuals, to find out which members of that group have either cancer or a precancerous condition that might benefit from early treatment. Screening is based on the principle that early disease will respond better to treatment than late disease.

There are three national cancer screening programmes in the UK—for breast, cervical, and colorectal cancers (➔ see NHS UK cancer screening, p. 47). There is no national prostate cancer screening programme, but an 'informed choice' programme of prostate risk management that includes the option for individuals to have a PSA test (➔ see Prostate cancer screening, pp. 57–8).

Criteria for screening

These criteria (see Box 4.2) are now widely accepted, and a screening programme should aim to satisfy them all. Many potential screening tests for cancer fail to do this, e.g. prostate cancer screening tests only fulfil the first criterion, i.e. it is an important health problem.

Harms and benefits

Screening may seem the right approach to take with many cancers. This is reflected in pressure from the public and the media in many countries to increase screening uptake.

However, screening can be potentially harmful for some individuals. It sometimes produces a false positive or a false negative result (see Table 4.1). At best, screening benefits only a few people. For example, in breast cancer, ~500 people are screened to reduce mortality by one. The risks and benefits of population screening are highlighted in Table 4.2.

Evaluating screening programmes

National screening programmes are expensive, and they divert resources away from other health-care activities such as primary prevention or treatment. It can be difficult to measure their cost-effectiveness.

A number of inherent biases come into play when evaluating screening tests. Tests tend to pick up the least aggressive cancers, as well as a number of cases that would have regressed naturally such as cervical dysplasia.

Diagnosis prior to clinical signs, i.e. a screening-detected disease, will improve survival statistics, even if those individuals do not live any longer than if they had found the disease through clinical signs at a later date. This is because the individual lives with the 'disease' for a longer period of time (known as lead time bias). Establishing the mortality rates of screened and unscreened groups is the only completely effective way of evaluating screening programmes.

Recall time intervals

Choosing the most effective time interval for some screening programmes is difficult. Reducing the recall interval will generally mean more positive screening results but will increase costs and the number of false positives. Another approach is more targeted programmes, aimed at those at highest risk (➔ see Cancer epidemiology and risk, p. 22).

Box 4.2 Criteria for screening
- The condition being screened for should be an important health problem.
- The natural history of the condition should be well understood.
- There should be a detectable early stage.
- Treatment at an early stage should be of more benefit than at a later stage.
- A suitable test should be devised for the early stage.
- To whom should the test be acceptable?
- Intervals for repeating the test should be determined.
- Adequate health service provision should be made for the extra clinical workload resulting from screening.
- The risks, both physical and psychological, should be less than the benefits.
- The costs should be balanced against the benefits.

Adapted from Wilson JMG and Jungner G (1968). *Principles and practice of screening for disease*.p.26–27 Geneva: WHO with permission from the World Health Organization.

Table 4.1 Screening sensitivity and specificity

		Disease status	
		+	−
Test	+	True positives (TP)	False positives (FP)
Result	−	False negatives (FN)	True negatives (TN)

Sensitivity: an effective test needs to be sensitive enough not to miss actual cases of cancer within the screened group (false negative cases).

Specificity: tests with a high specificity will send few individuals who do not have cancer for further diagnostic procedures, by producing as few false positives as possible.

Sensitivity = TP/(TP + FN)	Specificity = TN/(TN + FP)

Positive predictive value = TP/(TP + FP)

Even the best screening tests will produce more false positive results than true positive results. This is due to the low incidence of disease within screened populations. This leads to increased follow-up and anxiety for a large number of individuals.

Table 4.2 Risks and benefits of screening for cancer

Costs involved (cons)	Benefits (pros)
• Morbidity of screening test	• Life years gained for those with curable cancers
• Longer morbidity for those with unaltered prognosis	• Avoidance of morbidity from radical treatment
• Overtreatment of questionable abnormalities	• Reassurance with negative results
• False positives, giving unnecessary treatment	• Reassurance that the disease is at an early stage
• False negatives, giving false reassurance	• Avoid the cost of expensive treatment for advanced cancers
• Screening expenses	• Extra years of productivity
• Cost of additional cases treated	
• Cost of early treatment and extra follow-up	
• Diversion of resources from primary prevention and treatment	

Adapted from Chamberlain J (1988). Screening for early detection of cancer. In Tiffany R and Pritchard AP (eds). *Oncology for nurses and health care professionals*, Vol 1, pp. 155–73. New York: Harper Row.

Screening recruitment

A high uptake is required for an effective population screening programme, although a higher uptake will lead to still greater benefits from these programmes. In the UK, uptake and coverage for breast and cervical cancer screening are above 70%.

Screening uptake

Though overall uptake is high for breast and cervical screening, certain disadvantaged groups are under-represented such as older women, people from ethnic minorities, and those with high levels of deprivation. In some cases, these groups are at greatest risk of contracting the targeted disease, e.g. deprivation and cervical cancer are linked.

Reasons for the low uptake of screening in certain groups are complex and include socio-demographic characteristics, knowledge, attitudes and beliefs, social influences, and health factors.

Many methods have been tried to enhance recruitment. Recommended approaches include:
- Focusing efforts on those who have never been screened
- Telephone counselling to discuss barriers to screening
- Tagged notes in primary and secondary care
- Reducing economic barriers such as transportation costs and timing of screening visits to avoid working hours.

A trial, recruiting in Bristol and Manchester, explored whether giving women the opportunity to attend screening appointments outside of normal working hours improved uptake. The Out of Hours Study (OOHS) was randomized by birth date and offered:
- A normal working hours screening appointment
- An evening appointment
- A weekend appointment
- A normal appointment, but with the option to change to the weekend or evening.

The trial was published in 2014 and indicated that the optimum strategy for improving attendance at breast screening was to offer a traditional office hour appointment and to include in the letter of invitation an option to change to an evening or weekend appointment, if wished.

Information on this study can be accessed here (⅏ https://www.nature.com/articles/bjc2013377).

Informed uptake

Since screening can harm, as well as benefit, individuals, information available to those considering screening should clarify both the risks and benefits, including:
- The purpose of screening
- The likelihood of positive and negative findings, including false positive and false negative results (see Table 4.1)
- The risks of the screening process
- Follow-up plans, including counselling and support services.

NHS UK cancer screening

Information about the current UK cancer screening programmes, including recent statistics, current studies, and patient leaflets, can be accessed via NHS Cancer Screening Programmes at Public Health England (⌘ http://www.cancerscreening.nhs.uk/).

Future directions

The growing emphasis on prevention and early detection, coupled with changes in technology, knowledge of cancer development, and genetics, will all create new screening opportunities in the future. Current screening proposals that are ongoing include:

• The use of HPV testing in cervical screening: the Department of Health will roll out HPV testing across England as a triage for women with mild or borderline cervical screening test results and as a test of cure for treated women

• Comparison of faecal occult blood versus sigmoidoscopy for colorectal cancer: in the next 4 years, the Department of Health intends to invest £60 million to build flexible sigmoidoscopy into the current bowel screening programme.

Breast cancer screening

Breast cancer screening is done by mammogram. This involves taking an X-ray of each breast, whilst it is carefully compressed. Women generally say it is slightly uncomfortable, although about 1 in 14 women find it extremely painful. The radiation dose to the breast is about five times that of a chest X-ray (CXR).

A mammogram can detect small changes in breast tissue that are too small to be felt by the woman herself or by a doctor. Two views of the breast are taken at each screening—one from above and one into the armpit diagonally across the breast. Two views increase small cancer detection rates by up to 43%.

Research now suggests that out of every 1000 women screened, 5.7 lives will be saved.[1] The reduction in breast cancer deaths is attributed to:

• Diagnosis and treatment of asymptomatic pre-invasive disease (ductal carcinoma *in situ*)
• Diagnosis and treatment of early invasive breast cancer which would otherwise not present until systemic spread had occurred.

There has been concern in recent years that the breast screening service has led to 'overdiagnosis' of breast cancers, i.e. the screen detection of cancers that normally would not have been detected in a woman's lifetime. Recent research would indicate that the benefits of screening still outweigh the risk of overdiagnosis.[5]

To date, there is limited evidence that there is a mortality benefit in screening for women under the age of 50.

The NHS breast screening programme

This was set up in 1988. Around 2 million women are screened in the UK each year. Women aged between 50 and 70 are now routinely invited for screening every 3 years. From 2012, this will be extended to some women between the ages of 47–49 and 71–73 years as part of the extension randomization project. This is a randomized trial to determine if screening in these extended age ranges is effective or not. It is anticipated that a full rollout of the extension project will be complete in England by 2016. Screening is carried out in a specialized screening unit, which can be either mobile or hospital-based. It costs about £40 for each woman screened.

Why is there currently routine screening only for those of 47–73 years of age?

• Mammograms are not as effective in pre-menopausal women and show a far higher rate of false positives. The density of breast tissue makes it more difficult to detect problems, and these women also have a lower incidence of breast cancer.
• The breast tissue of post-menopausal women is increasingly made up of fat. This is clearer on the mammogram and makes interpretation of the X-ray more reliable.

Screening for other groups

- Women at moderate to high risk of breast cancer because of their family history should be offered annual mammography when they are aged between 40 and 50 years. A magnetic resonance imaging (MRI) scan may be of particular benefit in this group.
- Women aged over 70 are not routinely invited for screening, though they can continue to self-refer to the 3-yearly programme. Nurses have an important role in giving these women accurate information about the potential risks and benefits of continuing or stopping screening. A recent study has found that an intervention tool (based on a 10-minute structured interaction with a radiographer) used with women attending their final screening mammogram appointment increases the chances of timely presentation with a potential breast cancer.[6] Further studies are required to see if this results in improved survival in this group of women.
- Some European countries offer more frequent screening to try to reduce the number of interval cancers (those detected in between screening visits). The cost/benefit of this more frequent approach is currently being evaluated in several trials.[7]

Suspicious abnormalities

- If a suspicious abnormality is seen, the woman is recalled to the breast screening centre.
- A clinical examination is performed with further X-rays, an ultrasound (US) examination, a needle test for cytology, or a core biopsy if appropriate.
- Women thought to have cancer are referred promptly to a breast surgeon who will arrange appropriate treatment.
- Five per cent of women are recalled for further tests, though only five cases of cancer are found per 1000 women screened.

Breast self-examination

- Scientific evidence does not support teaching women to carry out ritualized breast self-examination.
- A more relaxed approach to breast awareness is just as safe and effective.
- Women should be encouraged to check their breasts for what is normal for them, but there is no recommended routine self-examination to a set technique.

References

5 Duffy SW, Tabar L, Helene A, et al. Absolute Numbers of Lives Saved and Overdiagnosed in Breast Cancer Screening, From a Randomized Trial and From the Breast Screening Programme in England. Discussed at: ℘ https://www.nhs.uk/news/cancer/breast-screening-is-beneficial/

6 Forbes et al (2011). Available at: ℘ http://www.kcl.ac.uk/innovation/groups/earlypres/assets/forbes.pdf

7 NHS Breast Cancer Screening. Available at: ℘ https://www.nhs.uk/conditions/breast-cancer-screening/

Cervical cancer screening

Cervical screening can prevent cancer by detecting and treating early abnormalities, which, if left untreated, could lead to cervical cancer. It is not a direct test for cancer but picks up early abnormalities on the cervix, which increase the risk of getting cancer. However, it will also detect cancer that is already present.

Liquid-based cytology testing

Screening is carried out using liquid-based cytology (LBC). A speculum is inserted into the vagina, and cells are taken from the cervix using a specially designed brush. Most women consider the procedure to be only mildly uncomfortable. The cells from the brush are placed in preservative fluid, spun, and cleaned, before being placed on a slide and examined by a cytologist.

Since 2008, LBC testing has replaced PAP (Papanicolaou) smear testing in the UK for cervical screening; this is because it was found to reduce inadequate tests from 9% to <2%.

National screening programme

The NHS cervical screening programme calls all women between the ages of 25 and 64 for a free cervical screening test every 3–5 years[8] (see Box 4.3).

The programme is carried out through a call-and-recall system of women who are registered with a general practitioner (GP). It tests over 3 million women a year, and the estimated cost is around £175 million a year in England. Women who have not had a recent test may be offered one when they attend their GP or family planning clinic on another matter.

Effective screening interval

There has been a lot of debate about the best interval for cervical screening recall. More frequent screening may slightly reduce the incidence of cervical cancer but will increase the cost of the programme substantially. It could also lead to many more women facing the anxiety of abnormal tests, without any actual benefit.

Exclusions

Younger women are not tested, as cervical cancer in this age group is very rare. In addition, because the cervix is still developing, there is a very high rate of false positives. Women who have never been sexually active are able to withdraw from the call-and-recall system due to their very low risk

---

Box 4.3 National cervical screening programme

Age group	Frequency of screening
25	First invitation
25–49	3-yearly
50–64	5-yearly
65+	Only offered to those not tested since age 50 or who have had recent abnormal tests

of cervical cancer. Older women are not routinely involved in the screening system, as they are statistically at very low risk for developing cervical cancer. Women who have had abnormal screening tests previously may still be followed up as part of a surveillance programme, and women over 65 who have never previously had a screening test are able to access one.

Women in same-sex relationships

Gay and bisexual women of screening age are now encouraged to actively take part in the normal 3-year screening programme. This is because HPV can still be transmitted during lesbian sex, and smoking (another risk factor in cervical cancer) has been shown to be more prevalent in gay and bisexual women.

Abnormal testing follow-up

The test aims to find abnormal cervical cells. Test results are graded as borderline (slight dysplastic changes, which normally return to normal), mild, moderate, or severe. Results may also be graded as cervical intraepithelial neoplasia (CIN) 1, 2, or 3. CIN 1 is where one-third of the cervical epithelium is affected. CIN 3 is where the full thickness is affected. Strictly speaking, CIN can only be diagnosed by a biopsy.

Women with a borderline result will be asked to have a repeat test in 6 months. After three borderline results or one mild, moderate, or severe result, women will normally be referred for colposcopy (using a low-powered microscope). Here the changes can be more closely observed, biopsies can be taken, and possible treatment offered.

The usual approach for CIN 2 and 3 disease is colposcopy and loop diathermy removing the abnormal cells. If CIN 3 disease extends into the endocervical canal or there is microinvasion, a cone biopsy is carried out.

Nursing support and prevention advice

If women have an abnormal smear, they will naturally feel anxious. It is important to talk through what the result actually means. CIN grades are not cancer, although many women may think they are. The nurse should clarify any ↑ risk of cancer and the purpose of follow-up. This can also be a good opportunity to talk through other risk factors, such as multiple sexual partners, non-barrier methods of contraception, and smoking, and to discuss risk reduction activities.

Human papillomavirus testing and triage

Nearly 100% of cervical cancer cases show signs of HPV infection. If women with borderline or mildly abnormal smears do not have high-risk HPV infection (HPV 16 or 18), they have an extremely low risk of developing cervical cancer.

HPV triage, or testing in combination with standard cervical screening, has been evaluated in the UK in women with mild or borderline cervical screening test results and also as a test of cure for treated women.

If women have a screening result which shows borderline changes or low-grade dyskaryosis, their sample is tested for HPV. If HPV is then found, the woman is invited for colposcopy to assess her cervix more closely. If the test is negative, the woman returns to the regular screening programme.

In addition to this, if a woman has had treatment for a cervical abnormality, she will be screened again for HPV 6 months later. If this test is positive, she will be recalled for colposcopy to check if further treatment is needed. If no HPV is found then, once again, the woman returns to the normal screening programme.

In some areas of the country, there is currently a pilot of 'primary HPV screening'. This is where cervical screening samples are tested routinely for HPV testing before going for cytology. This is thought to increase the accuracy of the screening test, and it also might mean HPV-negative women will not need to be screened as frequently.

Human papillomavirus vaccine

The use of HPV vaccines has a role in preventing cervical cancer disease. The national HPV immunization programme began in 2008 for schoolgirls aged 12–13, and a catch-up programme up to 18 years.

Uptake has been consistently very high, and it is believed that up to 400 lives every year could be saved by vaccinating young women before they become infected with HPV. The vaccine used is the Gardasil® vaccine, which is thought to be extremely safe and should remain effective for 7–8 years.

References

8 NHS Cervical Cancer Screening. Available at: ℘ https://www.nhs.uk/conditions/cervical-screening/

Bowel and prostate cancer screening

Bowel cancer screening

Bowel cancer is the second highest cause of cancer deaths, and trial results have suggested that bowel screening, when acceptable to the public with a high enough uptake, could reduce bowel cancer mortality by 16% in the targeted group.[9]

The faecal occult blood test (FOBT) is not a test for cancer; it tests for a high-risk sign of the disease. About 2% of FOBT tests end up positive. These will be followed up by diagnostic colonoscopy.

In Scotland, the FOBT screening test has already been replaced by the faecal immunochemical test (FIT), and across the rest of the UK, FIT will replace FOBT by the end of 2019. FIT offers an advantage in that it is specific to human haemoglobin. This means that, unlike FOBT, the result is not influenced by the presence of other types of blood in the stool such as that ingested in the diet.

National bowel cancer screening programme

The UK's bowel cancer screening programme started in 2006 using the FOBT. By 2010, it was fully rolled out throughout the UK, targeting men and women between the ages of 60 and 69 years. People older than 70 years can obtain a testing kit on request. Eligible people receive information and a testing kit through the post, with detailed instructions on how to carry out the test and return it to the screening laboratory, with positive tests resulting in the individual being invited for a colonoscopy.

Flexible sigmoidoscopy can also complement testing, and the NHS in England is now providing a 60% coverage of sigmoidoscopy screening in 55–64 year olds. The current pilot has been reported, with evidence that a single flexible sigmoidoscopy examination between 55 and 64 years of age confers a substantial reduction in colorectal cancer incidence and mortality.[10]

Prostate cancer screening

Currently, prostate cancer only fulfils the first screening criterion—that the condition is an important health problem. The natural history of prostate cancer is poorly understood. There are asymptomatic forms of the disease that either would never prove fatal or might produce symptoms only very late in disease development. Autopsy reports also suggest that more men die with prostate cancer than from it.

A national screening programme would therefore identify many men who would never benefit from treatment but who could be harmed both physically and psychologically.

Two methods of screening for prostate cancer exist:
- Digital rectal examination—this is easy to carry out but has low sensitivity and specificity. It is not recommended in asymptomatic men
- PSA testing.

There is considerable demand for PSA testing amongst men concerned about the disease, but there is currently no screening programme for prostate cancer; there is, however, an informed choice programme. This is called 'Prostate Cancer Risk Management' and provides men and GPs with information on the advantages and disadvantages of PSA testing. This highlights the risks and benefits and should enable men to make an informed choice.

Information leaflets are available for patients and health professionals via the NHS Cancer Screening site at: ℞ https://www.nhs.uk/conditions/cervical-screening/

Prostate-specific antigen

PSA is a protein found in a higher concentration in prostate cells than in blood. It is raised beyond its normal threshold (see Table 4.3) in about 75% of prostate cancers. It can also be raised in benign prostatic hyperplasia, prostatitis, and urinary tract infections (UTIs).

If PSA tests are found to be abnormal, then individuals could be referred for transrectal ultrasound (TRUS) and prostatic biopsy as a diagnostic test. About two-thirds of men having TRUS will not have prostate cancer detectable via biopsy.

Persistently elevated PSA

The best management for those men with a persistently elevated PSA, but who have had negative biopsies, is unclear. These men may face prolonged periods of follow-up and experience considerable anxiety.

Table 4.3 Normal PSA levels

There is some controversy about cut-off points for normal PSA levels. Some areas use 4ng/mL, whereas others use age-related ranges. The recommended ranges from the Prostate Cancer Risk Management Programme are as follows.

Age (years)	PSA cut-off (ng/mL)
50–59	>3.0
60–69	>4.0
70+	>5.0

Reproduced from Burford DC, Kirby M, Austoker J. Prostate Cancer Risk Management Programme: information for primary care; PSA testing in asymptomatic men. NHS Cancer Screening Programmes, 2009 © Crown Copyright, reproduced under the Open Government Licence v.3.0.

References

9 Hewitson P, Glasziou P, Erwig LM, Towler B, Watson E. Screening for colorectal cancer using the faecal occult blood test, Hemoccult. *Cochrane Database Syst Rev* 2007;1:CD001216.

10 Atkins W, Wooldrage K, Maxwell Parkin D, et al. Long term effects of once-only flexible sigmoidoscopy screening after 17 years of follow-up: the UK Flexible Sigmoidoscopy Screening randomised controlled trial. *Lancet* 2017;**389**:1299–13.

Dietary prevention

Diet has been clearly linked to colorectal, stomach, H&N, and prostate cancers. Obesity has been linked to post-menopausal breast and endometrial cancers. Inactivity, which can be linked to obesity, has also been directly linked to increasing risks of colon cancer. Regular alcohol use has been linked to the development of some cancers, specifically cancers of the H&N, breast, liver, colon, and oesophagus. Around 4% of all UK cancers can be attributed to alcohol use.[11]

There are clear links between poor diet and social deprivation, highlighting the inequalities that exist in cancer rates within the UK. Barriers to improving diet are:

- Access and availability—whether people have access to good-quality, affordable food locally
- Attitudes and awareness—knowledge, attitudes, motivation, and skills concerning the buying, preparation, and eating of healthy food.

Advice for improving diet

- Increase the intake of fruit and vegetables to at least five portions a day.
- Increase the intake of dietary fibre from bread and other cereals (particularly wholegrain varieties), potatoes, fruit, and vegetables.
- Maintain a healthy body weight [within the body mass index (BMI) range of 20–25].
- Keep the consumption of red meat and animal fat to a minimum (<140g per day). This will also have a preventative effect on heart disease.

Strategies for improving diet

Successful strategies include:

- Individual and small group counselling sessions aimed at behavioural change
- Changes to the local environment, e.g. in shops and catering outlets
- National media campaigns such as the five-a-day fruit and vegetable campaign and the national school fruit scheme.

These strategies can also help with obesity. Combining them with strategies to increase activity is probably more effective in sustaining weight loss than diet or exercise alone in adults.

Reduction in obesity is an important part of the UK government's strategy for improving health across the population as a whole. The document *Healthy Lives, Healthy People: A Call to Action on Obesity in England* was published in 2011 and lays out the evidence linking obesity with poor health. It also highlights projects which have been successful in promoting healthier lifestyles and how these can be embedded in communities.

The National Heart, Lung, and Blood Institute (NHLBI) provides a useful interactive website for both health professionals and patients. It lists a range of useful strategies to help treat obesity (℞ https://www.nhlbi.nih.gov/health-topics/overweight-and-obesity).

Alcohol

Approaches to reducing alcohol consumption include the following strategies:

- Taxation and pricing
- Licensing
- Targeted drink-driving campaigns
- Controlling the promotion of alcohol: advertising, broadcasting, sponsorship, and packaging
- Changing attitudes; campaigns to promote responsible drinking. Campaigning groups have recently included Cancer Research UK and Macmillan Cancer Care
- Support and treatment, via a range of voluntary and health-care organizations.

Brief interventions

'Brief interventions involve opportunistic advice, discussion, negotiation or encouragement. They are commonly used in many areas of health pro-motion, and are delivered by a range of primary and community care professionals.'[11]

For smoking cessation, brief interventions typically take between 5 and 10 minutes and may include one or more of the following:

- Simple opportunistic advice to stop
- An assessment of the patient's commitment to quit
- An offer of pharmacotherapy and/or behavioural support
- Provision of self-help material and referral to more intensive support such as the NHS Stop Smoking Services.

Brief interventions from health-care professionals have been shown to have an important role to play in dietary advice and smoking prevention, and in reducing alcohol consumption and improving alcohol-related problems.

All health professionals should consider the opportunities they have in their everyday practice to initiate brief health promotion activities.

Reflection points

- How might you introduce cancer prevention strategies into your own practice?
- What potential barriers exist?
- What resources, including training or education, might you require? Find out what resources exist in your own area that promote:
- Smoking cessation.
- Responsible alcohol use.
- Dietary advice.

References

11 National Institute for Health and Care Excellence. *Brief Interventions and Referral for Smoking Cessation in Primary Care and Other Settings.* Public Health Intervention Guidance No. 1. London: National Institute for Health and Care Excellence; 2006.

Smoking cessation

- Smoking is the main avoidable cause of premature death in the UK.
  People who stop smoking live longer than those who do not, and their
  risk of lung cancer diminishes with time. In 2009, Cancer Research UK
  estimated that around 25% of all UK cancer deaths were caused by
  smoking.
- Smoking rates in the UK have steadily declined over the last 30 years.
  However, this decline has slowed down in recent years. The decline was
  originally faster in men than women.
- Around 21% of adults now smoke in the UK (21% of men and 20% of
  women). Smoking amongst children ↑ in the 1990s but has now ↓ again
  to around 10%.
- Socio-economic trends in smoking behaviour are strong. In manual
  groups, smoking rates are around 28%, whilst in non-manual groups, it
  is 13%. The gap between socio-economic groups has ↑ since the 1970s,
  and this is one of the major causes of health inequalities between socio-
  economic groups within the UK, and a major cause in the differences in
  life expectancy.[12]
- NHS Stop Smoking Services: the local NHS Stop Smoking Services
  provides support to smokers wanting to quit. Most Stop Smoking
  advisers are nurses or pharmacists, and all have received training for
  their role. This service offers a combination of:
  - Group treatment and individual face-to-face counselling
  - Nicotine replacement therapies (NRTs) and drugs used to reduce
    cravings (bupropion and varenicline).

Evidence from clinical trials suggests that smokers are four times more likely
to quit smoking using this combined approach, than by willpower alone.

The 4-week quit rates for the service show about 35% of people remain non-smokers at 4 weeks. Smoking cessation treatment is extremely
cost-effective, compared with many other health service interventions. The
cost per life year of around £800 is much cheaper than most other medical
interventions, although smoking rates are currently only declining at <0.4%
per annum in the UK, and a faster decline is needed if national targets are
to be met.

Smoking cessation is now funded and organized at Clinical Commissioning
Group (CCG) level, replacing a previous ad hoc approach. The key aims of
the current service are to:

- Increase referral rates via GPs and other members of the primary care
  team, as these are a major source of recruitment
- Focus on low-income and pregnant smokers and ensure the needs of
  minority ethnic populations are catered for
- Improve links with acute hospital trusts to ensure patients receive help
  with smoking cessation whilst in hospital.[12]

Department of Health position/aims on tobacco use

- Reducing exposure to second-hand smoke—making smoke-free environments the norm at work and at leisure.
- Media/education campaigns.
- Reducing the availability of tobacco products and regulating supply—including action on shops that sell cigarettes to children and further reductions in tobacco smuggling.
- Further improvements to NHS Stop Smoking Services and ↑ availability of NRT to help smokers quit.
- Reducing tobacco promotion—the Standardized Packaging of Tobacco Products Regulations 2015 came into force in May 2016.
- Regulating tobacco, e.g. adding hard-hitting picture warnings to cigarette packets.

Useful resources for smokers for easy-access advice about giving up smoking

- NHS Smoking Cessation website: ℘ http://www.smokefree.nhs.uk
- NHS Smoking Cessation resources.
- Facebook: ℘ http://www.facebook.com/NHSSmokefree
- Twitter: ℘ twitter.com/nhssmokefree
- YouTube Channel: ℘ http://www.youtube.com/user/ smokefreevideos

References

12 Office for National Statistics (2012). *General Lifestyle Survey 2010* (overview: a report on the 2010 general lifestyle survey). Available at: ℘ http://webarchive.nationalarchives.gov.uk/ 20160107053724/http://www.ons.gov.uk/ons/rel/ghs/general-lifestyle-survey/2010/index. html

Skin cancer prevention

Skin cancer is a largely preventable disease. By taking simple measures to protect the skin from the sun, people can substantially reduce their risk of getting skin cancer. Because skin cancers are visible, they can also be detected early and removed, before they pose a threat to life.

Risk factors for skin cancer

- Fair skin which burns easily and tans poorly.
- Personal or family history of skin cancer.
- History of intense or prolonged sun exposure.
- Higher-than-average number of pigmented skin naevi (moles).

Use of sunscreens

Sunscreens do prevent sunburn, but they may not protect against skin cancer. They may reduce the amount of sunlight reaching the skin's surface, but if they are used to prolong the amount of time a person spends in the sun, they could potentially increase skin cancer risk.

More effective prevention behaviour is to wear a hat and shirt, stay in the shade, and avoid the summer sun in the middle of the day. From a socio-economic perspective, this approach is also much cheaper, as sunscreens can be prohibitively expensive if used as often as recommended.

NHS advice on preventing skin melanoma and other skin cancers

This can be summarized as:
- Avoid the sun when it is at its hottest.
- Wear clothes that protect your skin from the sun.
- Use sunscreen—at least sun protection factor (SPF) 15 is recommended.
- Avoid burning.
- Tan sensibly, and preferably do not sunbathe at all.
- Avoid sunbeds and sun-lamps. It is now illegal for under 18s to use sunbeds or lamps.
- Check your moles.

Skin cancer advice to give about changes in moles (ABCDE guide)

- A stands for asymmetrical—melanomas have two very different halves and are an irregular shape.
- B stands for border—unlike a normal mole, melanomas have a notched or ragged border.
- C stands for colours—melanomas will be a mix of two or more colours.
- D stands for diameter—unlike most moles, melanomas are larger than 6mm (1/4 inch) in diameter.
- E stands for enlargement or evolution—a mole that changes characteristics and size over time is more likely to be a melanoma.

Reproduced from Skin Cancer (melanoma) NHS choices (2017): ℘ https://www.nhs.uk/conditions/melanoma-skin-cancer/symptoms/ © Crown Copyright under the Open Government Licence v.30.

Cancer genetics

Since the completion of the entire mapping of the human genome in 2003, there has been a quantum leap forward in understanding the genetic basis of cancer. Every cancer arises due to genetic mutations that have occurred within a cell and altered the normal life cycle of that cell. These genetic mutations are usually acquired within a person's lifetime (➲ see Cancer biology, p. 32).

Currently, genetic testing tends to be used for people with an existing diagnosis of cancer (in order to target treatments) and in people with a high familial risk of cancers. Large-scale genetic testing of groups of people who are currently well has not been applied. This may be changing, however, with the advent of schemes such as 'Trusight', which is being run on a trial basis by Cancer Research UK, using genetic screening to identify over 100 cancer-predisposing genes in patients with cancer, but also their relatives.

Outside mutations which occur within a cell's life, about 5–10% of cancers are thought to be due to an inherited cancer-predisposing gene. A number of inherited genes have been identified that confer an ↑ predisposition to specific cancers. Generally, all people carry two copies of these genes. Predisposition to specific cancers occurs when a person inherits a mutated copy. If a person is known to carry a mutated gene that causes a cancer predisposition, then the risk of their offspring inheriting the predisposing gene mutation is 50%. This is called dominant inheritance (see Fig. 4.1).

Assessment of familial risk

Having one or more relatives affected with cancer raises anxiety for many people, suggesting an inherited tendency to cancer in their family. However, for most people, it is much more likely that the family history has arisen through chance due to:

- Shared environment
- Shared lifestyle
- Cancer being a common disease in the Western population.

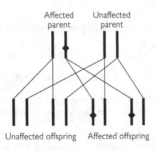

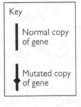

Key

Normal copy of gene

Mutated copy of gene

Affected parent   Unaffected parent

Unaffected offspring   Affected offspring

Fig. 4.1 Autosomal dominant inheritance.

A detailed family tree is important for this assessment and should take into account:
- The numbers and relatedness of affected relatives and age at diagnosis
- The number and relatedness of unaffected relatives
- The presence of other clues in the family history, e.g. related cancers, bilateral disease.

Key features pointing towards a possible inherited predisposition are:
- Multiple, closely related individuals with cancer
- Several generations in the family affected with cancer
- Early age of onset of cancer, e.g. pre-menopausal breast cancer, colorectal cancer at age <50 years, or childhood tumours
- Bilateral breast cancer
- >1 primary in an affected individual
- Rare cancers, e.g. ♂ breast cancer.

Through this risk assessment, families are usually grouped in one of three categories:
- Low genetic risk
- Moderate genetic risk
- High genetic risk.

Genetic testing

Currently, genetic testing can only be offered where there is an affected family member who is willing and able to provide a blood sample for testing. In many families, a causative mutation is not found. All individuals undergoing genetic testing are offered genetic counselling within Clinical Genetics Services to discuss the implications of possible testing outcomes.

In families where a causative gene mutation is found, predictive testing can be offered to at-risk relatives to clarify their personal risk of developing a related cancer. This allows surveillance and surgical interventions to be targeted at those individuals at high genetic risk. Predictive testing also raises ethical and practical considerations for those individuals considering testing, and therefore, predictive testing is offered through Clinical Genetics Services.

Common cancers with inherited predisposition

Breast cancer

Around 5–10% of breast cancers are thought to be due to a hereditary factor. Several genes are known to be involved in inherited predisposition—the two most common ones are *BRCA1* and *BRCA2*. A woman who inherits a mutated form of one of these genes will have a lifetime risk of developing breast cancer in the order of 50–80%.

There are other specific cancers that may be associated with inherited mutations in *BRCA1*/*BRCA2*:

• Ovarian cancer—lifetime risk of 20–60%
• ♂ breast cancer
• Prostate cancer
• Colorectal cancer
• Ocular melanoma
• Pancreatic cancer.

Both men and women can inherit mutations in the *BRCA1* and *BRCA2* genes; however, men are much less likely to develop an associated cancer than women in a family. Both men and women can pass on the mutated gene to their offspring (see Fig. 4.1).

Management of familial breast cancer

Individuals and families who fall into the low genetic risk group can be reassured; their risk of developing cancer is close to that for the general population.

In 2013, NICE published new guidelines on the management of people at high risk of developing breast cancer, which updated their guidance from 2004—individuals and families who fall into higher genetic risk groups should be counselled about their risk. Counselling often takes place in family history clinics within Breast Care Services for moderate-risk women. Counselling for high-risk families takes place within Clinical Genetic Services. Women and families at higher genetic risk are eligible for a number of interventions.

Early detection

• Offer annual mammographic surveillance to women aged 40–69 years with a known *BRCA1* or *BRCA2* mutation.
• Offer annual mammographic surveillance to all women aged 50–69 years who have or have had breast cancer who remain at high risk of the disease.
• Offering annual MRI surveillance to all women aged 30–49 years who have or have had breast cancer who remain at high risk of the disease, including those who have a *BRCA1* or *BRCA2* mutation.

Risk-reducing surgery

Women identified to be at high genetic risk for breast and/or ovarian cancer may choose to undergo prophylactic mastectomy to remove healthy tissue, in order to reduce the risk of developing cancer. There is evidence that such surgery does reduce the risk of developing these cancers, but the reduction in risk is not absolute, as not all the tissue can be removed. Women considering this intervention are offered genetic counselling within Clinical Genetic Services.

Drug treatment

A recent change in the NICE guidance recommends that women who are at moderate or high risk of breast cancer should be counselled and offered treatment with the hormone treatments tamoxifen or raloxifene. This is governed by the following guidelines.

- These drugs are not suitable for people who have had thrombosis or endometrial cancer, so other options for reducing risk should be discussed. If patients have had prophylactic bilateral mastectomy, the risk will now be very low and drug treatment should not be necessary.
- High-risk pre-menopausal women should be offered a drug called tamoxifen. High-risk post-menopausal women should be offered tamoxifen or raloxifene.
- Medium-risk pre-menopausal women may be offered a drug called tamoxifen. Medium-risk post-menopausal women may be offered tamoxifen or raloxifene.
- Tamoxifen or raloxifene should not be taken for >5 years.
- Further information is available at: ℘ https://www.nice.org.uk/guidance/cg164

Ovarian cancer

BRCA1 and *BRCA2* gene mutations may also predispose to ovarian cancer. A family in which there are two or more ovarian cancer diagnoses has a high chance of being related to a predisposing gene mutation.

Early detection

Currently, there is no surveillance method that has been proved effective in identifying early changes in the ovaries. A national trial called the UK Familial Ovarian Screening Study (UKFOCSS) considered whether women with a significant family history of ovarian cancer or breast/ovarian cancer or colorectal/ovarian cancer would benefit from annual US scan and CA-125 serum marker. Early results of this trial suggested that there may be a benefit in detecting early cancers if the screening takes place every 4 months. This second phase is now in progress.

Colorectal cancer

Several genes are known to be involved in inherited predisposition to colorectal cancer. The two most important genetic syndromes that predispose to colorectal cancer are:

- Hereditary non-polyposis colorectal cancer (HNPCC)
- Familial adenomatous polyposis (FAP).

HNPCC causes ~5–10% of colorectal cancers and confers a 75% risk of developing colorectal cancer by the age of 65 years. There are other specific cancers that may be associated with HNPCC:

- Endometrial cancer
- Ovarian cancer
- Small bowel cancer

- Stomach cancer
- Ureteric cancer
- Renal pelvis cancer.

FAP accounts for <1% of colorectal cancers. It confers a 100% risk of developing colorectal cancer by the age of 50 years. Individuals affected with FAP will develop hundreds of adenomatous polyps in the bowel during their teenage years.

Both men and women can inherit these colorectal cancer predisposing syndromes and can pass on the mutated gene to their offspring (see Fig. 4.1).

Early detection and management

Individuals identified as being at moderate or high genetic risk are offered regular surveillance, usually by sigmoidoscopy or colonoscopy.

HNPCC

- Colonoscopy every 2 years from the age of 25 years.
- Any polyps identified are removed at colonoscopy.
- Endometrial/uterine screening is not routinely offered, as there is little evidence of effectiveness.

FAP

- Sigmoidoscopy annually from adolescence.
- Upper gastric endoscopy in known gene carriers.
- Prophylactic colectomy is offered if extensive polyposis is identified.

Rare cancer syndromes

A number of rare genetic syndromes can predispose individuals to specific patterns of malignant and non-malignant tumours. Examples include:
- Li-Fraumeni syndrome:
  - Early-onset breast cancer
  - Childhood sarcomas
  - Leukaemias
  - Brain tumours
- Cowden syndrome:
  - Young-onset breast cancer
  - Non-medullary thyroid cancer
  - Uterine cancer
  - Multiple hamartomatous skin lesions
- von Hippel–Lindau syndrome:
  - Cerebellar haemangioblastomas
  - Renal cell carcinoma
  - Phaeochromocytoma
  - Retinal angiomas

Further reading

Eeles RA, Easton DF, Ponder BAJ, Eng C (eds). *Genetic Predisposition to Cancer*, 2nd ed. London: Hodder-Arnold; 2004.

Scotting P, Howard P. New methods of detecting cancer and identifying genetic risk of disease. *Cancer Nurs Pract* 2013;**12**:16–21.

Section 3

The Experience of Cancer

The Experience
of Cancer

Chapter 5

Living with and beyond cancer

Cancer survivorship

Cancer survivorship has become a very significant part of the way we understand how people live with cancer, and also how cancer services are organized. Increasing numbers of people are surviving cancer, due to more screening, earlier diagnosis, and more effective treatments. This has led to a change in our perception of cancer as a disease from a 'death sentence' to a long-term or chronic illness.

For the person living with cancer, cancer survivorship can represent an identity that is positive and enabling, and for cancer services, it marks a shift from treatment of the cancer alone to a focus on the longer-term effects of cancer on the whole person and their quality of life. In terms of cancer services, in the UK, developments have been led by the National Cancer Survivorship Initiative (NCSI), and in the United States (USA) by the National Coalition of Cancer Survivors.

Survivorship may have different meanings, depending on the context:
- Living beyond 5 years from diagnosis
- Living at any time after completing treatment apparently free of cancer
- Living with and beyond cancer.

The latter definition **living with and beyond cancer** is the most widely used. This means that anyone who has been diagnosed with cancer can identify themselves as a survivor.

Survivorship has been identified as having five particular attributes:[1]
- **Process**: survival can be seen as a personal journey from diagnosis onwards, e.g. the cancer journey
- **Uncertainty**: survivorship leads to loss of the certainties of life and the fear that life may be shortened by cancer
- **Life-changing experience**: leading to permanent changes and a reappraisal of life and personal priorities
- **Duality of positive and negative aspects**: people often have longer-term health problems after cancer but nonetheless may feel a sense of personal growth or transformation
- **Individual experience with universality**: each experience of living with cancer is unique, but it can also be a shared experience that has common features.

Living with and beyond cancer

Survivorship has a number of consequences for the individual, which can include:
- Fatigue, pain, and disability
- Feelings of abandonment or isolation after the end of treatment
- Changed relationships with partner, family, and friends
- Fear of recurrence
- Dealing with the unrealistic expectations of others that life is 'back to normal'.

This challenges assumptions about the nature of rehabilitation or a return to normal after cancer. Rather, life is unlikely to be the same, usually having both better and worse aspects, and the challenge of survivorship includes finding new priorities and a new lifestyle, finding a 'new normal', and moving on with a changed perspective on life.

Cancer can therefore be considered a long-term condition, with lasting effects on the person and their life. An important aspect of this is the late effects of treatment. These can be very severe and disabling in some cases, e.g. following pelvic radiotherapy, a significant proportion of patients experience bowel, urinary, and sexual disturbances.[2]

Services for cancer survivors

There are increasing numbers of cancer survivors; in 2009, there were 2 million people in the UK living with or beyond cancer, and over half of them had been diagnosed >5 years before. Many of these people will be living satisfying lives, often with a greater appreciation of life. However, there will also be a significant minority for whom ongoing care will be necessary. To meet their needs, a model of risk-stratified care pathways has been developed which has the following levels:

1. Self-care with support and open access for those whose lives are largely free of ongoing cancer-related problems, including information and health education
2. Planned coordinated care across different clinical teams, with identified key trigger points that initiate assessment or reassessment
3. Complex case management by MDTs for those with complex and enduring problems.

With each step, greater resources will be needed to support the cancer survivor. Cancer survivorship services are based on the following principles:

- A greater focus on recovery, health, and well-being
- A shift towards holistic assessment, information provision, and personalized care planning
- A shift towards support for self-management, based on individual needs
- A shift towards tailored support that enables early recognition of the consequences of treatment and the signs and symptoms of further disease plus tailored support for those with advanced disease
- A shift from measuring clinical activity to measuring experience and outcomes for cancer survivors, through routine use of Patient-Reported Outcome Measures (PROMS) (→ see Patient-reported outcome measures, p. 468).

The Recovery Package

Within the UK, Personalized Survivorship Care Plans, based on Holistic Needs Assessment (→ see Holistic needs assessment and care planning, p. 464), are part of the *Recovery Package*[3] for cancer survivors. This has the overall aim of improving the QoL through targeted interventions and lifestyle choices for survivors. The Package will include some or all of the following:

- Holistic Needs Assessment
- Cancer Treatment Summary
- Personalized Survivorship Care Plan
- Cancer Care Review (in primary care)
- Patient education and support events.

Ideally, this will also include information on the following:

- Key contacts in primary and secondary care
- Prevention advice and information on potential signs of recurrence
- Advice on long-term physical and psychosocial effects
- Options for psychosocial, nutritional, and other supportive interventions.

Implications for cancer nursing

All nurses working with people who have cancer, and particularly specialist nurses, need to be aware of their long-term needs and to support them in making positive adjustments after cancer treatment. Specialist nurses may be more actively involved in the process, e.g. by organizing well-being events. Key elements of the nursing role will include:

- Supporting survivors with diet, activity, and lifestyle choices
- Preparing survivors for, and dealing with, late effects of treatment and recurrence
- Providing psychosocial support.
- Helping patients to identify their sources of informal and professional support and manage their own condition as far as they are able to.

To review progress in this area of evolving practice, see: ℜ http://www.macmillan.org.uk/about-us/health-professionals/programmes-and-services/recovery-package

References

1 Doyle N. Cancer survivorship: evolutionary concept analysis. *J Adv Nurs* 2008;62:499–509.
2 Adams E, Boulton M, Horne A, *et al*. The effects of pelvic radiotherapy on cancer survivors: symptom profile, psychological morbidity and quality of life. *Clin Oncol* 2014;26:10–17.
3 Department of Health and Social Care (2013). *Living With and Beyond Cancer: Taking Action to Improve Outcomes*. Available at: ℜ https://www.gov.uk/government/publications/living-with-and-beyond-cancer-taking-action-to-improve-outcomes

Cancer survivorship and personal identity

For the person with cancer, survivorship can involve a new personal identity, linked to the cancer experience, though not necessarily defined by it. Personal identity is defined by the **continuity of memory** of who we are and our experience of **embodiment**, or who we are located within our body and any changes that take place to it.[4] We also experience life as a personal **biography**, a **narrative**, or a **life story** for ourselves, as we go through life, from the past, through the present, and into the future, making sense of personal experiences and memories. When we have extreme experiences like cancer, our biography or narrative may be severely disrupted and this challenges our sense of who we are. The identity of a cancer survivor therefore requires repairing of this disruption or a discontinuity of memory by making sense of what has happened and rebuilding the personal biography or narrative, a process which can be termed **narrative reconstruction**.

Narrative reconstruction involves finding meaning in the cancer experience. This can involve:

- Incorporating new and painful experiences into the sense of personal identity
- Reinforcing enduring personal values (e.g. moral or religious ones)
- Maintaining or resuming rewarding activities (e.g. work or hobbies)
- Adapting to a new body, possibly changed in appearance, function, or sensation (e.g. pain or fatigue)
- Reappraising personal priorities and finding growth in adversity.

For some people, this new narrative will include cancer survivorship, and being a cancer survivor will become central to their new sense of who they are.[5] Identifying yourself as a **cancer survivor** can have particular benefits:

- To replace an identity defined by illness (e.g. victim) with one that supports self-efficacy
- To support a new attitude to health and health-promoting behaviours
- To provide protection against preoccupation with worries about cancer and recurrence
- To feel part of a wider community of people who have overcome the challenge of cancer.

Adoption of the cancer survivor identity is associated with good treatment outcomes, fewer cancer-related symptoms, and a tendency to optimism.[5] It can lead to a greater sense of personal and interpersonal growth, acceptance, and life satisfaction.[6]

However, being a cancer survivor does not work for everyone. In one study, although the majority identified with the term cancer survivor, 40% preferred to see themselves as someone **who has had cancer**.[6] The reasons why some people do not feel comfortable with the term include fear of recurrence, not having felt close enough to death to be a survivor, and not wanting to be defined by the disease.[7]

References

4 Little M, Paul K, Jordens C, Sayers E-J. Survivorship and discourses of identity. *Psychooncology* 2002;11:170–8.
5 Deimling G, Bowman K, Wagner L. Cancer survivorship and identity among long-term survivors. *Cancer Invest* 2007;25:758–65.
6 Chambers S, Baade P, Meng X, Youl P, Aikeen J, Dunn J. Survivor identity after colorectal cancer: antecedents, prevalence and outcomes. *Psychooncology* 2012;21:962–9.
7 Kaiser K. The meaning of the survivor identity for women with breast cancer. *Soc Sci Med* 2008;67:70–87.

Cancer stories or narratives

Cancer stories or narratives help people make sense of their experience of illness and treatment. They usually include a problem, a plot, a cast of characters, and a location or locations in time and place. They also develop causal links between events and have an emotional quality. To the cancer nurse, these narratives have a particular value in helping them to make sense of what happens to people with cancer **in their own terms**. They have a role in giving a voice to the patient's experience in a health system that is often dominated by medical priorities.

We can identify certain themes that occur in narratives of illness, and thereby understand different types. Frank identifies three main narrative types:[8]

- Restitution narrative—a decline from health into illness, then a return to health
- Chaos narrative—life going out of control with illness
- Quest narrative—illness provides the opportunity for transformation.

These types of narrative help us to understand the experience of a person with cancer. Sometimes we will find these experiences in published research, based on interview. As an example of this, Thomas-MacLean's (2004) research identified how women's experiences of breast cancer could be understood, according to these narrative types. Restitution narratives signify returning to something like normal after overcoming the cancer, though often there are residual effects of the treatment, e.g. mastectomy:[9]

> 'I am fine. I am still the person I was before breast cancer, but I have changed.'

Reprinted from Thomas-MacLean, R (2004) Understanding breast cancer stories via Frank's narrative types. *Social Science & Medicine*, **58**(9), 1647–1657 with permission from Elsevier.

The chaos narrative may characterize someone's whole experience of cancer, and it often forms a part of it.[9]

> 'It's [breast cancer] always on your mind, the back of your mind, any little thing that goes wrong. And um, now this is my, I had a biopsy yesterday and that's my third biopsy.... You know I think this has worried me a bit because I got so I could relax and not think about it and all of a sudden this came up. I thought I could go the whole summer without having to have an appointment for a change with a doctor and this came up.'

Reprinted from Thomas-MacLean, R (2004) Understanding breast cancer stories via Frank's narrative types. *Social Science & Medicine*, **58**(9), 1647–1657 with permission from Elsevier.

The quest narrative is often represented in published accounts of cancer, of people who overcome the adversity of cancer and find new meaning in their lives.[9]

> 'And, as a result, I've done some things I never would have done.'

Reprinted from Thomas-MacLean, R (2004) Understanding breast cancer stories via Frank's narrative types. *Social Science & Medicine*, **58**(9), 1647–1657 with permission from Elsevier.

However, this is not the case for everybody, and some people feel that media reports of transformative experiences put pressure on them to be positive when they feel life is not fully within their control.

Another source of personal narratives is the website Healthtalk,[10] run by the UK-based charity DIPEx. This contains videos of interviews conducted with many people with different cancer types at different stages of their journey. The website has free and open access and can be used by professionals, people with cancer, or their carers, as a resource for learning about other people's experience of living with cancer. Quotations from people interviewed about their experience of cancer are used extensively in this chapter.

Personal accounts of cancer

Aside from research, other stories are accounts written by people themselves as a means of sharing their experience. Two well-known accounts from the UK were written by journalists:

- Diamond J. *Because Cowards Get Cancer Too*. London: Vermillion; 1998
- Picardie R. *Before I Say Goodbye*. London: Penguin Books; 1998.

Although these are personal accounts, written from personal experience of cancer, their appeal partly relies on the skill of the writer and they represent the experience of articulate, middle-class people.

Fictional accounts of cancer in books and films

Works of fiction, including films, with a theme about cancer can give us insights into the emotions associated with the disease, but they will also be selective in what they represent, aiming to construct a story with a particular purpose or to elicit a specific emotional response from the reader or viewer. For example, Aleksandr Solzhenitsyn's classic novel *Cancer Ward*, although based on personal experience, is widely interpreted as an allegory of life in communist USSR, so that cancer in the novel is a metaphor for communism. The film *50/50* (2011) is also based on personal experience of cancer but is more of an attempt to represent human experience, using both drama and humour.

References

8 Frank AW. *The Wounded Storyteller: Body, Illness, and Ethics*. Chicago: University of Chicago Press; 1995.
9 Thomas-MacLean R. Understanding breast cancer stories via Frank's narrative types. *Soc Sci Med* 2004;58:1647–57.
10 Healthtalk. Available at: ℳ http://www.healthtalk.org/peoples-experiences/cancer

The cancer journey

The term 'cancer journey' has become a popular and useful way of understanding personal experiences of cancer. It has the implication of being a whole experience and a process that has a beginning and an end. Identifying different stages of individual experience, including diagnosis, treatment, recurrence, dying, and death, can help us to focus on the needs of people at the different times on their cancer journey. Each stage will have particular meaning and implications for the person with cancer and their family and friends.

Diagnosis

A diagnosis of cancer can be experienced as a single event. However, for many people, it will be experienced as a process or as a series of confusing events, with new information arriving at unpredictable intervals, in an unfamiliar hospital environment and in an unfamiliar medical language. The period prior to diagnosis will have an impact on how it is experienced. For example, if there are pre-existing emotional or social problems, these may be at the forefront of the patient's mind and delay their response to diagnosis. Consider the following scenarios:

- Diagnosis of breast cancer by routine mammography: in this case, the patient may be unprepared or only partially prepared for the possibility of cancer. Diagnosis may be dominated by treatment choices and disruption of daily life.
- Diagnosis of lung cancer: this may be accompanied by a physical crisis, like breathlessness, making the time of diagnosis a period dominated by symptom distress and functional problems. Adjustment to the diagnosis is accompanied by profound changes to the daily life and outlook of the patient and their family.
- Diagnosis of bowel cancer: this may be precipitated by a change in bodily functions, e.g. finding blood in the faeces, raising concerns about health. After help is sought, treatment may be radical and disfiguring (e.g. colostomy), leading to profound changes in daily functioning and self-image.

Delay in diagnosis may occur either because the person does not think the problem is serious or because of a fear of being told the implications of diagnosis. Sometimes, cancers are not identified promptly in primary care. Delays will have an impact on how the diagnosis is experienced. The patient may feel regret at having delayed seeking help or anger towards health professionals for delays in starting treatment.

A major challenge for the patient at diagnosis is to begin making sense of the seriousness of the situation and what the implications will be for their future. Information is often framed in technical language that the patient may not understand. There is evidence to suggest that some physicians give overly optimistic interpretations of the patient's prospects of cure. We also know that some patients deny the seriousness of their condition. However, in many situations, the context of awareness may be ambiguous and contain contradictions. Patients may be told they have a serious illness but that their prospects for cure are good. Where the information is confusing or ambiguous, patients may 'fill in the blanks' for themselves. It can then be very difficult for the health-care professional, the patient, or their carer to know who knows what or what the most accurate information is.

Treatment

Treatment brings its own demands and can be very disruptive to existing life and routines. The person becomes a 'patient', a term that signifies passivity. One profound change that takes place is that treatment is managed by professionals, and this inevitably results in a loss of control by the patient and their carers. In spite of professional management, treatment can be a series of unpredictable and unforeseen events, including complications, stalls, and changes of plan.

Most people strive for their personal aspirations, for stability and personal control. Cancer disrupts both longer-term aspirations and plans and day-to-day routines. The effects of the illness on daily life and the demands of particular treatment regimens may come to dominate an individual's life and that of their family. Effective health care at this point can make a significant difference to a patient's experience of cancer, e.g. organized treatment pathways and MDT working.

However, we must bear in mind that these stages may not be the most significant experiences for individual patients. As health professionals, we may never know the details of individual lives and families, even if we think we know the patient well.

Reactions to diagnosis and treatment

Reactions to the early stages of diagnosis and treatment will be determined by a number of different factors. These include previous experiences of illness in the patient and others. People who have not experienced serious illness before may have no personal context within which to understand what is happening to them. On the other hand, experience of cancer in a close relative may predetermine their own reaction. For example, if a woman's mother died of breast cancer under circumstances of pain and distress, the same woman being diagnosed with cancer may fear that this will also happen to her, in spite of evidence to the contrary. Other social factors, like media stories of celebrities with cancer, can also have an effect.

Many people do not fully register the reality or implications of a life-threatening illness at the time of diagnosis. Initial reactions may be of shock, numbness, and disbelief. This can make it hard to take in the volume of new information being presented. For some, possibly as many as 20%, the trauma of diagnosis will lead to an acute stress reaction or disorder (➜ see Stress and trauma reactions, p. 578).

> 'It was a very strange experience. I felt as though I was sitting in the corner by the window, it was rather like an out of body experience, and when I came back, you know, I came back to reality, I kept trying to put myself back in the seat I was in but I kept going back to the window again. I think everybody thought I was taking it very well, I was very controlled.'

Breast Cancer in Women Interview 02. Transcribed from healthtalk.org
© DIPEx 2018 and University of Oxford 2018, all rights reserved.

Others will try to focus on the elements that they can control or that they feel are the most controllable within their lives. Getting on with the treatment may be the most effective way for the newly diagnosed patient to manage the new realities of their lives.

> 'I'm one of these people that's "Right, OK what are we going to do then?" I didn't, I didn't fall apart at all, I thought right OK what have we got to do. Do I, can I go to work, silly things go through your head, can I go to work, I've got to do this and I've got to do that and lets just get on with what, what's got to be done. I just wanted to get over it, I just wanted to sort it out and get rid of it. And because he told me that we caught it fairly early I just wanted to get on with it really.'

Cervical Cancer Interview CC13. Transcribed from healthtalk.org
© DIPEx 2018 and University of Oxford 2018, all rights reserved.

Taking in the full implications of a cancer diagnosis can take time. Whilst some people find it helpful to talk about their feelings, others can feel quite isolated and unsure how to deal with it.

> 'I was just in a daze the whole time. I was quite bottled up at the time. I didn't talk to people about my feelings. I coped. And everybody thought I was coping fine, which I was on the surface but underneath I was in agony. And I was lying awake in the nights thinking I would not see my children grow up, because the daughter who'd I'd just been weaning was,

she'd been born in 1981 so she was just over one year old when I found the lump. And my son was two-and-a-half coming up to three when I was having the treatment.

And when I say I bottled everything up, I bottled up my feelings. I didn't ask for help. I didn't talk to people about how upset I was. I didn't even tell my husband much, that I was lying awake in the night.'

Breast Cancer in Women Interview 14. Transcribed from healthtalk.org
© DIPEx 2018 and University of Oxford 2018, all rights reserved.

Many experience a 'rollercoaster' of new experiences, information, and appointments. For many, the full implications are felt when the rollercoaster ride stops at the end of treatment. Unfortunately, this is often the time when professional support is withdrawn, so the patient can feel isolated or abandoned.

'In fact the other thing I think that, once you've finished your treatment you're just left. Okay, so you've got a breast care nurse you can contact if you want to, but she's busy, she's got other more important things to do. You just feel as though, that you're just dumped basically, you know? That's it. Treatment's over. Finished, done with. Off you go. See you in four months. And it's a bit scary. Especially when you've got things like: "Oh God, that pain", you know? "Is that normal?" And things like that.'

Breast Cancer in Women Interview 05. Transcribed from healthtalk.org
© DIPEx 2018 and University of Oxford 2018, all rights reserved.

Reflection points

- Can you think of different ways that patients have managed their lives during treatment?
- What options are there in your area of work for supporting patients who have completed treatment?
- Can you think of ways in which these could be improved?

Living with cancer

Living with cancer inevitably leads to changes—some for the better, and some for the worse. The unpredictability of the course of the disease means that some degree of uncertainty about the future becomes a feature of life for those living with cancer.

' … I think is one of the hardest things is, wondering when the day's going to come when you're going to wake up and you're not, not going to feel as well as you did the day before. And you're going to wonder, "Is this the start of the end?" sort of thing. That's, that I suppose is probably the thing that sort of is constantly at the back of your mind. I mean they, they always talk about living with cancer, and it is, and it, you know you can sort of forget about it sometimes but really not, it's there, it's always there. And sort of it does affect whatever, any, whatever happens or things you know, you know things happening in a few months time. People ask you, "Would you like to do this?" And you always think, "Oh I wonder if I'm going to feel okay to do that," sort of thing. But you just have to get on and do it.'

Pancreatic Cancer Vicky - Interview 15. Transcribed from healthtalk.org
© DIPEx 2018 and University of Oxford 2018, all rights reserved.

Relationships with other people, family, and friends can get better or they can get worse.

'I mean some people were great but some people, and I mean it wasn't that people didn't want to help, they just didn't know what to say. And so they just avoided it. And avoided me, which was difficult. So I think it is more difficult when you're younger, probably. And certainly people's reactions to it are probably more marked.'

Breast Cancer in Women Interview 17. Transcribed from healthtalk.org
© DIPEx 2018 and University of Oxford 2018, all rights reserved.

Each person will cope differently with similar problems. For example, some people keep things to themselves, whilst others are keen to share their news with others, even if the response would be unpredictable.

'I came home and just phoned everybody. I just wanted, I just wanted to tell everybody. I don't know why, there was no sort of' "Oh dear poor me," or, there was nothing like that. I just wanted everybody to know. And that's when I had to deal with everybody else's emotions. And I think it was probably, I thought once everybody knows I can actually be myself, I can actually then start coping with it myself. If I've got to cope with everybody else for the next six weeks, it will be much more difficult.'

Breast Cancer in Women Interview 19. Transcribed from healthtalk.org
© DIPEx 2018 and University of Oxford 2018, all rights reserved.

Most people value information about the disease and treatment. However, they may also need other forms of information, e.g. about how to cope emotionally, and this is not always so readily available.

'I felt I'd got all the information I needed from this breast care nurse particularly, when she explained to me what was going to happen and *what was going on, just in my case. And I think I read a couple, you know, I read a couple of things. Now if I see anything to do with breast cancer I'll pick it up and read it. Or cancer generally, I will read it. But at the time it, that wasn't what I needed. It wasn't information, it was more sort of, I don't know, emotional sort of side of things that I was, I was after, and that's what I put my energies into, rather than the factual information. What I was looking for, I wanted to talk with people who had been ill and who were better, that's all I wanted to hear about. I wanted to get to see the other side, and I didn't want to sort of know about the in-between bit.'*

Breast Cancer in women Interview 10. Transcribed from healthtalk.org
© DIPEx 2018 and University of Oxford 2018, all rights reserved.

Living with cancer often involves a personal search for meaning within the cancer experience. The unavoidable question 'why me?' will seldom have a clear answer, though where there is a direct link between behaviour and cancer, e.g. lung cancer, this may be associated with considerable guilt. The question is more likely to result in a search for new or additional meaning in the person's life. This may involve a spiritual journey, a deepening of personal relationships, or a general re-evaluation of priorities and aspirations, resulting in deep changes in lifestyle.

'It's funny but I think, I think that happening to me wasn't so much of a bad thing when, you know, in retrospect, because it really did change me, it not just changed physically how, you know, what I eat and whatever and physically how I feel but it also changed my outlook.

... I just, life just had a whole new meaning and I just felt that I'd gotten a second lease on life and that it didn't, it didn't matter what the challenges were. I just felt that I could overcome them and that, you know, little squabbles, or little things that used to bother me just didn't bother me anymore.'

Colorectal Cancer Interview 03. Transcribed from healthtalk.org
© DIPEx 2018 and University of Oxford 2018, all rights reserved.

Reflection points

- How can we support patients through periods of uncertainty?
- How can we ensure that we do not provide false reassurance?

Fear of recurrence

The unpredictability of the disease course and the uncertain prognosis mean that a degree of uncertainty about the future becomes a feature of the lives of those living with cancer.

> 'Now the future, I'm not really sure what's going to happen. I've got another appointment at the hospital in another month's time just for a check-up to see how things are going. The cancer that I've got in the bones is incurable.... You can understand that in a way because it's there, it's, they say it's going to be controlled and contained, but nobody will actually tell me, and I think that that's because they don't know, whether I'm going to be back to walking absolutely normally, or whether this is ultimately going to be a further problem and it's going to kill me.'

Breast Cancer in women interview 01. Transcribed from healthtalk.org
© DIPEx 2018 and University of Oxford 2018, all rights reserved.

However, accepting a degree of uncertainty into one's life may be a step towards a more positive future.

> 'And I do feel very positive. I think, I don't know I don't think cancer will come back, or if it comes back I'll fight it again. So I'm very positive. I do feel very happy. I feel happier than before. And I don't complain about things like bills to pay or because it's cold or because it's raining, I do feel much happier. And I feel much healthier as well. I don't know why but I feel much stronger than before.'

Cervical Cancer Interview CC15. Transcribed from healthtalk.org
© DIPEx 2018 and University of Oxford 2018, all rights reserved.

The nursing role in supporting people with fear of cancer recurrence

Some degree of concern about recurrence is to be expected and should not be considered as abnormal. In addition, fear of recurrence should be viewed within context; it is often associated with concerns about the future of other family members, including children, and it may be linked with bad experiences of treatment, e.g. side effects, and other health anxieties.

The nursing role in supporting people with fear of cancer recurrence should involve:[11]

• Validating the fear of recurrence as a normal part of the cancer experience
• Helping patients to identify any common triggers for anxiety, e.g. hospital visits.
• Supporting patients in developing their knowledge of potential symptoms and how to deal with them, e.g. who to contact.
• Promoting self-efficacy and a positive approach to survivorship.
• Identifying those patients for whom this is a more serious or enduring problem and referring them on for psychological support or treatment (see Psychological support, p. 130).

References

11 Ziner KW, Sledge GW, Bell CJ, Johns S, Miller KD, Champion VL. Predicting fear of breast cancer recurrence and self-efficacy in survivors by age at diagnosis. *Oncol Nurs Forum* 2012;39:287–95.

Cancer recurrence and facing death

Cancer recurrence

Recurrence of disease after treatment brings a new set of challenges. Cure becomes less likely; additional and new effects of the illness may become apparent, and it signifies a new stage in the cancer journey. If there has been an extended period when the patient has been free of illness, then there may be new strains on family relationships. Cancer becomes a chronic illness or a terminal illness. Recurrence can be harder to deal with than the original diagnosis.

> 'I rang my sister straight away and told her. So she was upset obviously. And my husband, I didn't tell straight away, because he was in work and I didn't want him getting upset in work and then driving home, because it was quite a long drive. So I waited till he got home before I told him. So he was a little bit taken aback. But he was kind of philosophical about it and, "Well, we've done it once. We'll beat it again" you know, kind of thing. So he was like, "We, we, we'll deal with it. Don't worry about it." And I kind of, I kind of agreed with him, but at the same time I felt that that was it. It was back and this time it was going to try and get me. So that was, I, I did find it, that was more shocking to me than the first time. It, it, it was more frightening, far more frightening than the first time. So it was very difficult.'

Pancreatic Cancer Helen - Interview 04. Transcribed from healthtalk.org
© DIPEx 2018 and University of Oxford 2018, all rights reserved.

The full implications of cancer may be more apparent at recurrence than at diagnosis. Not everyone feels ill at diagnosis, but patients are more likely to be symptomatic at the point of recurrence. Patients can therefore feel much more vulnerable than they did previously. Recurrence may also trigger a loss of confidence in health professionals. This might lead the patient to express anger, frustration, or disappointment. It may also lead to a loss of faith in conventional medicine, and many people at this point turn to alternative or complementary therapies.

For some people with cancer, recurrence will lead to a referral to palliative care services and an open acknowledgement that death from the cancer is now inevitable. This transition can be very difficult not only for the patient, but also for their family and for the professionals who have been treating them (➔ see Referral to palliative care services, p. 150).

Within this transition to palliative care, nurses have a significant role of advocacy for patients and families. This includes addressing emotional reactions to the transition and the prospect of facing dying and death. Nurses need to draw on existing relationships with patients and families, and on their own communication and relationship skills in doing this.

Further reading

Broom A, Kirby E, Good P, Wootton J, Yates, P, Hardy. Negotiating futility, managing emotions: nursing the transition to palliative care. *Qual Health Res* 2015;25:299–309.
Vivar CG, Whyte DA, McQueen A. 'Again': the impact of recurrence on survivors of cancer and family members. *J Clin Nurs* 2010;19:2048–56.

Facing death

Facing death may be particularly hard if it challenges a person's assumptions about life and death.

> 'I think probably my attitude at the moment would be anyway, "How could God love me if you know he's made this happen to me?" And, 'Why should, why should this be me? Why me?' That must be the question that everybody that's younger must ask. We expect to live until we are in our 80s or even 90s and the thought I'm going to pre-decease my mother is not a good one. Just comes back to the fact of not being able to accept the fact that I'm dying, just can't accept it. I'm too young. I'm not ready to go. I've got all these lovely babies and it's just not fair but then you know nobody ever said life was going to be fair, I know.'

Living with Dying Interview 02. Transcribed from healthtalk.org
© DIPEx 2018 and University of Oxford 2018, all rights reserved.

Some people respond with anger and frustration.

> 'But anger yes, I get extremely angry and frustrated but it's anger with me and frustration. I mean I'm sat in this chair, now if I want something I've got to ask my wife, would you mind, would you pass me an apple or a cup of tea and I drink gallons of tea and the poor woman is in and out. I feel guilty about that and I get very angry. I think to myself why the hell can't I do that? You know, I should be able to do that, but I know I can't because I'd be on the floor and that would make things much worse. So anger is something that I think comes in the package but it's frustration as much as anger. Both perhaps. When I said to the consultant that I was very angry, his answer was, 'Well I can understand that'. They all understand my anger but it doesn't help it.'

Living with Dying Interview 27. Transcribed from healthtalk.org
© DIPEx 2018 and University of Oxford 2018, all rights reserved.

Other people feel that getting angry just makes things worse.

> 'I didn't get angry. I mean a lot of people ... I've spoken to a lot of people and they've said you know "why me?" and this, that and the other but I learned a long time ago that, that I have a certain amount of energy and to expend that energy on anger is just a waste of time because all, it doesn't, it doesn't achieve anything – all it does is make you more tired and more frustrated. Being ill is very tiring, being in pain and I'm in pain all the time, is very tiring. So I have to try and channel my energy into positive things.'

Living with Dying Interview 09. Transcribed from healthtalk.org
© DIPEx 2018 and University of Oxford 2018, all rights reserved.

For others, it is an opportunity for reflection and appreciation.

> 'Yes. Assess your own lives. Assess your life and what has been. What is it your life has been and it's all the positive things. All the times that you've enjoyed. Life is a mixture of all sorts of things. There are sad moments and there are moments when things have gone wrong and there are things when you can be upset and angry about things, but find the

positives. *And rejoice in those positives and rejoice in the life that you've had. Celebrate the life that you've had and come to terms with the fact that it will ultimately end. The only difference is that you now know and some people – well it comes to an end and they don't know about it. And I don't know which is worse.'*

Living with Dying Interview 14. Transcribed from healthtalk.org
© DIPEx 2018 and University of Oxford 2018, all rights reserved.

Reflection points

- How does your service manage the transition from active treatment to palliative care?
- Can you think of any ways of improving the support of patients who have recurrence and are facing the prospect of death for the first time?

Chapter 6

The social experience of cancer

Cancer and social identity

Identity has a social, as well as a personal, dimension—who we perceive ourselves to be is experienced within a social context. Roles within the family, friendship group, community, and society are all likely to change after cancer, and this will depend on choices the person makes about which groups they feel they belong to. We choose to identify with other individuals and groups who help us to maintain a positive self-image and self-esteem.

When a person is diagnosed with cancer, this will challenge the social identity they held before, e.g. of someone who is healthy and active. Most people under these circumstances will experience changes in their social life. For example, they are likely to encounter more people with cancer and so develop a sense of belonging to a group of people with cancer, or cancer survivors. This has the benefit of sharing new experiences with others, but it also carries the risk of being identified with the disease. For this reason, most people also aim for continuity of friendships and relationships, as far as this is possible.

People commonly experience a change in their friendship group during the course of diagnosis and treatment for cancer. Some friends find it difficult to cope with the cancer and withdraw, and others come forward to provide practical and emotional support. Additionally, many people make new friends who are going through the same experience, and they form new circles of friends specific to their cancer experience. This can include membership of a support group. It is likely then that the friendship group will change during the course of treatment for cancer.

The person's previous roles and lifestyle are likely to be disrupted by treatment. This can include work, which is a significant role in most people's lives, their family life, and their role within the family, as well as recreation, exercise, and social life. These roles and activities bring satisfaction and are part of the individual's social identity. Disruption can be distressing and lead to a sense of guilt, of letting people down. Most people aim to return to familiar roles and activities, and in the short term, this may not be possible. Longer-term adjustment may involve a return to 'normal' roles and activity or finding a 'new normal' that takes into account the changes that have taken place because of cancer. This may, for example, involve giving up work or working shorter hours, and making more time for family or interests outside of work.

Many people adopt the social identity of a **cancer survivor**. This can be preferable to being seen as a 'cancer patient' or victim. It provides a positive frame for the experiences associated with cancer and can promote positive health behaviours and a buffer against being preoccupied with worry about cancer getting worse or returning.

Cancer and the family, including children

Cancer is not only a personal experience, but a family one. It usually leads to changes in roles and new pressures on relationships. Adults may have to take on additional financial responsibilities, and if the person with cancer is the main wage earner, loss of income can lead to both financial pressures and loss of role and self-esteem.

Problems can emerge within the family as a result of the strain that the cancer puts on relationships. Family members often have to take on new or additional caring roles, and this can become a burden, particularly for children. There may also be less time and energy for social activities, and this can weaken supportive relationships outside of the family. Communication within the family can also become a problem. This can centre on the extent to which information is shared about the illness and prognosis. Feelings may be bottled up to avoid distressing other family members, and this can lead to distress and frustration. Also, any long-standing conflicts within the family may get worse under the strain of illness. Family members can experience disrupted sleep and fatigue and may develop a less healthy lifestyle, including for example alcohol misuse.[1]

Changes to the financial status of the family will have profound implications for all of its members. These include reduced income, the extra costs associated with treatment (e.g. transport, car parking), and also any continuing expenses (e.g. mortgage payments). The effects may be dramatic, like bankruptcy, but even relatively small changes can impact on activities and the QoL. For example, it may be more difficult to afford presents, holidays, or activities, and this could lead to guilt in parents and disappointment in children.[2]

Family resilience and cohesion

The ability of families to deal effectively with problems and grow together can be termed **family resilience**, and **family cohesion** refers to the bonding between family members that gives them a sense of strength and identity as a unit. A number of factors have been identified that promote resilience in the family unit in the face of adversity, including:

- 'Family cohesion: nurturance, education, and protection of family members, promoting a sense of identity and security
- Positive outlook: confidence, optimism, and sense of humour
- Shared values: shared understandings about life and the world
- Flexibility: family roles can adapt to new situations and circumstances
- Family communication: open expression of thoughts and emotions
- Financial management: ability to provide for the needs of family members
- Family time, shared activities, and recreation: develop cohesion and promote close family relationships
- Support network: individual, family, and community networks that support and share resources.'

Extracted from Black, K, Lobo, M (2008) A Conceptual Review of Family Resilience Factors. *Journal of Family Nursing*, **14**(1), 33–55 with permission from SAGE.

Nurses can promote resilience and cohesion in families by supporting open communication, reviewing successful coping patterns, affirming strengths and incorporating these into care plans, and providing additional professional support to vulnerable family members at times of crisis.[3]

Children

If an adult member of the family has cancer, children are likely to experience distress. Although parents naturally feel protective towards their children, keeping information from them will not necessarily reduce their anxieties. Children know when something is wrong, and even very young children will be aware that their parents have fears and concerns. They will need to understand why their parent or other family members are tired, in pain, or upset, and it is natural for them to fear that the person might die. A wide variety of reactions should be expected in children, e.g. a child may become withdrawn or angry, as well as overtly distressed and tearful.[4]

For these reasons, it is important for both family members and professionals to consider the needs of children and to communicate openly with them.

When supporting families with children, encourage them to:
• Think how they will talk to their children about the cancer
• Make time to talk and express feelings
• Be honest and open
• Provide information about cancer to the children and allow them to ask questions
• Consider their age—children over 6 tend to understand more fully what is going on, and younger children may need more reassurance.

It can help to use toys or stories about illness to help younger children (under 6) to understand what is happening. If treatment is likely to result in a visibly changed appearance, children should be prepared for this. It is important to recognize formal supports, including schoolteachers, and to liaise with the child's school. If children are being raised in single-parent households and the parent is ill or dying, professional support will be essential in giving the child a sense of continuity. If the parent is going to die, legal guardianship arrangements will have to be considered.

Websites

Macmillan Cancer Support. Talking to children and teenagers when an adult has cancer. Available at: ℜ https://www.macmillan.org.uk/information-and-support/coping/talking-about-cancer/talking-to-children

NHS Choices. Talking to children about cancer. Available at: ℜ https://modalitypartnership.nhs.uk/self-help/livewell/topics/cancer/talkingtokidsaboutcancer

References

1 Northouse L. Helping patients and their family caregivers cope with cancer. *Oncol Nurs Forum* 2012;39:500–6.

2 Amir Z, Wilson K, Hennings J, Young A. The meaning of cancer: implications for family finances and consequent impact on lifestyle, activities, roles and relationships. *Psychooncology* 2012;21:1167–74.

3 Black K, Lobo M. A conceptual review of family resilience factors. *J Fam Nurs* 2008;14:33–55.

4 Forrest G, Plumb C, Ziebland S, Stein A. Breast cancer in the family; children's perceptions of their mother's cancer and its initial treatment: a qualitative study. *BMJ* 2006;332:998–1003.

Caring for someone with cancer

Family members or friends who provide care to people with cancer are often referred to as 'carers'. A carer is someone who provides informal care, i.e. care that is not professional but may nonetheless be essential for the patient's well-being. Carers also share the experience of cancer. They may do this over periods of many years and for long hours during the day, often balancing other family and work responsibilities. Caring is a normal and natural part of family life, but care of the person with cancer may involve taking on a range of responsibilities and activities for which the carer feels ill-prepared. For example, they may have to:

- Cope with changes in the patient's condition and make risk assessments
- Manage symptoms
- Manage medications
- Find information and manage communications with health staff
- Provide intimate personal care
- Manage finances and the logistics of hospital visits
- Provide emotional support
- Adjust their working hours and deal with their own health problems.[5]

Carers are often thrown suddenly into a new world of medical language and personnel. They report difficulties in knowing who to contact about problems associated with the cancer, and how to contact them, how to broach difficult subjects, how to get support, and how to talk to other friends and family about the problems. Carers often feel a strong sense of responsibility to act as an advocate on behalf of the patient but may lack the confidence to do so or feel that they are not taken seriously. They may also find it very hard to express their own personal concerns or needs, as they feel the person with cancer is the priority.[6]

In terms of information, carers' needs are broadly comparable to those of people with cancer.[7] They tend to be given information on medical aspects of cancer but are less likely to be given information on psychosocial and supportive care. Most information is also offered in the earlier stages of disease and treatment, and carers may experience unmet needs for information in the longer term.

The partners of people with cancer may find it the hardest, as they see their relationship change in the face of illness, and there is some evidence that their QoL suffers as a result of their caring role. On the other hand, many people find that the shared experience of suffering brings them closer together, and some discover a personal sense of growth as a result of their experience.

To help carers, nurses can:

- Identify who the main carer for the patient is and assess their ability to provide the necessary care
- Provide training where this is appropriate for them to take on caring roles
- Provide access to information at all stages of the cancer journey, including the roles and contact details of key members of the professional team

'Because you see your husband as a patient and when they're really sick it's really hard to see them in the role of your husband ... you're doing things for them that you wouldn't normally do, it changes. You're viewing them in a different way.... That's really hard because that's your husband, but you're doing the job that a doctor or a nurse would do, and it's just really hard because it's like you've met a new person.'[8]

'I was impressed with [surgeon] because he actually took the time to find out who I was, make sure I was all right, and introduced himself to me; when we came out of there, even though we had probably some of the worst news you could be told, we felt good.'[9]

Extracts reprinted from Ussher, J, Wong, T, Perz, J (2010) A qualitative analysis of changes in relationship dynamics and roles between people with cancer and their primary informal carer. *Health: An Interdisciplinary Journal for the Social Study of Health, Illness & Medicine,* 15(6), 650–667 with permission from SAGE and from Morris, SM, Thomas, C (2001) The carer's place in the cancer situation: where does the carer stand in the medical setting? *European Journal of Cancer Care,* 10, 87–95 with permission from Wiley.

- With the patient's permission, invite them to take part in consultations and decisions
- Recognize the contribution of carers to the process of caring and their importance to the patient's well-being
- Recognize that being a carer is a process that makes particular demands on the person
- Recognize that carers have needs too, including their own health problems, and direct them to sources of support.

References

5 Given B, Given C, Sherwood P. Family and caregiver needs over the course of the cancer trajectory. *J Support Oncol* 2012;10:57–64.

6 Sinfield P, Baker R, Ali S, Richardson A. The needs of carers of men with prostate cancer and barriers and enablers to meeting them: a qualitative study in England. *Eur J Cancer Care* 2012;21:527–34.

7 Adams E, Boulton M, Watson E. The information needs of partners and family members of cancer patients: a systematic literature review. *Patient Educ Couns* 2009;77:179–86.

8 Ussher J, Wong T, Perz J. A qualitative analysis of changes in relationship dynamics and roles between people with cancer and their primary informal carer. *Health (London)* 2010;15:650–67.

9 Morris SM, Thomas C. The carer's place in the cancer situation: where does the carer stand in the medical setting? *Eur J Cancer Care* 2001;10:87–95.

Employment and finances

Disruption to employment

A diagnosis of cancer can have a major impact on the work life of both patients and their carers. People with cancer are more likely to be unemployed than members of the general population, and given that work is an important source of financial independence and general well-being, there is an undisputable need to provide effective work support services for people with cancer.

Work support needs to be an integral part of every stage of the patient's treatment. Health professionals need to be alert to potential work problems and to encourage patients to think positively about work, as set out by the '5 Rs':

- **Raise** work issues with patients early in the treatment pathway in a sensitive and acceptable manner. Asking 'what things in your life are affected by your diagnosis and how can we help you with these?' is likely to elicit more useful information than 'is work a problem?'
- **Recognize** the risk factors for poor work outcomes. Patients might not recognize potential problems, and it is therefore helpful for health professionals to be on the lookout for these. Some examples would be: Has the patient made contact with their employer? What is the relationship with their employer like? Is there about to be major restructuring at work? How flexible is the job—will it be possible for modifications to be made to the workplace and to work responsibilities?
- **Respond** effectively to the straightforward work problems that patients identify.
- **Refer** patients who have more complex difficulties to the appropriate specialist services. It is important that in each local area, the services to provide help and support are identified and made available. Cancer information centres can be key to ensuring that this happens.
- **Revisit** work issues at intervals during treatment—particularly around (but not limited to) the time of diagnosis, the commencement of treatment, towards the end of treatment, and at the time that the patient is discharged from active management.

Patients might need encouragement to:
- Make contact with their employers and keep them updated on treatment schedules
- Start to think about the adjustments that might be needed to facilitate returning to work.
- Ask their health professionals about the likely impact of the treatment on work
- Avoid making hasty decisions about withdrawing from work.

Macmillan Cancer Support has helpful advice for patients to think about managing their work situation, which can be accessed here: ℘ https://www.macmillan.org.uk/information-and-support/organising/work-and-cancer

Patients with complex work problems are likely to benefit from vocational rehabilitation. This would include:
• Detailed assessment of the person's capacity for work and the workplace requirements
• Rehabilitation interventions to build work skills and confidence
• Education on managing specific symptoms (such as fatigue) in the workplace
• Liaison with employers, e.g. to negotiate a phased return to work
• Psychological interventions
• Information on employment rights and responsibilities
• Supported withdrawal from work where appropriate
• Liaison with other work support services
• Careers advice and guidance.

The provision of vocational rehabilitation varies from area to area. It is generally (although not exclusively) provided by occupational therapists and physiotherapists, and local referral routes can be identified through rehabilitation departments and cancer information centres (➲ see Rehabilitation of the cancer patient, pp. 138–40).

Further reading

Eva G, Playford D, Sach T, et al. *Thinking Positively About Work: Delivering Work Support and Vocational Rehabilitation for People With Cancer.* London: National Cancer Survivorship Initiative; 2012. Available at: ℘ https://www.macmillan.org.uk/documents/getinvolved/campaigns/workingthroughcancer/ncsivrevaluationfinalreport-fullfinalversionjuly2012.pdf

Culture, the media, and the meaning of cancer

Cancer occupies a powerful place in public consciousness. As well as being a dreaded disease, cancer can also act as a metaphor for death. In her analysis of cancer as a stigmatizing condition, Susan Sontag observed that cancer took over the role previously occupied by tuberculosis, as the mysterious bringer of death.[10] Cancer was generally viewed by the public as an incurable illness and representing moral failure on the part of the person with cancer, leading to them being shunned. The use of military metaphors, such as the 'fight' against cancer, suggests that cancer is an enemy to be fought. Within this military vision of cancer, the patient is potentially cast as a victim or hero.

More recently, as personal stories or narratives of cancer emerge, the nature of the cancer experience is presented with greater complexity and a range of other metaphors. Examples of recent terminology are 'struggle' and 'survival'. This suggests a challenge to be overcome, rather than a war to be fought. Combined with terminology changes, charity fundraising campaigns have emphasized living with cancer, rather than defeating cancer. This acknowledges the reality that, although not all cancers are curable, many are and much can be done to help people live with its effects.

Media reporting of cancer, e.g. in newspapers and magazines, continues to emphasize the fear of the disease and the dominant position of medicine in overcoming it and returning people to fulfilling lives. The cancer survivor is portrayed as courageous and sometimes as proud, strong, triumphant, and happy. Stories are framed in the language of struggle, and sporting metaphors are common, e.g. climbing mountains, the 'race for life'. Other metaphors are the journey or ordeal of cancer. Cancer is sometimes portrayed as transformative, developing character traits like altruism, stoicism, courage, and inspiration.[11] The experience of celebrities, including their death, can be portrayed as a narrative of heroism, transformation, and redemption, played out on a public stage before a mass audience, with reference to religious imagery.[12]

The media also reinforce gender stereotypes within society. Women are more likely to be shown reacting with strong emotions, making extensive use of support groups and helping others. Men show strength of character in withstanding the trauma of cancer, but not communicating their emotions so readily.[11]

References

10 Sontag S. *Illness as Metaphor; and AIDS and Its Metaphors*. London: Penguin; 1991.
11 Seale C. Cancer heroics: a study of news reports with particular reference to gender. *Sociology* 2002;36:107–26.
12 Walter T. Jade and the journalists: media coverage of a young British celebrity dying of cancer. *Soc Sci Med* 2010;71:853–60.

Gender, age, and cancer

Gender and cancer

Both personal and social identities are associated with the physical attributes of sex and the social construction of gender. Within the Western cultural context, men are perceived as less emotionally expressive and less likely to ask for, and receive, help. To what extent this is the result of cultural stereotypes of $\male$ and $\female$ roles or physical differences is debatable. However, there is evidence to support different patterns of help-seeking and of accepting help amongst women and men. It is important to bear in mind that women are often over-represented in research, with breast cancer providing much of the background for studies of emotional reactions to cancer, and psychological interventions.

The perception of gender identity may be altered as a result of treatment and associated changes to the body, e.g. after surgery or as a result of hormone treatments. This can impair the individual's ability to carry out their perception of their gender role, impact negatively on self-esteem, and cause significant distress. This is more likely when the cancer and treatment affect the sexual parts of the body, e.g. the breasts and ovaries in women and the testicles and prostate in men (❥ see Sexuality and cancer, p. 606). However, this can also happen when there are impairments to the social role, e.g. work and caring activities.

Age and cancer

Cancer raises particular survivorship issues for older patients. Ageing is associated with declining health and multiple morbidities, so that cancer must be considered alongside other illnesses, treatments, and changes in QoL. Declining health can lead to loss of autonomy, greater dependence on others, and a consequent erosion of personal and social identity. The active maintenance of dignity and self-esteem may become more prominent features of care.

With greater technical advances, older patients are also receiving more active forms of treatment, and this reinforces the need for effective supportive care. Consideration should be given to the risks of dehydration, anaemia, depression, fatigue, insomnia, and also bone health.[13] Older patients are at greater risk of cognitive impairment and confusional states (❥ see Acute confusional state or delirium, pp. 594–5), and it is important to monitor the effects and side effects of all medications, but particularly systemic treatments.[14]

Decision-making about treatment for older adults can be different for both clinicians and patients. Clinicians may be more cautious in older patients who have comorbidities and are less physically robust. There is some evidence to suggest that older patients are more likely to trust health professionals to make decisions on their behalf, although this is subject to individual differences. Patients of all ages should always be actively engaged in the decision-making process.

Younger adult patients with cancer may face the particular challenges of long-term illness, disability, and the prospect of dying at a time of life they would not have expected or predicted them. They may experience more loneliness, as there are fewer people of their age with cancer. For younger people, cancer may be more disruptive to life and work plans, including changes in body image, sexuality, fertility, and childcare. There is also evidence to suggest they are more likely to be distressed and anxious about the course of their disease and its outcome, particularly fear of cancer recurrence.[15]

Further reading

Chapple A, Ziebland S. Prostate cancer: embodied experience and perceptions of masculinity. *Sociol Health Illness* 2002;24:820–41.

Moynihan C. Men, women, gender and cancer. *Eur J Cancer Care* 2002;11:166–72.

References

13 Naeim A, Aapro M, Subbarao R, Balducci L. Supportive care considerations for older adults with cancer. *J Clin Oncol* 2014;32:2627–34.

14 Mandelblatt JS, Jacobsen PB, Ahles T. Cognitive effects of cancer systemic therapy: implications for the care of older patients and survivors. *J Clin Oncol* 2014;32:2617–26.

15 Lebel S, Beattie S, Arès I, Bielajew C. Young and worried: age and fear of recurrence in breast cancer survivors. *Health Psychol* 2013;32:695–705.

Ethnicity, culture, and cancer

Ethnicity, or identification with a racial and cultural group, can be central to social identity. Differences have been identified between ethnic groups in different countries in terms of use of cancer screening, access to treatment, and survival. In the UK, for example, there is evidence of higher mortality due to breast cancer in people of South Asian or black Caribbean and black African women, compared to white British women.[16] The reasons for this are complex but include stage at diagnosis and deprivation. Immigrant groups are more likely to have lower socio-economic status and educational level. These factors, along with language barriers and cultural beliefs about illness, may lead to delays in presentation and diagnosis, with poorer outcomes.

Cultural beliefs about cancer may be in contradiction to conventional medical opinion. It is important therefore that nurses seek to understand patients' health beliefs where this is relevant to enabling access to services. As part of the cancer nurse's health education role, they should also provide information to vulnerable groups to raise awareness about cancer detection and treatment. The extent to which communication about diagnosis and prognosis is shared openly also varies between cultures.

The lack of a common language or common understandings about health can lead to miscommunication, and people from minority communities can experience a perception of poorer care and less self-efficacy.[17] Some studies have highlighted a perception of medical discrimination within ethnic minorities.[18] This will lead to mistrust and make it harder to develop effective long-term working relationships between the professional and the patient. Nurses will need to develop the capacity to respond to culturally diverse populations. This will involve developing cultural self-awareness and the necessary knowledge and skills to meet the needs of patients representing all parts of society.

Reflection point
How can I ensure that cultural diversity is respected within my practice?

Websites
African Caribbean Leukaemia Trust (ACLT). Available at: ℜ https://aclt.org
Asian Women Cancer Group. Available at: ℜ http://www.asianwomencancergroup.co.uk
Cancer Black Care. Available at: ℜ http://www.cancerblackcare.org.uk

References
16 Jack RH, Davies EA, Moller H. Breast cancer incidence, stage, treatment and survival in ethnic groups in South East England. *Br J Cancer* 2009;100:545–50.
17 Palmer NRA, Kent EE, Forsythe LP, *et al*. Racial and ethnic disparities in patient-provider communication, quality-of-care ratings, and patient activation among long-term cancer survivors. *J Clin Oncol* 2014;32:4087–94.
18 Campesino M, Saenz DS, Choi M, Krouse RS. Perceived discrimination and ethnic identity among breast cancer survivors. *Oncol Nurs Forum* 2012;39:E91–100.

Threats to personal identity—stigma

A person's social identity may be threatened if their interactions with others lead to them being 'labelled' with an undesirable or abnormal stereotype associated with cancer. This can, for example, result from them feeling judged, discriminated against, or rejected by other people. This is referred to as social stigma.

Stigma can include the experience of discrimination (enacted stigma), the fear or perception of discrimination (felt stigma), or the adoption of negative stereotypes (self-stigma).[19] It can create additional problems for the individual—they may adopt a negative self-image and lose self-esteem, they may feel a burden of responsibility for being different, or they may feel inhibited in interaction with others.

This can be a particular problem for two groups of people with cancer: those whose appearance is changed as a result of the cancer treatment, e.g. H&N cancers, and those who are perceived to bear some responsibility for their cancer, e.g. lung cancer linked to smoking.[20] Stigma is associated with depressive symptoms, and this can occur in any cancer, e.g. colorectal cancer.[21]

Patients with lung cancer may experience guilt, regret, and self-blame if they have previously smoked and if they continue to smoke. They can also feel that others, including health professionals, judge them for their behaviour.[22] This is reinforced by public health campaigns against tobacco use. It is therefore important that nurses show acceptance of patients as they are, and that they also encourage patients to talk about their fears or experiences of stigma and discrimination.

The following can help to prevent or ameliorate the experience of stigma:[20]

• Maintaining valued roles and activities supporting health, family, occupation, and recreation
• Feeling safe to discuss uncomfortable feelings and difficult experiences
• Correcting misconceptions about the causes of cancer
• Finding benefits in the illness experience.

References

19 Brown C, Cataldo J. Explorations of lung cancer stigma for female long-term survivors. *Nurs Inq* 2013;20:352–62.
20 Lebel S, Castonguay M, Mackness G, Irish J, Bezjak A, Devins GM. The psychosocial impact of stigma in people with head and neck or lung cancer. *Psychooncology* 2013;22:140–52.
21 Phelan SM, Griffin JM, Jackson GL, *et al*. Stigma, perceived blame, self-blame, and depressive symptoms in men with colorectal cancer. *Psychooncology* 2013;22:65–73.
22 Lehto RH. Patient views on smoking, lung cancer, and stigma: a focus group perspective. *Eur J Oncol Nurs* 2014;18:316–22.

Supportive and Palliative Care

Supportive care

Supportive care and palliative care

Supportive cancer care is a broad term describing all of the activities that help patients and their families to cope with the cancer and its treatment. Importantly, this involves active collaboration with those who use cancer services, i.e. patients and families, to make the best use of both formal and informal resources. Its aim is to maximize the benefits of treatment, but equally to enable the patient and family to live as well as possible with the disease and its effects, achieving an optimal QoL.

Supportive care should be provided at every stage of the patient's cancer journey, from before diagnosis, through diagnosis and treatment, to the outcome of treatment, and including care of the dying and bereavement where necessary. It includes: user involvement and self-help; coordination of care; communication and information-giving; psychological, social, and spiritual support; rehabilitation; complementary therapies; general and specialist palliative care; and services for families, including bereavement care.

Supportive care is therefore not a specialty in itself but describes a range of activities and services, some of which are general and some of which are specialist. It falls within the remit of all of the professional groups working with cancer and requires a range of skills, from, e.g. basic communication skills to advanced and specialist psychological skills. It also requires effective communication and continuity of care across different parts of services, and between service users (patients and their families) and service providers (professionals). Palliative care can be seen as a specialist element of supportive care, but there is considerable overlap, and they are frequently used together, i.e. 'supportive and palliative care'.

Further reading

The National Council for Palliative Care. Available at: ℘ http://www.ncpc.org.uk/palliative-care-explained

National Institute for Health and Care Excellence (2004). *Improving Supportive and Palliative Care for Adults with Cancer.* London: National Institute for Health and Care Excellence.

National Institute for Health and Care Excellence. Available at: ℘ http://www.nice.org.uk/

Communication in cancer care

Communication is a central aspect of cancer care. Effective communication not only facilitates high-quality nursing care, but also enables early detection of cancer and self-management, reduces emergency admissions and inequalities of access to care and treatment, and supports longer-term adjustment and survivorship.[1]

However, communication can be a problem in all groups of health professionals. They may avoid difficult topics, particularly the most emotional ones, or find it difficult to break bad news. Poor communication makes assessment, information giving, and emotional support more difficult.

Advanced communication skills training

Training in advanced communication skills has become a high priority in trying to address these problems. It is important to deal with the emotional aspects of communication and to address the attitudes and beliefs underlying practice. Training may focus on eliciting patient concerns and breaking bad news. Training programmes often use audio and video recording and feedback, role-play involving actors, and small group work. Effective communication involves not only skills, but also knowledge and the right attitudes to enable it to take place.

SAGE & THYME™

Some nurses also find it helpful to use communication models. One example of this is SAGE & THYME™ (see Box 7.1), which has been developed specifically to enable nurses or other staff to identify and address the emotional concerns of people with cancer and their carers.[2]

Box 7.1 The SAGE & THYME™ model

Setting – If you notice concern – think first of the setting, create some privacy – sit down.
Ask – 'Can I ask what you are concerned about?'
Gather – Gather all of the concerns – not just the first few – 'Is there something else?'
Empathy – Respond sensitively – 'You have a lot on your mind.'

and

Talk – 'Who do you have to talk to or support you?'
Help – 'How do they help?'
You – 'What do YOU think would help?'
Me – 'Is there something you would like ME to do?'
End – Summarize and close – 'Can we leave it there?'

Reproduced from Connolly, M, et al (2010) SAGE & THYME™: A model for training health and social care professionals in patient-focussed support. *Patient Education and Counseling*, **79**, 87–93 with permission from Elsevier.

Reflection points
• Have I had adequate communication skills training for my role?
• What sort of training is available for me in my practice area?
• Are there any models that I could use to support my communications with patients and carers?
• Who do I talk to in my organization to get on a communication skills training course?

The context of communication

One factor that clearly affects the practice of communication skills is the context within which it takes place. The nursing environment is frequently busy and unpredictable, and nurses are subject to multiple conflicting demands. The type of nursing role is a significant factor in the way a nurse communicates. Ward-based nurses generally care for groups of patients who may have different levels of dependency, whereas clinical nurse specialists often work with a single patient at a time.

Consider the following factors that influence communication in your practice area:
• Staffing levels and workload
• Distractions and interruptions
• The need to prioritize different aspects of care
• Organizational policies and procedures.

Reflection point
• Are there factors in the environment where I work that make it harder for me to communicate effectively?
• What can I do to manage these?

A culture of communication

The social environment of care is another significant factor in the style and use of communication skills. If the dominant culture is one of task, rather than relationship, orientation, then nurses may feel discouraged from communicating with patients on an emotional level.

The attitude of senior colleagues, such as ward managers or consultants, is a critical factor in determining communication style; and this will also influence the sort of support and supervision that is available. Nurses will not elicit patient concerns if they do not feel able to deal with them or if they feel they will not be supported with the consequences of emotional disclosure. Openness and free sharing of information both promote effective communication.

Reflection points
• Do I feel supported in my communications with patients and carers?
• What sort of support do I need to communicate effectively?

The patient's view

It is important to be aware of the patient's contribution to communication. It is recognized that nurses give 'cues' to their availability or their willingness to discuss sensitive or emotional issues, and the same is true of patients. Not all patients wish to disclose their personal feelings to nurses, and they may give subtle cues that discourage questioning. Both nurses and patients may want to keep conversations emotionally 'safe'. There is evidence that what patients value most in nurses are professional competence and knowledge, warmth, availability, approachability, and good communication skills, both verbal and non-verbal.[3]

Reflection points

- How can I find out what patients value about the way that I communicate with them?

Further reading

Gysels M, Richardson A, Higginson IJ. Communication training for health professionals who care for patients with cancer: a systematic review of effectiveness. *Support Care Cancer* 2004;12:692–700.

Williams AM, Irurita VF. Therapeutic and non-therapeutic interpersonal interactions: the patient's perspective. *J Clin Nursing* 2004;13:806–15.

References

1 Department of Health. *Improving Outcomes: A Strategy for Cancer*. London: Department of Health; 2011. Available at: ℘ https://www.gov.uk/government/uploads/system/uploads/attachment_data/file/213785/dh_123394.pdf

2 Connolly M, Perryman J, McKenna Y, *et al*. SAGE & THYME™: A model for training health and social care professionals in patient-focussed support. *Patient Educ Couns* 2010;79:87–93.

3 Roberts D. *Psychosocial Nursing Care: A Guide to Nursing the Whole Person*. Maidenhead: Open University Press; 2013.

Types of communication

Verbal communication

Verbal communication is the use of language in the form of words to convey information, best seen as a dialogue between the people involved. In cancer care, communication importantly involves the giving of information about cancer and its treatment, eliciting information to form the basis of assessment, sharing of feelings and concerns, and the provision of emotional support.

Verbal communication involves asking questions, listening and attending, giving clear verbal messages, and checking that the message has been understood.

- **Questions** may be open (e.g. 'how are you today?'), which invites the patient to say how they are feeling, or closed (e.g. 'are you in pain?), which invites a yes or no answer.
- **Listening** is demonstrated partly through verbal responses (e.g. 'that sounds very painful for you') and partly through non-verbal signs like eye contact and facial expression. Listening should also allow pauses and time for the patient to think, absorb information, and consider their own response.
- Responses to patients can involve **paraphrasing** (e.g. 'so, you've been feeling very tired this week') that show you are engaged with the conversation, **checking for understanding** (e.g. 'when you said you'd had enough, did you mean … ?'), and **summarizing** (e.g. 'you've been so tired this week that you haven't felt like doing anything'.

Non-verbal communication

Non-verbal communication is an essential part of the communication process. It includes eye contact and facial expression, body posture, and gestures. Proximity, the use of interpersonal space, is also a very important aspect of non-verbal communication nursing, and it needs to be used carefully to ensure that the patient feels comforted, and not threatened, by the presence of the nurse. Touch is a fundamental aspect of nursing and can be used as a therapeutic tool, as well as a means to achieving physical care. It can provide comfort, express warmth, and develop rapport with the patient. Paralanguage (how things are said) is also important. This includes the tone, pitch, volume, and speed of speech. Emotions are often communicated non-verbally.

Cues

Cues are the communication of mutually understood and subtle messages, often conveying emotions, emphasis, or comfort. Cues can be:
- Heard (e.g. a pause in speech or a change of tone)
- Seen (e.g. a smile, a gesture of the hand)
- Felt (a touch).

Factors to consider in your practice
- Clarity of verbal expression, framing questions carefully, and paraphrasing, summarizing, and checking for understanding.
- Allowing pauses and silences in conversation.
- Sensitivity in the use of personal space when providing intimate care.
- Engaging in eye contact and adopting a warm facial expression.
- Adopting a sensitive orientation in relation to the patient, e.g. being face-to-face or on a similar level, not above.
- Using body movements and gestures that are purposeful, but non-threatening.

Telephone communication

Telephone communication can occur at many points in the patient's care. Access to specialist advice over the phone can enable patients to feel supported, whilst living independently in their own homes. Families will frequently make enquiries by phone, and this should be encouraged as a means of keeping in contact. It is useful to establish with the patient in advance if there is information that they do or do not wish to be transmitted to the family. Significant news about diagnosis or test results should not be given by telephone.

The challenge of communicating by phone is that non-verbal aspects of communication are absent, and this can make it hard to judge the emotional quality of the conversation or the emotional state of the person. It becomes more important to note paralanguage, like the person's tone of voice, as a sign of how they are feeling. It is also important to check for understanding regularly.

Telephone triage

This system enables patients to gain rapid access to expert advice and assessment. Nurses who carry out telephone triage need to develop a range of skills, including clinical knowledge, assessment skills, communication skills, and effective decision-making ability. Ideally, staff should be trained for this purpose and have access to written guidelines or a protocol.

These are guidelines for good practice:
- Clearly state who you are and what your role is.
- Obtain the caller's name and contact number.
- Speak to the person who has the problem.
- Take a detailed history of the presenting problem.
- Give clear advice on the phone, either on what the person can do to deal with the problem at home or whether they should go to hospital or contact their GP.
- Ensure that the person clearly understands their priorities and options, and what they should do next.
- Document details of the call, including any advice given and any follow-up required, and liaise with relevant colleagues.
- Ask if there are any further concerns that need to be dealt with.

Use of the Internet

E-mail and texting are popular media for patients to keep in touch with cancer services, particularly if they lead busy work lives. They also enable photographic images to be sent that aid assessment. They lack non-verbal and paralinguistic elements that are effective in communicating emotion, so care needs to be taken to ask about, and respond to, emotional concerns.

The Internet enables patients to access information on cancer from sources all over the world. This can include personal accounts of cancer, support groups, technical information on research and treatments, and alternatives to conventional treatments. Patients and carers can share experiences of cancer and seek advice and support. Around two-thirds of cancer patients reported going online to search for information.[4] In the UK, organizations such as Macmillan Cancer Support, Cancer Research UK, and Breast Cancer Care have very well-developed websites providing information on treatment, psychosocial aspects of care, and online communities where people affected by cancer can offer real-time support for each other.

Less formally, patients and carers can establish their own online support and advice groups via social media sites such as Facebook and Twitter. Sometimes these online communities can be open to all, or alternatively they may be restricted to patients who have experience of a particular cancer or treatment modality. There is some evidence to suggest that this type of support site is particularly useful to patients who experience stigma such as those with lung cancer.[5]

For patients and carers, it is often hard to establish the status of information on the Internet, how accurate or reliable it is, or whether it is a commercial site. Patients and families should be encouraged to consider the credibility of any websites they use, e.g. who funds the website, what its purpose is, and what the original source of its information is.

Additionally, providers of health care, such as hospitals and community services, use an online presence to provide information on their own services or keep users updated. They may use their own websites and/or use social media sites to do this. Some of the more trustworthy sites can be identified by their domain name—British government websites end in gov. uk, and academic websites in ac.uk. In the USA, university sites end in .edu, and in Australia in edu.aus. Charities, which can be excellent sources of information, use .org, but this can also be used by commercial groups who may have a financial interest in people using their services. Other business domain names include .co, .com, and .net.

Use of the Internet is limited to those who have access to the necessary technology, and this can exclude those with limited financial resources. However, many information centres in hospitals enable patients to have access.

Social media and the nurse

Social media are now part of daily life for most people, including nurses and people with cancer. Professionally, nurses can use social media to enhance professional networks and professional development. However, they also pose potential risks. For example, patients may wish to be 'friends' with the nurse who cares for them, and this could compromise the professional role of the nurse. Nurses are advised not to use social media to pursue friendships with patients or other service users.[6] For this reason, nurses should consider using different social media for different purposes, e.g. one for personal friends and one for professional use. Also, social media are public platforms, and nurses should use caution in what they post, avoiding references to work, and particularly avoiding mention of patients. Photos of patients should never be posted online. Nurses should also be aware of their privacy settings to ensure private information is not inadvertently made public. Online posting is immediate, so it is important not to post if you are angry or upset, but to take time to calm down and think about the best way to respond. Many employers have their own media policy to which employees should adhere, and the Nursing and Midwifery Council (NMC) has issued guidance for nurses on the use of social media, which emphasizes the professional Code of Practice.[6]

Further reading

Adams E, Boulton M, Watson E. The information needs of partners and family members of cancer patients: a systematic literature review. *Patient Educ Counsel* 2009;77:179–86.

National Institute for Clinical Excellence (2004). Supportive and palliative care: research evidence; user Involvement in planning, delivering and evaluating services. In: National Institute for Clinical Excellence. *Improving Supportive and Palliative Care for Adults with Cancer: The Manual*. pp 29–45. Available at: ✆ https://www.nice.org.uk/guidance/csg4/resources/improving-supportive-and-palliative-care-for-adults-with-cancer-pdf-773375005.

Peterson E, Shen JM, Weber J, Bylund C. Cancer patients' use of the internet for cancer information and support. In: Kissane D, Bultz B, Butow P, Noble S, Bylund C, Wilkinson S (eds). *The Oxford Textbook of Communication in Oncology and Palliative Care*, 2nd ed. Oxford: Oxford University Press; 2017. pp. 51–55.

Royal College of Nursing (2009). *Legal Advice for RCN Members Using the Internet*. RCN Publication code: 003 557. ISBN: 978-1-906633-28-8.

Warren E, Footman K, Tinelli M, McKee M, Knai C. Do cancer-specific websites meet patient's information needs? *Patient Educ Counsel* 2014;95:126–36.

References

4 Castleton K, Fong T, Wang-Gillam A, *et al*. A survey of Internet utilization among patients with cancer. *Support Care Cancer* 2011;19:1183–90.

5 Rains S, Peterson EB, Wright KB. Communicating social support in computer-mediated contexts: a meta-analytical review of content messages shared on-line among individuals coping with illness. *Communication Monographs* 2015;82:403–30.

6 Nursing and Midwifery Council. *Guidance on Using Social Media Responsibly*. Available at: ✆ https://www.nmc.org.uk/globalassets/sitedocuments/nmc-publications/social-media-guidance.pdf

Promoting effective communication

Communication is most effective if the nurse demonstrates warmth, empathy, genuine concern about the patient, and a non-judgemental attitude. A warm and confident tone of voice is important.

The following factors and behaviours promote effective communication:
• Space, time, and availability
• Active listening and attention
• Assessing and focusing on how the patient is feeling
• Open questions
• Focusing, probing, and paraphrasing
• Clarifying or summarizing.

Inhibiting effective communication

Communication is least effective if the nurse demonstrates a lack of time or attention through their behaviour, is focused inwards on personal feelings such as stress or anxiety, lacks warmth, or is judgemental. The following behaviours can inhibit communication:
• Leading or closed questions
• Premature or false reassurance
• Advising or blaming
• Changing the topic or being defensive
• Judging or placating
• Focusing on a physical assessment to the exclusion of a psychological assessment
• Using medical terminology when everyday alternatives could be used.

Imparting significant news (breaking bad news)

Imparting significant information, or breaking bad news, about diagnosis, treatment, and prognosis can be a problematic issue in cancer care, for a number of reasons. Health professionals may:
• Lack confidence, experience, or training in communication skills
• Feel personal discomfort dealing with sensitive issues
• Wish to promote hope but be unrealistically optimistic.

Most people want to be told the truth. Patients value when professionals:[7]
• Allow them time to deal with new information
• Are able to acknowledge when they are afraid
• Provide a balance of honesty and hope
• Acknowledge the limits of their own knowledge.

If professionals are not clear, consistent, and open, or do not give sufficient information, there can be a loss of confidence and trust on the part of the patient and their family.

Role of the cancer nurse in giving significant news

At many points, the doctor will give the patient any significant news about cancer and its treatment. However, nurses, particularly specialist cancer nurses, will frequently give information that can have a significant impact on a patient's view of their future or on their QoL.

Nurses will often be asked to see a patient after they have been given some news by a doctor. The nurse will also have an important role in ensuring continuity of care between departments or services, and may need to clarify information.

A fairly simple and straightforward model for breaking bad news is SPIKES (see Box 7.2).[8] Used well, this model makes the process feel less stressful for the professional and promotes patient participation in difficult treatment decisions. It addresses six main aspects of the bad news consultation.

The following are guidelines for giving significant information or bad news:
• Ensure there is privacy, time, and space for the consultation.
• Make sure that the patient knows who you are and what your role is in their care.
• Establish what the patient currently understands their circumstances to be (e.g. diagnosis, prognosis) and with whom they have discussed it.

Box 7.2 SPIKES: steps in breaking bad news

Step 1: S—SETTING UP the interview
Step 2: P—Assessing the patient's PERCEPTION
Step 3: I—Obtaining the patient's INVITATION
Step 4: K—Giving KNOWLEDGE and information to the patient
Step 5: E—Addressing the patient's EMOTIONS with empathic responses
Step 6: S—STRATEGY and SUMMARY

From Baile et al (2000) SPIKES—A Six-Step Protocol for Delivering Bad News: Application to the Patient with Cancer. *The Oncologist*; 5(4), 302–311, included with permission from Wiley.

- Allow the patient to express their own narrative of events up to the present, in their own terms, as this will help to establish their context for understanding the new information.
- Inform them that there has been a new development, and give them an initial indication of the nature of the news.
- Note their reaction, and ask them what they now need to know.
- Give information in response to their expressed needs, respecting their preferences about the nature and amount of information they require.
- Allow the patient and their family to air their feelings, to express distress, fear, frustration, or anger at the circumstances in which they find themselves, without entering into any blame or attribution of fault (unless there is clear evidence of negligence or poor practice).
- Consider what meaning this news has for this patient and their family at this time, and invite them to discuss the implications as they see them.
- Offer additional sources of information if these are available, e.g. information leaflets.
- Ensure that the patient knows and understands the next step in their care or treatment, and with whom they will next have contact.
- Liaise with all relevant colleagues on the outcome of the interaction, and document this.

It is important to remember that reactions to bad news are hard to predict. You should keep an open mind and try to understand the impact of the news on the particular circumstances and priorities of this patient and their family.

Further reading

National Institute for Health and Care Excellence (2004). *Improving Supportive and Palliative Care for Adults with Cancer*. Cancer service guideline [CSG4]. Available at: ℗ https://www.nice.org.uk/guidance/csg4

References

7 Stajduhar K, Thorne S, McGuinness L, Kim-Sung C. Patient perceptions of helpful communication in the context of advanced cancer. *J Clin Nurs* 2010;19:2039–47.
8 Baile WF, Buckman R, Lenzi R, Glober G, Beale EA, Kudelka AP. SPIKES—a six-step protocol for delivering bad news: application to the patient with cancer. *The Oncologist* 2000;5:302–11.

Patient information and involvement

Patient information

Patient involvement in cancer services operates at two levels:
- Providing information and involving patients and carers in decision-making about their own care
- Involving patients and carers in decisions about the development and management of cancer services.

Information giving is a very important aspect of cancer care. The amount and type of information that an individual patient wants will depend on a number of factors, including their age, gender, education, and personality. Their needs may also change at different stages of their illness. The priorities for most people are:
- Extent of the disease
- Outcome of treatment and prognosis
- Types of treatment available
- Side effects of treatment
- Effects of treatment on social life and activities
- Personal autonomy and return to normal life.

Ways of providing information

Verbally

In cancer care, information is usually given verbally and face-to-face with the patient. This allows interaction between the patient, family, and nurse. The patient can ask questions and gain clarification and support. It also allows the health professional to adapt information to the needs of the patient, to monitor their response, to give explanations, and to respond to questions.

In writing

There is a wide range of information now available in written form. Some of it is provided by charitable organizations and is written in everyday language. Many cancer services have information centres where patients can access written information or information on video, CD, or the Internet. Some cancer services provide written information on their own services.

There are advantages of written information is that it can be taken away, studied at leisure, and shared with family and friends. It is important to match the nature or level of written information with the needs of the audience, although this can be more difficult than giving information verbally.

Patient-held records

In some areas, patients are offered their own record of their illness and treatment. This offers the opportunity for written information to be accumulated, for professionals to make entries in the record, and for patients to record their own experiences in diary form.

Reflection points
- What sources of information do you offer your patients?
- How can you match the information to their needs?

Information technology

The Internet enables patients to access information on cancer from sources all over the world. This can include personal accounts of cancer, support groups, technical information on research and treatments, and alternatives to conventional treatments. However, it is often hard to establish the status of information on the Internet, how accurate or reliable it is, or whether it is a commercial site. Patients and families should be encouraged to consider the credibility of any websites they use, e.g. who funds the website, what its purpose is, and what the original source of its information is. Some of the more trustworthy sites can be identified by their domain name—British government websites end in gov.uk, and academic websites in ac.uk. In the USA, university sites end in .edu, and in Australia in .edu.aus. Charities, which can be excellent sources of information, use .org, but this can also be used by commercial groups who may have a financial interest in people using their services. Other business domain names include .co, .com, and .net.

Use of the Internet is limited to those who have access to the necessary technology, and this can exclude those with limited financial resources. However, many information centres in hospitals enable patients to have access.

Chat rooms are another way that the Internet can be used. Both patients and carers can correspond with people in a similar position and use them as a source of support.

The Independent Cancer Taskforce's Strategy for England 2015–2020 recommends that patient experience is as important as clinical effectiveness and safety. To this end, it encourages shared decision-making and proposes maximizing the use of digital technology, giving consenting patients online access to test results and communications.

Further reading

Adams E, Boulton M, Watson E. The information needs of partners and family members of cancer patients: a systematic literature review. *Patient Educ Couns* 2009;77:179–86.

Independent Cancer Taskforce (2015) *Achieving world-class cancer outcomes: a strategy for England 2015–2020.* Available at: ℳ https://www.cancerresearchuk.org/sites/default/files/achieving_world-class_cancer_outcomes_-_a_strategy_for_england_2015-2020.pdf

National Institute for Clinical Excellence (2004). Supportive and palliative care: research evidence; user Involvement in planning, delivering and evaluating services. In: National Institute for Clinical Excellence. *Improving Supportive and Palliative Care for Adults with Cancer: The Manual.* pp 29–45. Available at: ℳ https://www.nice.org.uk/guidance/csg4/resources/improving-supportive-and-palliative-care-for-adults-with-cancer-pdf-773375005.

Warren E, Footman K, Tinelli M, McKee M, Knai C. Do cancer-specific websites meet patient's information needs? *Patient Educ Couns* 2014;95:126–36.

Patient and family involvement in decision-making

The evidence suggests that most people want to take an active role in making decisions about their care and treatment. However, this varies from person to person. More people want to be fully informed than to be fully involved in the decision-making process itself.

It is the responsibility of all nurses working in cancer care to involve the patient and their family as fully as possible in the process of clinical decision-making.

Consent and competence

Consent is the most basic level of involvement in decision-making. To give informed consent, the patient needs sufficient information and needs to be free from coercion and be competent. Competence means that the patient must be able to understand the nature and purpose of the treatment and its risks and benefits, and be able to retain the information for long enough to make the decision (➔ see Mental capacity, p. 164).

Choice and shared decision-making

Shared decision-making is likely to result in patients feeling more involved, improved patient–professional relationships, and better outcomes. Choices should always be offered where these are possible, although it is also important to be clear when choices are limited. Decision-making should be viewed as a shared responsibility. For example, the patient and their family need to be involved in decisions about whether to proceed with adjuvant therapy. However, care needs to be taken to ensure that they do not feel decisions are being pushed onto them, creating an additional burden for the family. The extent to which a patient wants to be involved will be influenced by a number of personal factors. They may have other concerns that distract them, or they may have difficulty taking in the information offered.

Conditions that impair decision-making
- Anxiety.
- Pain.
- Nausea.
- Fatigue, malaise.
- Depression.
- Drowsiness—may be due to sedation.
- Family conflict.

Key issues

- Be clear what the treatment or care options are.
- Outline the implications of the options in terms of likely outcomes and any risks involved.
- Offer additional sources of information, e.g. support groups, websites.
- Advise on what to do when the patient is feeling tired or unwell, e.g. focus on current priorities.

Key questions

- What information do you need in order to make this decision?
- How would you like to be involved in the decision-making process?
- What sort of support do you need to help you make this decision?
- Who is the key person to contact for information/support?

Decisions can be particularly difficult when active or curative treatment is no longer an option. This can represent a difficult period of transition for the patient and family. At times of transition, it can be particularly important to 'have someone on the end of the phone', to talk things through and offer support. Specialist nurses are often best placed to provide this support.

Further reading

Coulter A. Patient information and shared decision-making in cancer care. *Br J Cancer* 2003;89(Suppl 1):S15–16.

Shepherd H, Tattersall M, Butow P. The context influences doctors' support of shared decision-making in cancer care. *Br J Cancer* 2007;97:6–13.

Thorne S, Oliffe J, Stajduhar K. Communicating shared decision-making: cancer patient perspectives. *Patient Educ Couns* 2013;90:291–6.

Ziebland S, Evans J, McPherson A. The choice is yours? How women with ovarian cancer make sense of treatment choices? *Patient Educ Couns* 2006;62:361–7.

Patient involvement in evaluating and managing health care

The Department of Health document *Patient and Public Involvement in the New NHS*[1] identified the benefits of user involvement as '*promoting the individual's perspective, improving services, improving public understanding,* and *improving health*'. In addition, the Independent Cancer Taskforce's Strategy for England 2015–2020 promotes the use of the annual National Cancer Patients Experience Survey to monitor patients' experiences and improve services.

What level of involvement?

Basic levels of involvement include providing information, seeking feedback on services, and consulting on developments to services. This can be done through questionnaires, surveys, meetings, or focus groups.

Participation or partnership involves service users as participants in the process of planning, managing, or evaluating services. This can be achieved through having service users as members of committees or employing them as consultants to services.

User involvement: issues to consider

Meaningful involvement

In order for involvement to be meaningful, the role of the service user must be clear, with an agreed sharing of responsibilities between the service and the service user. Otherwise there is a danger of only token involvement.

Representativeness

Individuals best represent their own personal experience. Service user groups will be better able to represent a range of views. When involving a service user, consider how representative their voice will be.

Education and payment

User representatives may require preparation and payment for the role.

Minority or disadvantaged groups

Special efforts may be needed to involve groups such as ethnic minorities who may not feel fully integrated into the systems that manage health care. Efforts should also be made to involve the physically ill and the socially and financially disadvantaged groups, such as the homeless, who often feel disempowered.

Language

This should be inclusive, avoiding medical jargon and technical terms, wherever possible.

Reflection points

- What level of involvement do service users have in your service?
- How could you improve user involvement?

Further reading

Attree P, Morris S, Clifton M, Hinder S, Vaughan S. *Exploring the Impact of User Involvement on Health and Social Care Services for Cancer in the UK*. London: Macmillan Cancer Support; 2008.

Attree P, Morris S, Payne S, Vaughan S, Hinder S. Exploring the influence of service user involvement on health and social care services for cancer. *Health Expectations* 2010;14:48–58.

Cotterell P, Harlow G, Morris C, et al. Service user involvement in cancer care: the impact on service users. *Health Expect* 2010;14:159–69.

References

1 Department of Health. *Patient and Public Involvement in the New NHS*. London: Department of Health; 1999.

Psychological, social, and spiritual support

The value of the nurse–patient relationship

Nursing is a unique combination of close interpersonal relationships and physically intimate care, delivered within a framework of personal and professional values.[1] Effective nursing involves the use of subtle and complex interpersonal skills, blending a focus on both task and relationship, integrating physical and psychological care. This can help the patient feel secure and cared for, and part of a warm and supportive environment. Many nurses also feel that the interpersonal relationships they have with patients are the most satisfying and rewarding aspect of their work. Increasingly, compassion is seen as integral to cancer nursing care. Although it may be a personal attribute of the nurse, the capacity and skills for compassionate care may be learnt through education and positive working practices.

Empathy, closeness, and intimacy

A close relationship with the patient requires the nurse to experience empathy for them. Empathy is the capacity to understand what the patient is feeling and to communicate this to them. Expressions of empathy go beyond sympathizing with the patient, to real emotional connection based on mutual understanding. There is some evidence that self-disclosure or personal openness on the part of the nurse aids this process, though only when it remains focused on the needs of the patient.[1]

Nurses build close working relationships with people who have cancer, often during times of distress, pain, and insecurity for the patient. Demonstrations of empathy, combined with confidence in the nurse's technical competence, will lead to trust. This can involve the skilled use of touch, humour, and metaphor, using physical proximity and a relaxed posture to enable a sense of closeness. The skilled nurse can make a potentially embarrassing situation comfortable, enhancing the patient's sense of well-being.

Advocacy for the cancer patient

Advocacy can be viewed as a moral or an ethical dimension of nursing care. It involves the nurse representing the patient's interests or providing care that respects their wishes or interests. It acts in different ways, depending on the level of dependency and the participation of the patient. It can involve protecting, supporting, or educating the patient, or empowering the patient and promoting self-determination.

Reflection point

How do I know when to be protective towards a patient and represent their interests, and when to change the emphasis to empowering them to make their own decisions?

Further reading

Bramley L, Matiti M. How does it really feel to be in my shoes? Patients' experiences of compassion within nursing care and their perceptions of developing compassionate nurses. *J Clin Nurs* 2014;23:2790–9.

Dowling M. The meaning of nurse–patient intimacy in oncology care settings: from the nurse and patient perspective. *Eur J Oncol Nurs* 2008;12:319–28.

References

1 Roberts D. *Psychosocial Nursing Care: A Guide to Nursing the Whole Person*. Maidenhead: Open University Press; 2013.

Emotional labour and stress

Nurses are expected to be warm and caring with patients, whatever their own personal feelings, to produce an outward appearance to the patient of being cared for. The cost of this act of caring in nursing may be the suppression of the nurse's own personal feelings.

The management of feelings when working as a carer can be described as **emotional labour**. This involves a form of acting within the professional role. Surface acting requires the presentation of a suitable expression to fit the situation, e.g. warmth and concern. Deep acting requires self-monitoring and the modification of inner feelings, e.g. smiling, whilst suppressing feelings of discomfort in the presence of pain or distress.

Although emotional labour is often recognized as a feature of nursing, it is not formally taught and it is not always valued by health-care employers. It may be seen as an extension of the traditional role of women in society—both undervalued and emotionally demanding. For some nurses, this emotional aspect of the role can seem limitless—where does the role end? Therefore, emotional labour also means that the nurse needs to manage the boundaries of their role and the work/home boundary, to feel secure and to be able to enjoy their work.

Managing stress

It is clear that working with patients who are distressed, in pain, or dying can be very stressful for nurses. In terms of occupational demand, three factors are significant in predicting the ability to cope: work demands, the degree of control over demand, and personal and professional support. In addition to the emotional demands of the work, sources of stress can include:
- High turnover of staff and vacancies
- Conflicts with colleagues
- Poor management or leadership
- Role ambiguity or role conflict
- Lack of support.

Working environments that are supportive and where caring relationships are valued are likely to be less stressful for nurses and emotional labour more effective.

Compassion fatigue, secondary traumatic stress, and burnout

The negative effect of the stresses of caring on the nurse has been described by different terms. Compassion fatigue and secondary traumatic stress refer to the effects, particularly on health professionals, of working long term with people who are in pain, traumatized, or suffering.

Burnout refers to long-term loss of energy and interest in work. It can include:
- Emotional exhaustion
- Demoralization and personal isolation
- Loss of job satisfaction.

Compassion fatigue, secondary traumatic stress, and burnout can lead to:
- Poor sleep, poor concentration, chronic tiredness
- ↑ reliance on drugs such as alcohol, cannabis, tobacco, and coffee

- Tension and irritability
- Work problems spilling over into the home and social life.

On the other hand, emotional labour does not usually lead to personal problems and may be very rewarding in the long term. Experiencing and exercising compassion for others can be a cause of personal and professional satisfaction, and exposure to trauma may lead to personal growth, i.e. post-traumatic growth.

How to cope with stress and prevent burnout

Developing support systems
- Work stresses should be dealt with at work—teams should develop systems for mutual support and dealing with stress. Examples include regular individual or group supervision (➔ see Psychological support, pp. 130–1) or discussion during handover periods. This helps to reduce any sense of personal isolation.
- Debriefing, a meeting of those involved in a difficult or distressing incident, preferably with a facilitator, provides an opportunity to air feelings, share support, and learn lessons for future practice.
- It is also important to take breaks during the working day.

Personal autonomy and control of workload
When work demands are high, having a sense of personal control over your own workload helps the coping process. Individuals should be able to monitor their own workload and regularly appraise this in consultation with their manager.

Role clarity
Role ambiguity, e.g. having a role with ill-defined limits, is associated with burnout. Roles should be defined, with any overlap between roles clarified.

Manage the work/home boundary
Take care not to use friends as the primary means of coping with work. Develop interests and social contacts that are separate from work. Live a healthy lifestyle, with adequate exercise, and monitor the use of drugs, including alcohol and coffee.

Education and personal development
Having regular access to education that fits with an overall plan of personal development keeps practice fresh and motivates the individual.

Reflection points
- Have I ever had problems coping with work?
- How did I deal with this at the time, and what helped most?

Further reading
Jackson D, Firtko A, Edenborough M. Personal resilience as a strategy for surviving and thriving in the face of workplace adversity: a literature review. *J Adv Nurs* 2007;60:1–9.
Professional Quality of Life Scale (ProQOL) (measures: compassion satisfaction, burnout, secondary traumatic stress). Available at: ℛ https://proqol.org/ProQol_Test.html

Psychological support

The NICE *Guidance on the Supportive and Palliative Care of Adults with Cancer* identifies four levels of professional assessment and support.[2] This is a useful model for understanding the contribution of different professionals. There is the potential for overlap between levels, and individuals may function on different levels at different times (see Table 9.1).

Psychological support: level 1

All health professionals should be able to provide basic psychological support: listening and communicating effectively, developing supportive relationships with patients and carers, and responding to distress.

Psychological support: level 2

Professionals with additional training, experience, or supervision may provide more specific or skilled support. This can include dealing with adjustment difficulties and loss, offering supportive counselling, problem-solving, and supporting the patient's ability to cope.

Psychological support and psycho-oncology services: levels 3 and 4

Level 3 involves a working knowledge of specific counselling or psychotherapy models. This may be done by a CNS with additional training or by psycho-oncology services.

Psycho-oncology is the term used to describe psychological services specializing in the care of people with cancer. It may be provided by individuals or teams. These teams will typically comprise some of the following: a psychiatrist, a clinical psychologist, a mental health nurse, or a social worker. Some of these may only work part-time within psycho-oncology.

Psycho-oncology services operate on levels 3 and 4 of the NICE model of psychological assessment and intervention, and typically provide:

• Psychological assessment and psychiatric diagnosis
• Psychological treatments, typically counselling and cognitive behavioural therapy (CBT)
• Consultation and liaison—advising on the management of psychological problems in cancer services
• Clinical supervision of cancer care staff
• Education in psychological aspects of care.

Counselling and psychotherapy in the cancer care setting

• Counselling is frequently available within cancer services. Many services are provided by professional counsellors with training and supervision, practising at NICE level 3. However, there can be considerable variation in the level of training or experience of individual counsellors.
• Within the UK, counselling is not a statutorily regulated profession, and therefore, the title of counsellor is not protected by law. However, there is a voluntary system of registration.

Table 9.1 Levels of psychological support

Level	Group	Intervention
1	All health-care professionals	Effective information giving, compassionate communication, and general psychological support
2	Professionals with additional expertise	Psychological techniques such as problem-solving
3	Trained and accredited professionals	Counselling and specific interventions, e.g. anxiety management and solution-focused therapy, delivered according to an explicit theoretical framework
4	Mental health specialists	Specialist psychological and psychiatric interventions such as psychotherapy, including CBT

Data sourced from NICE (2004) *Improving supportive and palliative care for adults with cancer.*
National Institute for Health and Care Excellence: ℘ http://www.nice.org.uk/guidance/csgsp

- Many nurses have undertaken some form of counselling training, but it can be very difficult to practise as a counsellor within a nursing role. There are a number of reasons for this:
  - Counselling is characterized by clear boundaries—contact takes place at set times and places, without interruption. A nurse's contact with patients is usually more fluid than this; it is harder to keep to set times or to guarantee privacy.
  - Nurses usually see their patients either on hospital wards, in busy outpatient departments, or in the patient's home.

For these reasons, it is more common for nurses to use counselling skills, such as active listening and attending, or to see counselling as an aspect of their role (e.g. breast care nurses) than to work specifically as a counsellor.

Websites

British Association for Counselling and Psychotherapy. Available at: ℘ http://www.bacp.co.uk/

References

2 National Institute for Health and Care Excellence (2004). *Improving Supportive and Palliative Care for Adults With Cancer.* Cancer Service Guideline [CSG4]. Available at: ℘ https://www.nice.org.uk/guidance/csg4

Specific psychological interventions

Cognitive behavioural therapy

CBT, or cognitive therapy, was developed initially for treating mood disorders like anxiety and depression. It is based on the idea that people develop characteristic patterns of thinking and feeling about life, which can become a problem. The therapist works collaboratively to help the patient develop more positive ways of dealing with the problems they encounter in life. It is widely used in treating people with cancer who have psychological problems, including adjustment to the disease and its treatment.

Problem-solving

Problem-solving is a specific cognitive behavioural technique that aims to help people clarify what their problems are and what potential solutions there may be, and how to overcome these. It has been proven to be very effective in the treatment of depression in people with cancer, and it can be administered by cancer nurses with suitable training and supervision.

Mindfulness

Mindfulness, or mindfulness-based cognitive therapy (MBCT), involves exercises that help us to experience mental life in a non-judgemental way without the distracting thoughts that can lead us to having problems. It has proved to be very helpful to people who experience recurrent depression and long-term problems like cancer.

Psycho-educational interventions

These usually combine education about cancer and its effects, group support, and help with coping strategies such as relaxation training and stress management.

Further reading

Bartley T. *Mindfulness Based Cognitive Therapy for Cancer: Gently Turning Towards*. Oxford: Wiley-Blackwell; 2011.

Moorey S, Greer S. *Oxford Guide to CBT for People with Cancer*, 2nd ed. Oxford: Oxford University Press; 2012.

Walker J, Hansen CH, Martin P, et al. Integrated collaborative care for major depression comorbid with a poor prognosis cancer (SMaRT Oncology-3): a multicentre randomised controlled trial in patients with lung cancer. *Lancet Oncol* 2014;15:1168–76.

Social support

Social support is composed of the following elements.

Emotional support

This involves the expression of positive feelings, like concern and affection, resulting in feeling that one is cared for, loved, or esteemed. Mostly, patients will get this from their family and friends, but nurses can help by acknowledging the patient's feelings and encouraging the open expression of emotions. Consideration should be given to people who have no clear supportive network, bearing in mind their personal preferences. Questions about the patient's social support should be included as a part of assessment (→ see Introduction to assessment, pp. 462–3).

Informational support

Informational support is usually sought and valued from professionals, and may take the form of advice or guidance, in addition to information about the illness, treatment, side effects, etc. (→ see Patient Information, pp. 118–19).

Instrumental support

This includes material or financial aid and services. Professionals frequently overlook these areas; they may simply attend to, and prioritize, the medical aspects of the patient's life when this type of support may be the highest priority for the patient and their family. It is therefore important to be sensitive to the full range of patients' concerns (→ see Employment and finances, pp. 95–6).

Social work support

Social workers are trained to provide support to the family as a system and to see the patient's needs within the social and family context. They will often work as part of the specialist oncology or palliative care team; and, to some extent, their role will overlap with others, in that they provide general psychosocial support.

Specific aspects of the social work role include:
- Supporting families with particular social problems or with young children.
- Helping to prepare families for bereavement.
- Arranging packages of care or access to specialist social facilities.
- Advice on finances and benefit entitlements.

Priorities for referral to a social worker
- Families or family members believed to be at risk.
- Individuals or families who lack social support or have clear financial difficulties.

Financial entitlements

Patients' needs for financial assistance can be considerable as they lose income and have additional expenses over the course of their treatment, e.g. transport, diet. There are a number of sources of advice on benefits and entitlements for people with cancer, many of which are charity-based and some of which act at a national UK level, including Macmillan Cancer Support, Maggie's Centres, and the Citizen's Advice Bureau.

The range of potential benefits is regularly reviewed but currently includes:
- **Attendance Allowance**: this helps with the costs of personal care for people aged over 65 with disabilities or long-term illness
- **Personal Independence Payment** (replacing Disability Living Allowance): this helps to pay for daily living and mobility costs for people aged under 65 with long-term illness
- **Carer's Allowance**: a benefit for adult carers who spend over 35 hours a week caring for someone
- **The Hospital Travel Costs Scheme**: this can help towards the costs of travel for people attending hospital for NHS treatment, if they are already receiving benefits because of low income
- **Prescription charge exemption**: this can be issued by doctors treating any person who has cancer.

See the Macmillan Cancer Support webpage, available at: ℘ http://www. macmillan.org.uk/

Further reading

Macmillan Cancer Support (2011). *Social Workers in Cancer Care: An Evidence Review*. Available at: ℘ http://www.macmillan.org.uk/documents/aboutus/health_professionals/socialworkers-anevidencereviewoctober2010.pdf

Spiritual support and chaplaincy

Spirituality

The experience of spirituality includes personal faith and religious affiliation, a sense of inner strength, hope, or purpose in life, and a search for meaning at times of illness or loss or when facing death. The term spirituality can have different meanings, e.g. there can be an overlap between spiritual and psychological care. Spirituality may concern personal distress, total pain (➲ see Classifications of pain, p. 558), and attitude towards dying, as well as matters of faith.

Support for spirituality can be seen as an essential part of cancer nursing. It is also a specialist activity that is undertaken by trained professionals such as chaplains.

Spiritual aspects of care should be based on good communication, an ability to listen to the patient, and being with them at times of pain, distress, and fear. This can be similar to other aspects of psychological and social support but deals with a less tangible area of human experience. Suffering and spiritual pain are two terms often used to describe personal experiences of existential distress, fear, despair, or hopelessness in the face of illness. These can include the person's whole being and transcend the physical or material aspects of life.

A person who is suffering may need to re-examine their inner sources of strength and their most fundamental beliefs about life. Supporting someone through this requires the nurse to make time and space, to be available, but without preconceptions, to affirm the patient's beliefs, but not to impose their own.

To do this requires an understanding of one's own beliefs and spirituality, a degree of self-awareness, and an ability to learn and grow in response to the experience of suffering in others.

Assessment of spiritual needs should include questions that open up the subject of spirituality for the patient, exploring the personal meaning of events, and allowing them space to discuss their concerns. Rather than being a single structured event, spiritual assessment is best seen as part of an ongoing relationship, in response to the patient's perception of their needs (➲ see Holistic needs assessment and care planning, p. 464).

Religious faith and chaplaincy

Religious faith is an important part of how people may cope with illness, so access to specialist spiritual support is an important aspect of care. In doing this, it is important not to make assumptions about faith or religious practices. People with no regular religious affiliation may wish to have support from a chaplain, whilst members of a religion may not always want to practise it. Helping people to practise their faith can include helping them to make a place for religious symbols within a ward setting, e.g. icons, books, or pictures. Some patients will have religious dietary requirements, need to observe religious festivals, or need uninterrupted time for prayer or meditation. Many hospitals and hospices have a chapel, or a multifaith room, which serves as a place of peace and contemplation for all.

Hospital and hospice chaplains often represent one of the main Christian denominations but will make themselves available to all patients who need spiritual support. It is important that contact details are maintained for members of different faiths. Hospital chaplains usually see their role as going beyond religious ministry, to providing support to both patients and staff and providing counselling.

Further reading

Holloway M, Adamson S, McSherry W, Swinton J. *Spiritual Care at the End of Life: A Systematic Review of the Literature.* Department of Health/University of Hull; 2011.

Marie Curie Cancer Care. *Spiritual and Religious Care Competencies for Specialist Palliative Care.* London: Marie Curie Cancer Care; 2003.

Taylor E, Mamier I. Spiritual care nursing: what cancer patients and family caregivers want. *J Adv Nurs* 2005;49:260–7.

Rehabilitation of the cancer patient

Rehabilitation of the cancer patient

Disability is a major, but often under-recognized, problem for people with cancer. The illness itself and the treatments given can cause short-term problems, such as restricted shoulder movements following mastectomy, as well as more severe disabilities such as paraplegia from spinal cord compression.

Most cancer patients are likely to need rehabilitation at some point in their illness. With an emphasis on self-management, rehabilitation enables patients to take on an active role in managing their lives and maintaining their independence. For patients with advanced disease, the focus of rehabilitation will shift from improving function to finding alternative ways to achieve satisfaction and fulfilment in daily activities. At the end of life, rehabilitation interventions must take account of rapidly changing needs and be led by the priorities of patients and their families. At all times, rehabilitation aims to maximize the potential for health and to support adaptation to changes and limitations imposed by the illness and its treatment.

The importance of rehabilitation in cancer care

Many cancer patients find the thought of progressive disability and future dependence on their carers worrying and distressing. Rehabilitation can engage patients and their families in an active process of achieving goals that are meaningful to them, so that decline does not have to be associated with helplessness and hopelessness.

With increasing numbers of people living with and beyond cancer, it is important that cancer survivors are able to maximize their potential to return to independent and fulfilling lives. Patients returning to work need the tools to stay healthy via a variety of local rehabilitation programmes.[1] These are outlined within the Recovery Package for cancer survivors (➔ see The recovery package, p. 73).

The process and aims of rehabilitation

The process of rehabilitation includes:
- Assessment to identify the nature and extent of functional difficulties and factors that will contribute to their resolution
- Working with the patient to set goals
- Identifying and implementing strategies to achieve these goals
- Constantly monitoring progress and adapting plans to incorporate changes.

Rehabilitation aims to:
- Maximize social participation—role, function, and social status
- Maximize well-being—physical and emotional
- Achieve satisfaction—adaptation to disability
- Minimize carer stress and distress.

Allied health professionals

Rehabilitation is a multiprofessional activity carried out by a range of AHPs, nurses, doctors, and other health and social care professionals. The AHPs involved could include, for example, occupational therapists, physiotherapists, speech and language therapists, dieticians, therapy radiographers, and lymphoedema therapists. Effective rehabilitation is a team effort which cannot be accomplished by any one professional working in isolation. Each discipline will have its own contribution; those of the occupational therapist and physiotherapist are outlined in ➲ Occupational therapy, p. 139 and ➲ Physiotherapy, p. 139.

Occupational therapy

Occupational therapists address the impact of disability on the patient's everyday life.

This involves:

- Assessment and analysis of the person's activities—those which are necessary for everyday living and those which are creative and enjoyable
- Working with the person to develop alternative ways of managing or providing resources, such as equipment or a wheelchair, that might make life easier.

Physiotherapy

Physiotherapists use a range of treatment approaches to reduce the effect of symptoms such as pain, fatigue, dyspnoea, and neurological impairment on the patient's QoL. These include:

- Maximizing the person's potential in terms of functional ability and independence through physical activity and exercise.
- Non-pharmacological approaches to pain management such as transcutaneous electrical nerve stimulation (TENS) (➲ see Transcutanous electrical nerve stimulation, p. 567).
- Manual therapies such as joint mobilization and manual lymphatic drainage (➲ see Lymphoedema, pp. 626–8; ➲ see Complementary therapies, pp. 142–4).

Both physiotherapists and occupational therapists are involved in teaching patients how to manage fatigue, breathlessness, and anxiety, using the techniques mentioned above.

Referrals for rehabilitation

Any patient whose ability to carry out daily activities is compromised by their illness should be referred to a suitable therapist for rehabilitation. Rehabilitation takes place in a variety of settings, including hospitals, hospices, the community, and specialist rehabilitation units, as well as those forming part of local programmes designed to promote independence and self-care.

In inpatient settings, discharge planning might supersede rehabilitation as the focus of care. Once the patient is at home, it is important to consider their longer-term rehabilitation needs and to make the appropriate referrals to community-based primary care rehabilitation teams.

Referral to a specialist rehabilitation unit may be considered for patients who need to adapt to living with a long-term disability and are motivated to engage in a structured rehabilitation programme. For example, a patient who has hemiplegia with cognitive and perceptual problems as a result of a brain tumour may benefit from the input of a physiotherapist to work on mobility, and an occupational therapist to develop strategies for managing daily occupations such as self-care and work.

Nurses play an active part in the rehabilitation process and can contribute by making appropriate rehabilitation referrals when the need for specialist intervention is identified, and by working with AHPs to encourage and enable patients to maintain their independence and control in their daily activities. This can involve goal setting and working collaboratively in the management of specific problems such as breathlessness.

Patients' rehabilitation needs vary from straightforward to complex, and Table 10.1 gives an indication of the roles and responsibilities of different members of the MDT at different levels.

Table 10.1 Recommended model of rehabilitation

Level	Recipients	Service providers	Intervention
Level 1 Information and support	Anyone with a cancer diagnosis where the illness or its treatment is likely to affect the person's ability to manage their everyday activities	All health and social care staff and support workers	• Identification of the need for further information and support through holistic assessment • Provision of information with signposting and referral to other services where necessary
Level 2 Routine rehabilitation	Patients with identified straightforward rehabilitation needs	Health and social care staff with skills and experience in rehabilitation	Assessment of specific rehabilitation needs Provision of straightforward rehabilitation interventions, e.g. advice on post-operative exercises
Level 3 Specialist rehabilitation	Patients with complex rehabilitation needs	Rehabilitation specialists with specific expertise in cancer rehabilitation	Detailed assessment and interventions for complex problems, e.g. the functional and psychosocial consequences of disability resulting from spinal cord compression or H&N cancer

Further reading

Rankin J, Robb K, Murtagh N, Cooper J, Lewis S. *Rehabilitation in Cancer Care*. Chichester: Wiley-Blackwell; 2008.

Taylor J, Simader R, Nieland P. *Potential and Possibility: Rehabilitation at the End of Life*. Munich: Elsevier; 2013.

References

1 Macmillan Cancer Support. *The Recovery Package*. Available at: ℘ https://www.macmillan.org.uk/about-us/health-professionals/programmes-and-services/recovery-package

Chapter 11

Complementary therapies

Complementary therapies

Complementary therapies are gaining popularity with both the public and health professionals in a number of areas of health-care provision, including cancer care. Up to 50% of patients with cancer make use of a range of therapies, including acupuncture, homeopathy, aromatherapy, reflexology, and massage.

Complementary therapies are used in addition to, and to complement, conventional therapies for cancer. They are sometimes grouped together with alternative therapies, under the umbrella term 'complementary and alternative medicine (CAM)'. However, alternative therapies aim to work as a distinct alternative, rather than a complement, to conventional therapies. In contrast, the term **integrated or integrative health or medicine** is increasingly used to describe an approach that combines elements of both complementary and conventional therapies, providing a 'total approach to care' that includes mind, body, and spirit. Many cancer centres offer integrated care, providing complementary therapies alongside conventional treatments for cancer.

In the UK, a variety of models are in operation to provide complementary therapies. For example, in hospices, volunteer therapists give treatments, and in some hospital settings, nurses with specialized training integrate therapies within their nursing role. However, people living with cancer commonly access complementary therapies via independent practitioners.

Why are complementary therapies popular?

Patients choose complementary therapies because:
- They improve psychological and emotional well-being.
- They provide a more personal and holistic approach than conventional medicine.
- They give patients a greater sense of personal control and empowerment than a health system that sometimes seems inaccessible, technological, and impersonal.
- Therapists spend more time with them, listening to and addressing their concerns.
- They help to manage side effects of conventional cancer treatments.
- They provide a more natural and gentle balance to conventional cancer treatments.

Where is the evidence?

However, complementary therapies have been criticized for having no evidence base. Though an evidence base is emerging for some therapies, they face challenges, meeting the same rigorous standards that would be expected for conventional cancer treatments. Complementary therapy outcomes are often highly subjective and difficult to measure, making randomized controlled trials, the 'gold standard' of treatments, hard to apply. Some would argue that patient choice alone is sufficient evidence for effectiveness. Both the Cochrane Library and NICE have a growing body of evidence on the effectiveness of different complementary therapies with different conditions (➔ see Websites, p. 146).

Holistic care

Given concerns about evidence and possible interactions with conventional treatments, attitudes towards complementary therapies vary between individuals and across professions. Some doctors are either reluctant to discuss the use of complementary therapies with patients or are hostile to their use, and this can lead to patients not disclosing when they are using them.[1,2] This can result in lost therapeutic opportunities, because patients value medical approval and advice on the safety of their choices. Nurses, on the other hand, have been more supportive of the use of complementary therapies, often based on their own commitment to holistic care. Specialist nurses may be uniquely well placed to act as 'gatekeepers' in the use of complementary therapies, both advocating for their use and supporting patients in making informed choices about which therapies are safe and likely to be of most benefit to them.[2] All health professionals need to take a pragmatic approach to the use of complementary therapies, as these therapies' popularity continues to grow.

Alternative therapies, e.g. Gerson Therapy™ or shark cartilage, are often viewed with suspicion by health professionals, as using them may delay the start of conventional medical care, reducing treatment options and chances of survival. They may also raise false hopes, which can lead to cruel disappointments. For this reason, it is important to distinguish between complementary and alternative therapies. It is also important to encourage patients and their families to talk about any alternative treatments they are taking or are thinking about taking.

Commonly used complementary therapies

These are some of the most commonly reported therapies used in cancer care, though this is not an exhaustive list.

Acupuncture

Acupuncture has been used quite extensively for control of chronic and treatment-related cancer pain. Use of the traditional point PC6 on the inside of the wrist seems to be an effective anti-emetic technique in the early stages during chemotherapy. There is also some evidence to show that acupuncture can relieve dyspnoea, and patients taking tamoxifen have found acupuncture helpful in reducing hot flushes.

Aromatherapy

Aromatherapy is a therapy that systematically uses essential oils derived from plants in treatments to improve physical and emotional well-being. Most of the evidence suggests that essential oils applied via massage can be helpful in a number of ways, including reduced anxiety and improved relaxation and emotional symptoms. QoL enhancement has also been reported. Despite the lack of a clear evidence base for the effects of aromatherapy, it remains one of the most widely used therapies in cancer care.

Massage

Massage is a term for a number of techniques that include touching, kneading, and manipulation of soft tissues for therapeutic purposes. The use of massage within cancer care is often integrated within nursing as skillful touch and a technique to enhance communication. It has been shown to be effective, although only short-term, in reducing anxiety and pain perception. Foot massage has been shown to have a positive effect on reducing pain and nausea and encouraging relaxation. An important aspect of this therapy is the element of focused touch. Patients have described relief from suffering, feeling good in spite of the cancer and its treatment, and feeling 'special' and empowered. The process of massage also contributes to the development of a positive relationship with the nurse.

Reflexology

This therapy is based on the principle that there are areas in the feet that correspond to all glands, organs, and parts of the body. The language of reflexology is not easily understood within orthodox health care and may be more readily accepted if it is viewed as a specific system of touch. Patients have reported benefits that include relief of pain and anxiety and improved quality of life. As with massage, the benefit of focused touch by the practitioner is probably a significant part of the therapeutic process.

Homeopathy

This is the treatment of illness by using remedies prescribed according to the principle that 'like cures like'. The remedies are derived from plant, animal, and mineral sources, which, through a process of serial dilution and agitation, become extremely dilute. There is limited evidence of effectiveness, but some patients show high levels of satisfaction when homeopathy is included in their package of care. Some of the symptoms that have been helped are the adverse dermatological effects of radiotherapy and anxiety and depression, positive effects on mood disturbance, and improvement in QoL.

Herbal medicines

Herbal medicines are readily available over the counter, but there are potential risks concerning the safety of remedies and the possibility of interactions with conventional drug regimens. Patients are encouraged to inform their health-care practitioner about any herbal preparations they are taking.

Reiki

Central to this system of healing that originated in Japan is the concept that an energy flow exists within living beings which supports life by helping to maintain homeostasis. This energy is known as Ki, and when diminished, ill health can arise. Alongside this is the concept that Ki can be channelled from its originating source by a Reiki practitioner and passed on to a recipient. Treatment consists of the practitioner placing their hands either on or just above certain points on the patient's body.

Spiritual healing

This is the channelling of healing energies through the healer to the patient. Healers do not generally relate to disease-specific symptoms but aim to help the patient in more general terms such as increasing well-being. Despite a lack of evidence for its effectiveness, spiritual healing remains a popular therapy with people living with cancer.

Regulation and training for complementary therapies

The House of Lords Select Committee on Science and Technology produced a report in 2000 that provided a framework for the potential integration of complementary therapies into orthodox care. A range of areas was covered, including research, regulation, training, and delivery models. Lack of an evidence base is one of the biggest hurdles to integration, but successive surveys have shown that, in spite of this, patients remain keen to have access to complementary therapies.

Safety was an important focus of the Select Committee report, and this is a key factor in the development of appropriate regulatory systems to protect the patient. Many therapies are working towards voluntary self-regulation, and this process includes a review of the quality of education and training.

The Complementary and Natural Healthcare Council (CNHC) is a UK voluntary regulator for complementary therapists, whose register was approved in 2013 by the Professional Standards Authority for Health and Social Care.

Therapies currently registered are: Alexander technique teaching, aromatherapy, Bowen therapy, craniosacral therapy, healing, hypnotherapy, massage therapy, microsystems acupuncture, naturopathy, nutritional therapy, reflexology, Reiki, shiatsu, sports therapy, and yoga therapy.

The NICE Guidance *Improving Supportive and Palliative Care for Adults with Cancer* (2004) recommends that NHS and voluntary sector providers and user groups work together to review the evidence of best practice on the use of complementary therapies, to agree on policies to ensure safe practice, and to develop complementary components of service directory.

Provider organizations should also ensure that:
- Patients have access to high-quality information on complementary therapies and where to access them
- Facilities are made available for complementary therapies
- Complementary therapists in the NHS conform to best practice
- Complementary therapists contribute to evaluation and research.

The nurse's role in complementary therapies

The key role that nurses have in relation to complementary therapies is to provide support to people who are exploring ways of coping with the symptoms of cancer. Nurses need to be comfortable in discussing therapies and be able to direct patients to the best sources of information. There may also be a need to modify unrealistic expectations, i.e. to be clear about the benefits and limitations of therapies.

Popular websites on complementary and alternative therapies for cancer offer information of variable quality. Many websites endorse unproven therapies, and some have the potential to be dangerous. Nurses have a valuable role in helping patients to make sense of the information. Getting to know, and build trust in, local practitioners and organizations will enable the nurse to give an informed opinion on who and what may help if patients seek advice on how to access complementary therapies.

When patients are admitted to hospital, it is important to find out if they are using any complementary therapies, in particular any supplements and/or herbal medicine. This is important from a safety perspective and is helpful in understanding how the patient is coping.

Patients' reasons for using complementary therapies include seeking an alternative to conventional medicine or they may wish to improve the quality of their lives. An advantage of complementary therapies is that they are generally perceived as treating the whole person. Making a positive decision to access a complementary therapy can facilitate empowerment and a sense of control and choice.

Professional accountability and complementary therapies

Where nurses provide a therapy within clinical practice, they must be confident that the training they have undertaken is suitable and that they are fit to practise. It can be difficult to determine the quality and standard of training courses, e.g. in areas such as aromatherapy and reflexology. Nurses need to be clear about what they want to achieve in delivering a therapy or part of a therapy and then make diligent enquiries. Nurses also have a duty to ensure that the patient gives informed consent before a therapy is given.

Significantly, the patient–practitioner relationship appears to be an important component of the therapeutic process, and the use of complementary therapies serves a variety of functions beyond the explicit relief of symptoms. Many patients report that the process of receiving complementary therapy from an independent practitioner makes them feel cared for. There are therefore significant potential benefits for the patient in seeking and making use of complementary therapies where these are safely delivered by a suitably trained person and ideally where there is a sound evidence base for their use.

Websites

The following organizations offer information on a variety of therapies and on the effectiveness of therapies:

Cochrane Library. Available at: ℜ http://www.cochranelibrary.com

College of Medicine and Integrated Health. Available at: ℜ https://www.collegeofmedicine.org.uk

Complementary and Natural Healthcare Council (CNHC). Available at: ℜ http://www.cnhc.org.uk

National Institute for Health and Care Excellence. Available at: ℜ https://www.nice.org.uk

Penny Brohn UK (Penny Brohn Cancer Care). Available at: ℜ https://www.pennybrohn.org.uk

Further reading

Barraclough J (ed). *Enhancing Cancer Care. Complementary Therapy and Support.* Oxford: Oxford University Press; 2007.

House of Lords Select Committee on Science & Technology (2000). *Complementary and Alternative Medicine.* HL Paper 123. Available at: ℜ http://www.parliament.the-stationery-office.co.uk/pa/ld199900/ldselect/ldsctech/123/12301.htm

Shneerson C, Taskila T, Gale N, Greenfield S, Chen Y-F. The effect of complementary and alternative medicine on the quality of life of cancer survivors: a systematic review and meta-analyses. *Complement Ther Med* 2013;21:417–29.

References

1 Smithson J, Paterson C, Britten N, Evans M, Lewith G. Cancer patients' experiences of using complementary therapies: polarization and integration. *J Health Services Res Policy* 2010;**15**, 54–61.

2 Tovey P, Broom A. Oncologists' and specialist cancer nurses' approaches to complementary and alternative medicine and their impact on patient action. *Soc Sci Med* 2007;64:2550–64.

Palliative care

Palliative care

Palliative care aims to improve the quality of life of patients and their families facing the problems associated with life-threatening illness, through the prevention and relief of suffering by means of early identification and assessment and treatment of pain and other problems—physical, psychosocial, and spiritual. Palliative care:

- Provides relief from pain and other distressing symptoms
- Affirms life and regards dying as a normal process
- Intends neither to hasten nor to postpone death
- Integrates the psychological and spiritual aspects of patient care
- Offers a support system to help patients live as actively as possible until death
- Offers a support system to help the family cope during the patient's illness and in their own bereavement
- Uses a team approach to address the needs of patients and their families, including bereavement counselling, if indicated
- Will enhance the QoL and may also positively influence the course of illness
- Is applicable early in the course of illness, in conjunction with other therapies that are intended to prolong life, such as chemotherapy or radiation therapy, and includes those investigations needed to better understand and manage distressing clinical complications.*

Palliative care services utilize the skills and knowledge of a multiprofessional team to support people who are experiencing a life-threatening illness, and their family members. This care may start at the diagnosis of an illness and continue during treatment until death, and for the family, into the bereavement period. One of the key themes of palliative care is working in partnership with people and their family members, to enable their remaining life to be as fulfilling as possible. The philosophy of palliative care can be applied across a variety of illnesses, settings, and contexts. Within practice settings, palliative care will be provided by:

- Staff who provide palliative care as part of a more general role
- Specialists who have particular expertise in the provision of palliative care.

General palliative and end-of-life care

General palliative and end-of-life care refers to a core set of skills and knowlege, based on a philosophy of care which can be used by any health and social care professional. Given that people with life-threatening illnesses and at the end of life can be cared for in any setting, these skills and knowledge should be part of any health or social care professional's repertoire. Practitioners utilizing this approach will include staff working on oncology or surgical wards in an acute hospital setting, or community nurses for whom palliative care is part of their work. General palliative care will include: holistic assessment and effective communication, basic symptom control, and psychological, social, spiritual, and practical and carer support.[1]

* Reproduced from World Health Organization (WHO). *WHO Definition of Palliative Care*: 🔊 https://www.who.int/cancer/palliative/definition/en/ with permission from the World Health Organization.

Specialist palliative care

Specialist palliative care refers to services for patients and their families with moderate to complex needs provided by practitioners with specialist qualifications and experience, e.g. clinical nurse specialists in palliative care. Specialist palliative care services are multiprofessional and include hospice inpatient care, community palliative care, and acute hospital teams, or teams with a particular focus, e.g. paediatric palliative care. This care may take place within the acute hospital, the community, nursing homes, or in a hospice setting. In the UK, some specialist palliative care services will be NHS-funded; others will be voluntary or charity-funded and have an independent status.

Specialist palliative care services may be provided on a consultation or an advisory basis, or can involve direct care of the patient and family. Although originally focused on cancer patients, specialist palliative care is provided for people with any life-threatening illness who have complex needs. Individuals with difficult-to-manage pain and symptom problems, complex family dynamics, and spiritual or psychosocial distress may require referral to the specialist services.

References

1 World Health Organization. *WHO Definition of Palliative Care*. Available at: ℜ https://www.who. int/cancer/palliative/definition/en/

Interface between cancer and palliative care services

Specialist palliative care services can be introduced at any stage of the illness, from diagnosis to the end of life, when patients would benefit. In the UK, it is not uncommon for patients to have palliative and cancer care in tandem.

Referral to palliative care services

A key part of the specialist palliative care role is to support the delivery of palliative care to patients and families in non-specialist settings (e.g. hospital or community). Referrals can be made to specialist palliative care services by GPs, nurses, or other professionals, or by patients themselves. Most services will have clear referral criteria, often specifying the reason for the referral. This might, for example, be pain or symptom management, family support, or spiritual support.

Specialist palliative care may involve regular visits to specific clinical areas, like oncology wards. In this way, good working relationships can be built up over time and referral pathways established. Ideally, specialist palliative care professionals will provide consultation, i.e. discussing general management problems and specific patient issues, and also education on aspects of palliative and end-of-life care. A referral will usually lead to a full assessment, resulting in either advice on management or, if ongoing contact is needed, in the teams working in partnership to meet the needs of the patient and family.

Referrals should be encouraged as early as possible to facilitate good working relationships and an effective transition to palliative care, and, if necessary, to prepare patients and families for end-of-life care. However, there are a number of factors that can prevent or delay referral (see Box 12.1).

Box 12.1 Barriers to timely referral

Factors in the individual referrer or medical specialty:
- Continuing treatment for too long; not accepting failure of treatment
- Avoiding uncomfortable conversations about death and dying
- Difficulties handing over or 'letting go' of patients.

Patient or family characteristics:
- Younger age of patient
- Patient or family resistance.

Organizational constraints:
- Lack of understanding or knowledge of specialist palliative care services
- Lack of onsite palliative care services or lack of effective working relationships with palliative care specialists
- Difficulty navigating service bureaucracy.

Data sourced from Broom, A, Kirby, E, Good, P, Wootton, J, Adams, J (2012) Specialists' Experiences and Perspectives on the Timing of Referral to Palliative Care: A Qualitative Study. *Journal of Palliative Medicine*; **15**(11), 1248–1253.

End-of-life care

The end of life is a unique moment for each individual, which will stay in the memory of family members and carers. Caring well for the dying provides an opportunity to enhance the experience and to promote dignity and comfort for the patient and their family. It is an important time to prepare for the death of a loved one, as the nature of the death can contribute positively or adversely to the bereavement experience.

The key aims of care at the end of life are:
- To enable the person to die with dignity and, wherever possible, in their preferred place of care
- To manage pain and distressing symptoms
- To enable the family to make the most of the time left and to minimize regrets
- To meet the needs of both the dying person and their family, including emotional and spiritual needs, and to make the memory of the death as positive as possible
- To honour a patient's wishes with respect to organ and tissue donation.

Recognizing the end of life

Recognizing the end of life helps practitioners to meet the patient's needs and prepares their family for the reality of death. However, there is commonly a reluctance to 'diagnose dying' or to state verbally that someone is dying. If it is thought that the patient is entering the dying phase, it is important to review the following:
- The person's physiological, psychological, social, and spiritual needs
- Current clinical signs and symptoms
- Medical history and the clinical context
- The person's goals and wishes (including advance statements and decisions) (➲ see Advance care planning, pp. 165–6)
- The views of those important to the person about future care.

The following can be signs of approaching death:
- General deterioration in condition
- Reduced communication or social withdrawal
- Agitation
- Gaunt appearance
- Pallor
- Mottling
- Cool or clammy skin
- Diminished intake of fluid and food
- Reduced fluid output
- Profound weakness
- Loss of appetite and difficulty swallowing
- Changes in breathing pattern
- Reduced consciousness
- Person becomes bed-bound.

If these signs appear suddenly in a person not expected to die, it is important to rule out other potentially reversible causes of deterioration, e.g. infection, hypercalcaemia, or haemorrhage. Patients showing these signs may stabilize or improve, and the situation should be monitored at least every 24 hours, avoiding investigations that are unlikely to directly affect clinical care (➔ see Symptom management at the end of life, p. 570). All members of the MDT should be consulted, and in situations of uncertainty, advice should be sought from more experienced or specialist colleagues. The Gold Standards Framework provides prognostic indicator guidance (➔ see Websites, p. 153).

Communication at the end of life

The focus of communication at the end of life is on providing opportunities for, and demonstrating a willingness to talk about, issues related to death and dying. It is also an opportunity to clarify what the patient's key concerns are. For example, this may be concern about their family and what will happen after their death, or it may be concerns about physical symptoms and the actual process of dying, or it may be concerns around unfinished business related to relationships. It is important to ask for the person's views on any care or treatments during the dying phase that may take place after they are no longer able to make decisions themselves (➔ see Advance care planning, pp. 165–6). Anxiety and fear associated with the process of dying are common. Voicing these anxieties and fears and breaking them down into specific issues are helpful. Specific issues to consider are:

- Identifying where the person wishes to be cared for (preferred place of care)
- Involving the person in decision-making for as long as possible
- Assisting the dying person to put their affairs in order, involving other members of the team who have specific expertise
- Considering spiritual needs (➔ see Spiritual support and chaplaincy, pp. 135–6)
- Letting the dying person know that their family will be supported in bereavement and what support is available
- Answering any questions honestly and being prepared to repeat any explanations
- Providing privacy and the opportunity for families to be together and make the most of the final days or hours
- Clarifying needs during dying, at death, and after death.

Caring for families in end-of-life care

A common concern of families when a family member is dying is meeting their needs for comfort, in particular, in ensuring that everything possible has been done to manage pain and distressing symptoms. If there have been problems and unmet needs around the time of the death, this may make the subsequent bereavement more difficult. It is therefore important to try to meet the needs of both the person who is dying and their family.

Inevitably, there comes a time at the end of life when the focus of care shifts from the patient to the family's needs. As the dying person deteriorates, the family's and practitioner's role in advocating on behalf of the person becomes greater. Families will have their own needs for information and support and will need to be informed when death is close. Some family members will wish to be actively involved in the physical care of the dying person, whilst others may find this very difficult. Support should be given to the decisions made by family members, in an inclusive and non-judgemental way. Consideration should be given after death to the personal, cultural, and religious beliefs and preferences of both the patient and family. This may include how the body is handled and where it is stored.

Good practice in end-of-life care

People die in a variety of ways in different settings, with a wide variation in levels of professional support, expertise, training, and confidence, and it is difficult to establish standards that can be applied universally. Guidance on best practice in end-of-life care has been reviewed in England and Wales in the light of problems with care pathways. At the time of writing, NICE guideline NG31 *Care of Dying Adults in the Last Days of Life* gives guidance on care in the last few (2–3) days prior to death. Important principles of care at the end of life include:

- Effective communication and provision of information
- Ensuring that patients and their families are fully involved in all aspects of decision-making, taking into account their mental capacity
- Care should be individualized and based on their personal goals and wishes, preferred care setting, and current and anticipated care needs
- Hydration should be maintained, based on their preferences and wishes, an assessment of their hydration needs, and including clinically assisted hydration where this fits with their needs and wishes
- Pharmacological and non-pharmacological methods should be used, in accordance with their needs and wishes, balancing potential benefits and harms, to achieve effective symptom management and pain relief.

(➔ See also End-of-life care, pp. 151–3.)

Websites

Gold Standards Framework. Available at: ℘ http://www.goldstandardsframework.org.uk/ (the Gold Standards Framework provides training and service improvement programmes tailored to many specific settings).

Further reading

Broom A, Kirby E, Good P, Wootton J, Adams J. Specialists' experiences and perspectives on the timing of referral to palliative care: a qualitative study. *J Palliat Med* 2012;15:1248–53.

Leadership Alliance for the Care of Dying People. *One Chance to Get it Right: Improving People's Experience of Care in the Last Few Days and Hours of Life.* Gateway Reference 01509. London: Leadership Alliance for the Care of Dying People; 2014.

National Institute for Health and Care Excellence (2015). *Care of Dying Adults in the Last Days of Life.* NICE guideline [NG31]. Available at: ℘ https://www.nice.org.uk/guidance/ng31

Bereavement

Bereavement is the experience of loss, particularly of someone close, and grief is the associated emotional reaction. Mourning describes the behaviours associated with death, which are usually culturally determined and involve social events and rituals, including funeral practices. Bereavement and the grief response are features of the cancer experience at many different stages of the journey. There are numerous losses associated with treatment (e.g. altered body image), the effects of the illness (e.g. loss of energy and fatigue), and the overall effects on the patient's life (e.g. loss of function, social activity, occupation).

Within the context of palliative care, bereavement is frequently encountered in the families of patients in the period prior to and after death. Effective end-of-life care involves care after death, including the need to attend to the family's needs, to provide information on what to do after the death, and to identify services that can help where these are available.

Features of grief

Grief is commonly associated with the following features:

- Yearning and pining for the lost loved one
- Being preoccupied with the deceased, or feeling they are seeing them or hearing their voice (which can involve hallucinations)
- Feelings of shock, disbelief, numbness, and derealization (feelings of unreality)
- Feeling sad and tearful
- Feelings of anger or guilt
- Physical feelings of anxiety, emptiness, tiredness, breathlessness, and sighing
- Disturbed sleep and appetite
- Social withdrawal, restlessness.

These can be considered to be normal reactions to the death of a loved one. The nature and scale of these features vary from person to person, and the duration varies considerably. Acute grief can last for up to 6 months following the loss. The process of grieving can be complex. It involves both letting go and moving on, whilst also maintaining a continuing link with the loved one. It involves a reinterpretation of the relationship, and its implications for the life of the bereaved. It is also a period of adjustment to a new reality that has long-term consequences for the assumptions the person has about their world.

Anticipatory grief

If death is anticipated, this gives the family some time to prepare emotionally for the death. Some family members go through features of bereavement prior to the death, and this may help with the later bereavement process. Nurses can work with the family to prepare for the process of dying and support emotional adjustment. This involves communicating effectively about dying and helping the patient and family to make decisions about care. Advance care planning can be an important part of this process (➜ see Advance care planning, pp. 165–6).

Complicated grief

As grief is a normal reaction to the experience of loss, it should not be seen as a problem, unless the intensity, duration, or effects of the grief cause difficulties for the bereaved person. Complicated grief, which can also be called abnormal, extended, or prolonged grief, involves an extended period of grieving, beyond 6 months, with intense feelings and disruption of usual life and activities.

Features of complicated grief can include:
- Persistent and intense yearning or longing for the lost person
- Preoccupation with the person, with rumination or thoughts or images that intrude into daily life and interfere with usual activities
- Feelings of disbelief and problems accepting the death
- Problems with moving on with life, resuming activities, or starting new ones
- Excessive bitterness related to the death
- Not being able to trust others since the death, or feeling detached from them
- Feeling that life is now meaningless or unbearable
- Persistent agitation.

Complicated grief is associated with worse health outcomes, and people may try to cope by using alcohol and drugs. There is a high rate of depression in complicated grief, often with suicidal feelings (→ see Depression, pp. 581–2). It also has some features of traumatic stress disorder, including intrusive memories and avoidance of associations with the deceased (→ see Stress and trauma reactions, p. 578). Complicated grief is more common where the lost person was a child or if the death was traumatic.

Screening and assessment for complicated grief

The majority of bereaved people do not require specialist support, so screening and assessment are intended to identify those at risk or in need of specialist interventions. A public health model of bereavement needs predicts that 60% of bereaved people will cope with support from family and friends. They will also benefit from information about the grieving process. Thirty per cent will be at risk of a complicated grief reaction and will need additional support, e.g. a peer support group. The remaining 10% will experience a complicated grief reaction and should be given access to professional support.[2]

There is a range of tools that can be used to assess risk before or after bereavement (→ see Further reading, p. 157). These take account of factors like the nature of the relationship with the deceased, the circumstances of the death, the availability of social support, and the personal vulnerability or resilience of the bereaved person. Screening enables specialist bereavement resources to be targeted on those in greatest need.

References

2 Sealey M, Breen LJ, O'Connor M, Aoun SM. A scoping review of bereavement risk assessment measures: implications for palliative care. *Palliat Med* 2015;29:577–89.

Bereavement support

Most people find their personal resources, combined with support from family and friends, are sufficient to enable them to manage their distress and adjust to life following their loss. If they seek help, it is usually to check that the feelings they are experiencing are 'normal', and most people will not require further professional help. Support for the bereaved person requires a sensitive, facilitative approach, indicating the availability to listen and talk about the deceased and encouraging the expression of feelings.

It is important to let the bereaved person know that everyone grieves in their own way and in their own time. There are a number of local and national support groups for the bereaved, e.g. Cruse (➔ see Websites, p. 157), which can be accessed directly by individuals. Many hospices also offer commemorative services and events that provide support and put bereaved people in touch with others in a similar position.

NICE recommends a four-stepped approach to bereavement support, becoming more complex and specialist with each successive step (see Box 12.2).[3]
People with more complex needs, including complicated grief reactions, will benefit from referral for specialist interventions, delivered by trained counsellors or therapists. Specialist bereavement services are usually based in hospices, and they sometimes involve volunteers who have been trained to support the bereaved. In the absence of specialist bereavement support, or in more severe cases, the bereaved person may be referred for specialist psychological support, including, for example, CBT (➔ see Psychological support, pp. 130–1).

Children and bereavement

Children will have particular needs after the death of a loved one. This will depend on their age, any previous experience of losses, and the ongoing relationships within the family. As with adults, children will benefit from being given time and space to adjust to changes and may also need answers to questions that the bereavement raises for their understanding of the world

---

Box 12.2 A stepped approach to bereavement support

- Information about local support services
- Practical support such as advice on arranging a funeral and information on what to do with equipment and medication
- General emotional and bereavement support, including support from health and social care workers or from voluntary, community, and religious groups
- Referral for specialist support from trained bereavement counsellors or mental health workers

Reproduced from NICE (2011) *Quality statement 13: Care after death – bereavement support. End of life care for adults.* NICE quality standard [QS13]: ℳ https://www.nice.org.uk/guidance/qs13 All rights reserved. Subject to Notice of rights.

NICE guidance is prepared for the National Health Service in England. All NICE guidance is subject to regular review and may be updated or withdrawn. NICE accepts no responsibility for the use of its content in this product/publication.

(➲ see Websites, p. 157 for Child Bereavement UK and Winston's Wish). Where possible, when an adult is dying, it is helpful to include children in discussions, and helping them to prepare memory boxes may help in their bereavement. Organizations such as *Daisy's Dream* are available to work with families to help prepare children for loss. Where child-focused bereavement services are available, they may work with families or individual children or in a group format.

Websites

Bereavement UK. Available at: ℛ http://www.bereavement.co.uk

Child Bereavement UK. Available at: ℛ http://www.childbereavementuk.org

Cruse Bereavement Care. Available at: ℛ http://www.cruse.org.uk

Daisy's Dream. Available at: ℛ http://www.daisysdream.org.uk/

The Compassionate Friends. Available at: ℛ https://www.tcf.org.uk

Winston's Wish. The charity for bereaved children. Available at: ℛ http://www.winstonswish.org.uk

Further reading

Diamond H, Llewelyn S, Relf M, Bruce C. Helpful aspects of bereavement support for adults following an expected death: volunteers' and bereaved people's perspectives. *Death Stud* 2012; 36:541–64.

Relf M, Machin L, Archer N. *Guidance for Bereavement Needs Assessment in Palliative Care*. London: Help the Hospices; 2008.

University of Nottingham (2011). *Bereavement Care Services: A Synthesis of the Literature*. Department of Health and Social Care. Available at: ℛ https://www.gov.uk/government/publications/bereavement-care-services-a-synthesis-of-the-literature

References

3 National Institute for Health and Care Excellence (2011). *End of Life Care for Adults*. Quality standard [QS13]. Available at: ℛ https://www.nice.org.uk/guidance/qs13

Ethics in cancer care

Introduction and overview of ethical guidance

Ethical and moral values affect all aspects of cancer care, including treatment, management of symptoms, end-of-life care, and participation in research. With advancing medical technology and developing evidence-based practice, ethical issues in cancer care are increasingly complex.

Much of our understanding of ethics in the practice of cancer care is based on the 'four principles' of biomedical ethics[1] (see Box 13.1).

It can be difficult to apply these principles within the complexity of everyday practice. For example, conflict can arise between two or more of these principles. Does the benefit of a treatment (beneficence) outweigh the risks (non-maleficence)? Beneficence alone can lead to paternalistic attitudes, and it should be balanced with the principle of autonomy. So are judgements on the patient's best interests based on medical criteria alone or do they fully respect the patient's own view of their best interests? It is important therefore to take into account the personal preferences of patients, their own values, and their social context.

Other ethical approaches include **virtue ethics**, which emphasizes individual values, such as compassion, as a basis for ethical action, and **feminist ethics**, which rejects paternalism and prioritizes caring and relatedness. Challenges to Western biomedical ethics have led to a revision of some traditional ethical principles. For example, **relational autonomy** suggests that individual interests must be considered within a family and social context.

Box 13.1 Four principles of biomedical ethics

- Autonomy—self-determination, the capacity to think, decide, and act on the basis of such thought, freely and independently. A person has the right to have control over his/her life, including decisions about how it should end. It is therefore acknowledged that a person should be able to refuse lifesaving or life-prolonging treatment.
- Beneficence—to do good; the principle refers to the moral obligation to act for the benefit of others. In treatment decisions, for example, at the end of life, this principle revolves around what will be in a person's best interests and being able to balance the benefit and harm of continuing treatment. A person's perception of their QoL is essential in determining best interests.
- Non-maleficence—not to harm; the principle asserts an obligation to not intentionally inflict harm. The harmful effects of a treatment may outweigh the benefits, leading to a debate about the benefit or futility of treatment.
- Justice—to be fair and equitable and to provide appropriate treatment in light of what is due or owed to a person. The distribution of resources is central to the debate about justice in the context of cancer care.

Adapted from Beauchamp, T and Childress, J (2013) *Principles of Biomedical Ethics*, 7th Edition. New York: Oxford University Press with permission from Oxford University Press.

Nursing ethics may be considered as supplementary to biomedical ethics or as separate **ethics of caring**, sharing many features of feminist ethics. It emphasizes human values expressed through caring relationships, and practical approaches to dilemmas based on specific circumstances, rather than abstract principles. This promotes a person-centred and reciprocal approach, with active participation of patients and their families in decision-making and the process of care (➔ see Patient and family involvement in decision-making, pp. 120–1).

Ethical decision-making

Decision-making in practice requires a balance of different elements. These include not only ethical principles, but also legal and professional frameworks, alongside the patient's and family's wishes. This will involve consideration of issues of informed consent and competence. In the UK, the law now requires doctors to take reasonable care to ensure that the patient is aware of any material risks involved in any recommended treatment and of any reasonable alternative treatments.[2] Nurses acting in advanced practice roles should be aware that they would be expected to work to the same standards of practice expected of doctors.

Involving the patient and family is an important part of any process of ethical practice. This will involve:

- Teamwork that incorporates the patient, the family, and the professional
- Open communication and the development of a therapeutic relationship that promotes the expression of individual values and preferences
- Attention to the patient and family experience of illness and their feelings about this.

What to do in situations of conflict or uncertainty?

Initially, any ethical dilemmas should be discussed within the MDT, ensuring that senior members of the clinical and managerial staff, who carry responsibility, are actively involved. It is important to keep communications within the team open. Further advice may be sought from colleagues with particular expertise (e.g. in some areas, medical ethicists are available for consultation). If the situation is ongoing or represents a recurring ethical dilemma, it may be possible to consult the local clinical governance department or ethics committee.

Ethics of cancer treatments and research

In providing treatments for cancer, there is a moral obligation to provide the best treatment available, and not to deprive patients of a treatment that would benefit them. This can present difficult ethical issues when patients are involved in clinical research, particularly phase 1 trials. Clinical researchers, when testing new treatments through clinical trials, will be unsure of which arm of a trial (i.e. the control or experimental group) would have advantages over another. This balance of uncertainty is termed **clinical equipoise**.

It is commonly believed in medical practice that this uncertainty can only be resolved when a body of evidence has been gathered from several trials and medical opinion is in agreement. This means that a treatment given in clinical research may not be the best treatment for an individual patient.

Considering this, it is important to appreciate that the aims of treatment and the aims of research are different:

- **Clinical medicine** aims to give the best treatment for the individual patient, based on a balance of the ethical principles of beneficence (do good) and non-maleficence (do no harm), and the best available evidence.
- **Clinical research**, however, may not aim to treat patients individually; rather it seeks to develop scientific knowledge that can be used for the benefit of groups of patients in the future, and to generate evidence of effectiveness. Indeed, patients who volunteer to participate in clinical research run the risk of not being given the optimal treatment for their condition or of being harmed by it.

Failure on the part of the patient to understand the risks of clinical research and to see only its potential therapeutic effects is termed **therapeutic misconception**. The different aims of treatment and research can make it difficult to apply the same ethical principles to both. The ethical conduct of clinical trials requires that the research should be of high scientific quality and subject to independent review, that there should be a favourable risk–benefit ratio, and that participants should be selected fairly, with informed consent, and treated with respect.[3] Equally, all patients involved in research, whether it is clinical, service evaluation, or qualitative research, should be involved as fully as possible and seen as partners in the research process (➔ see Patient involvement in evaluating and managing health care, pp. 122–3).

Implications for nursing care

Participation in clinical trials can be a difficult decision for patients, when the outcome of the treatment is uncertain. It may be offered to patients when other treatments have failed and they may feel they have limited options. Patients under these circumstances are in a very vulnerable position. They need help to understand both the risks and potential benefits of experimental treatments for them, in addition to the potential benefits for others (➔ see Clinical trials in the cancer setting, pp. 268–9).

Funding cancer treatments

The rising cost of cancer treatment poses difficult ethical questions for health services. Increasingly, demand outstrips resources, particularly for cancer drugs, with their very high development costs. The rising demand for cancer treatments is based on three main factors:

- The ageing population
- Technological developments
- Rising patient expectations.

This demand has led to higher expenditure—governments in the developed world have been under increasing political and media pressure to spend more on cancer drug treatments. With rising demand and rising costs, does this mean that services have to be rationed, or is it possible to set priorities for expenditure and allocate resources fairly, according to demand?

It is clear that some implicit forms of rationing take place, through individual treatment decisions by doctors and through waiting lists. This has been described as the **Postcode Lottery**. However, rationing has become more explicit through the operation of systems to decide on the fair allocation of treatments. The UK government has established NICE, whereby part of its job is to decide on which treatments have been proven to be cost-effective, based on the cost per quality-adjusted life year (QALY). NICE currently has a ceiling of £30,000 per QALY, above which a drug would not be approved to be used within NHS resources, though this may be exceeded under some circumstances where life expectancy is short.

However, a drug may have proven effectiveness but cost more than £30,000 per QALY. This poses a challenge to the health service—how can it provide the optimum treatments for cancer, whilst ensuring fair and equitable access to expensive drugs? Is it fair for pharmaceutical companies to charge so much for lifesaving and life-extending treatments? Patients have increasingly sought information on treatment options through the Internet and used the law to gain access to drugs deemed too expensive to prescribe. Some people who have the ability to pay themselves can access these drugs, though at the risk of losing rights to treatment under the NHS.

A partial, temporary solution to the problem of fairness of access was found in the establishment of the Cancer Drugs Fund in England in 2011. This allows funding of cancer drugs that exceed the NICE threshold or are yet to be approved by NICE, if they are judged to be the best treatment available for an individual patient. This has extended cancer treatments to tens of thousands of patients. However, the overall cost of the NHS drugs budget is currently capped through an agreement between the Department of Health and the pharmaceutical industry. This means that larger cancer drugs expenditure is likely to raise the prices of other drugs, potentially reducing the options to treat other diseases. In this way, cancer patients may benefit unfairly from the political weight placed on cancer drug availability, to the detriment of other health conditions. The future of the Cancer Drugs Fund in England is uncertain, and there are differences in how decisions are made about cancer drug availability in the four countries of the UK. The ethical, political, and financial arguments for and against explicit rationing of cancer treatments will continue to be debated for a long time to come.

References

1 Beauchamp T, Childress J. *Principles of Biomedical Ethics*, 7th ed. New York, NY: Oxford University Press; 2013.
2 Sokol DK. Update on the UK law on consent. *BMJ* 2015;350:h1481.
3 Miller FG, Brody H (2003). A critique of clinical equipoise. Therapeutic misconception in the ethics of clinical trials. *Hastings Cent Rep* 2003;33:19–28.

End-of-life care issues

Ethical issues are prominent in end-of-life care. Patients and families face significant challenges about the meaning of life and death. There are difficult decisions to be made about how best to provide care at the end of life. This requires a sensitive, holistic, and comprehensive approach that involves the patient, family, and health professional.

Mental capacity

Mental capacity, also known as competence, refers to a person's ability to make decisions about their care and treatment, based on an ability to understand and retain information, to weigh up the information and make a decision about it, and to communicate their decision. A lack of capacity means that the person is not able to make a particular decision at the time the decision needs to be taken.

In England and Wales, the Mental Capacity Act 2005 defines the absence of capacity as an inability to make or communicate a decision due to impaired mental functioning. In Scotland, the Adults with Incapacity (Scotland) Act 2000 similarly defines mental incapacity due to impaired mental or physical functioning, though in Northern Ireland, definitions of capacity are based in case law.

Under the terms of the Mental Capacity Act 2005, the lack of capacity requires two conditions to be present: an impairment of mental functioning and an inability to make a decision at a particular point in time. If a person has been assessed as lacking capacity to make a specific decision about their care or treatment, a decision may be made on their behalf, based on their best interests, and the following where they are applicable:

- An advance decision about treatment and care options (➔ see Advance care planning, pp. 165–6).
- Power of attorney. In England and Wales, a mentally competent person may appoint someone to hold Lasting Power of Attorney—or in Scotland, Welfare Power of Attorney—to make decisions about their health and social care on their behalf, in the event that they no longer have capacity. This can include decisions about accepting or refusing care and treatment. Anyone acting in a legal capacity on behalf of another person is also known as their legal proxy.
- A decision made by professionals, in consultation with family members, and incorporating the patient's wishes where these are known.

The Mental Capacity Act 2005 is based on five statutory principles:
- **Presumption of capacity**. All adults aged over 16 years are presumed to be capable of making their own decisions. unless it can be proven otherwise.
- **Support for the individual**. All practical steps should be taken to support an individual to make their own decisions.
- **Unwise decision**. Making an unwise decision does not prove a lack of capacity.
- **Best interests**. Any decision made on behalf of someone who lacks capacity must be made in their best interests.
- **Least restriction**. Any decision made on behalf of someone who lacks capacity must be based on the option that is less restrictive of their rights and freedom of action.

Advance care planning

Advance care planning is the formal process of making decisions in advance about future care by mentally competent individuals, in the event that they lose capacity. It is a way of ensuring that their wishes are respected and followed when they are no longer able to express them. It is most commonly used where the person with cancer is approaching the end of life, though it can be done at any stage of the cancer journey. It is a voluntary process, which involves discussion of future options if their condition deteriorates. It can include decisions about care and treatment choices, and whether to accept or refuse a treatment in specific circumstances. It may take the form of:

- **Advance statements**. These are statements about issues that are important to the individual and that they wish to be considered as a basis for any subsequent decisions about their best interests. This may include, for example, personal goals and values relating to care and discussion of care and treatments choices or the preferred place of care
- **Advance decisions to refuse treatment**. An advance decision will be legally binding in England and Wales, and potentially legally binding in Scotland and Northern Ireland, if the person making the decision is over 18 and has mental capacity, and it is valid and applicable to the circumstances. It can be given verbally, but it must be in writing if it includes the refusal of life-sustaining treatment. Patients cannot refuse basic care in advance, e.g. oral nutrition and hydration, repositioning in bed, but may refuse an active intervention like cardiopulmonary resuscitation (CPR) (➔ see Cardiopulmonary resuscitation, p. 167)
- **Appointment of Lasting Power of Attorney** (➔ see Mental capacity, p. 164). This must be recorded in the prescribed form and registered with the Office of the Public Guardian.

Patients may wish to have informal discussions about their preferences and about who would be best to represent their interests if they lose capacity. However, advance statements and advance decisions to refuse treatment are more formal and should be written down and kept in a place that is accessible to those who would need to use it, e.g. at the person's home and in their medical notes. Many services have local policies about the keeping of advance care plans. They should include full details of the person making it, clear statements about the purpose of the document, the circumstances under which it should be used, and the nature of care or treatments to be preferred, accepted, or refused, and it should be signed, witnessed, and dated. There are templates (see, for example, *Say it Once*—available at: ℘ http://www.sayitonce.info), and in some places, electronic options will be available.

It is important that **advance care planning** is seen as part of an **overall process of care planning** that deals with those aspects of care and treatment that may be needed if the individual loses capacity, in addition to those that concern them now. Initiating a discussion about advance care planning should, as far as possible, emerge out of routine discussions, ideally initiated by the patient. All advance care planning discussions should be documented and regularly reviewed, and key staff should be involved and informed about them. All staff involved should understand the professional and legal context, have a good knowledge of the patient and their circumstances, and be able to communicate effectively and sensitively (➔ see Communication in cancer care, pp. 107–9).

Reflection point

Consider what you might write in an advance care plan for your own end-of-life care. What would your personal priorities be?

Withdrawing and withholding treatment

Towards the end of life, treatment and care decisions can become particularly complex, challenging, and distressing. Professional, ethical, and legal considerations will need to be balanced with the wishes of the patient and family in deciding the best forms of care. The ethical principles underlying the withdrawal or withholding of treatment are no different from other aspects of care and include issues of consent and capacity. However, these decisions can be the most difficult, involving consideration of potential benefits or risks to the patient, and distress to the patient and their family. There is an established principle that life should be prolonged where this is consistent with the wishes and values of the patient and family, and unless it would lead to additional distress or risks for the patient.

In deciding on the best care and treatment options for the patient, the professionals involved should consider the following in deciding what the best overall benefit to the patient is:

• Whether the patient has mental capacity
• The expressed wishes of the patient where they have capacity
• Advance statements or decisions if they do not have capacity, or the views of the person with powers of attorney or other legal proxy whom they have appointed to make decisions on their behalf
• The wishes of family members, particularly where the patient lacks capacity and no legal proxy has been appointed
• Assessment of the patient's condition, including their experience of pain and other symptoms, their psychological state, and social and spiritual concerns
• Their own professional knowledge, skills, and experience, and the best available evidence and clinical guidelines for managing the specific condition of the patient
• The advice of any other colleagues or experts who are involved in, or can contribute to, their care and treatment.

The potential care and treatment options should be explained and discussed, and the preferences of the patient, family, and any legal proxy taken into account. The professionals should be guided by these but might judge that their wishes are not in the best interests of the patient. In conditions of uncertainty or disagreement, the nature of the dilemma should be discussed fully with the patient, their family, or legal proxy, and advice may be sought from a third party or other expert.

Decisions about the withdrawal or withholding of treatment are very sensitive and can be very emotional for all concerned. It is very important therefore to communicate fully, honestly, and openly about the nature and effects of these decisions, providing any information that is needed for the patient and family to be informed and involved.

Artificial hydration and nutrition

Hydration and nutrition are basic human needs and form part of basic care. Effective care and treatment can only be provided if the patient is adequately hydrated and fed, and these needs should form part of ongoing assessment. In the event of the patient becoming unable to take food and drink independently, or with assistance, then it may be necessary to provide this artificially. Artificial, or clinically assisted, nutrition and hydration can be provided via the following routes:

- Intravenous (IV) or subcutaneous (SC)
- Nasogastric (NG) tube
- Percutaneous endoscopic gastrostomy (PEG)
- Radiologically inserted gastrostomy (RIG).

From a legal point of view, these are treatments, rather than basic care. Any decisions to initiate them should involve thorough consultation with the patient and, where necessary, the family and legal proxy. Although artificial hydration and nutrition can prolong life, they may also place additional burdens on the patient (including, for example, fluid retention), so their initiation or continuation requires careful consideration. When the patient is close to the end of life (i.e. hours or days), it may be felt to be in the patient's best interests not to initiate them, or to withdraw them, if the benefits are likely to be outweighed by the burdens or risks. The wishes of the patient, where known, e.g. through an advance decision or the family or proxy, must be taken into account.

For family members, the provision of food and drink is a very basic expression of caring and sustaining individual and family life. The withdrawal of nutrition and hydration can be a very emotional event for the family, signifying the closeness of death, and it may even feel like the patient is being abandoned. For these reasons, clear explanation and discussion, along with emotional support, are an essential part of care. Members of staff can also find it difficult, and effective team communication is also very important.

Reflection points

- Have you been involved in the withdrawal of treatment from a patient at the end of life?
- How did the family feel about this and how did you feel?

Cardiopulmonary resuscitation

CPR is an emergency intervention when someone has a cardiac or respiratory arrest, aimed at restarting their heart or breathing and restoring circulation. It can involve compressing the chest, injecting drugs, defibrillation, and artificial ventilation. Under favourable circumstances, CPR can be very effective. However, it is less likely to be successful where the patient's condition is already poor due to serious illness. Even if successful, it carries numerous risks, including damage to chest and internal organs, organ failure, and consequent disability. In the event of an unsuccessful attempt at CPR, then the patient's death may be traumatic and undignified.

Because of these risks, and the possibility that CPR may lead to a worse quality of life for the patient, careful consideration should be given to initiating CPR in the seriously ill. An advance decision not to initiate CPR in cardiac or respiratory arrest is known as a Do Not Attempt CPR (DNACPR) or a Do Not Attempt Resuscitation (DNAR) order. Allow Natural Death (AND) provides a more positive alternative. In a person with advanced cancer, this can be incorporated into advance care planning.

A DNACPR order may be considered in the following circumstances:

• If, because of the patient's condition, there is no prospect of a successful resuscitation
• If the patient's QoL is already very limited and likely to be further worsened by CPR
• If their condition is so poor that there is little prospect of being able to consult them in the event of an arrest
• Where the patient is in the last few days of life and cardiac or respiratory arrest may be anticipated as part of the process of dying.

Under these circumstances, or at any point when advance care planning is taking place, the option of a DNACPR order may be raised with the patient and family. Sometimes they will raise it themselves, though others may choose not to discuss it. A decision not to attempt CPR does not require the consent of the patient or family, but every effort should be made to inform them about the decision. An advance decision by the patient to refuse CPR must be respected.

If the decision has been made, for sound clinical reasons, not to attempt CPR, the patient or their family or proxy may not necessarily agree. They may feel that every effort should be made to prolong life. Under these circumstances, it is essential to have a full and detailed discussion about the options and anticipated outcomes of CPR. If there is an ongoing lack of agreement, then a second opinion should be sought. Doctors are not under a legal obligation to give treatment against their clinical judgement, but they should consider the possibility of giving CPR, even with a limited chance of success, if it is the patient's wish.

Decisions about CPR should always be based on a careful assessment of the individual patient and the situation, and be reviewed if circumstances change. DNACPR decision should always be documented, and there are some formats that patients may use to record their own decisions.

Euthanasia and physician-assisted suicide (assisted dying)

Euthanasia is the act of taking another's life at their request, and physician-assisted suicide is where a doctor gives the means to someone to take their own life at the latter's request. These are usually considered to be a last resort where the person has a terminal illness which causes them unbearable suffering. Both euthanasia and physician-assisted suicide are illegal in most countries of the world, including the UK where it is illegal to encourage or assist suicide. Euthanasia is legal in the Netherlands, Belgium, and Colombia. Assisted suicide is legal in Switzerland, Germany, Japan, Albania, and in some states of the USA. In each case, there are legal constraints to its practice. In the Netherlands, for example, the following conditions must be present for the act of assisted dying to be legal:[4]

• The physician must be convinced that the request from the patient is voluntary and well considered.

- The patient's suffering is lasting and unbearable.
- The physician must inform the patient about their situation and prospects.
- The physician agrees with the patient that there is no other reasonable alternative.
- The physician consults with at least one other independent physician.
- The termination of life is carried out with due care.

Euthanasia and physician-assisted suicide are different from active symptom management which has the side effect of shortening life, and from the practice of deep continuous sedation or palliative sedation, which aims to reduce suffering but not shorten life. Data from the Netherlands, where euthanasia and physician-assisted suicide have been legal since 2002, suggest that the majority of deaths are directly affected in some way by medical decisions, including:[5]

- 36% of deaths involving alleviation of symptoms with a possible life-shortening effect
- 18% of deaths with abstention from potentially life-prolonging treatment
- 0.6% of patients terminate their own lives supported by proxies—either by stopping nutrition (0.4%) or by taking medication (0.2%)
- 0.2% of terminations of life without an explicit request from the patient
- 2.8% of euthanasia
- 0.1% of physician-assisted dying.

As can be seen from these data, both euthanasia and physician-assisted dying are rare events, even where they are legally sanctioned. It is important to note that assisted dying also takes place in countries where the law does not permit it.[5] However, both in countries where it is legal and in those where it is illegal, it continues to be very controversial and hotly debated. There are fundamental and conflicting principles behind the debate: the sanctity of life and the wrongness of killing, the need to act in the patient's best interest (beneficence), and the right to personal autonomy and freedom of choice. Underlying questions include: what is unbearable suffering, what is a good death, and should anyone other than the patient decide? Could euthanasia be used to avoid the high costs of medical care? Is legalization a slippery slope that could lead to the loss of rights of people with chronic illness and disabilities?

Aside from the ethical questions about assisted dying, there is the fundamental problem that people suffer as a result of illness and the process of dying, and how we should help them. Palliative care has developed specifically in response to this problem, so there is a strong argument that assisted dying should not be necessary where palliative care services are well developed and readily accessible. Patients may, for example, be concerned about being a burden on their families in their last days and so aim to avoid this by speeding their end. They may fear a loss of control over their lives and their bodies, or a descent into pain and indignity as they approach death. With adequate support for the patient and family, and adequate symptom control, these can be avoided.

What to do if a patient requests assistance to die

Any nurse working with a patient who faces the prospect of dying should be willing to listen to their concerns and aim to support them through their own process of deciding what their priorities are for their future. This is the basis for discussions leading to advance care planning. It is common for people with cancer to consider the possibility that they might not want to go on living if they felt that their life were to become unbearable. Most people need help to think about the process of dying and need information about the services and support that will be available to them. Common concerns when facing death include:

• Will I be in pain and will painkilling drugs speed up my death?
• Will I be able to maintain my sense of identity and dignity in the face of death?
• Will I still be able to make decisions about my care?
• Will I be a burden on my family?
• What will happen to me when I am dying?

In response to any approach from a patient about the possibility of assisted dying, you should:

• Take the patient and their concerns seriously and aim to identify their greatest anxieties
• Be prepared to talk about the process of dying and provide information about end-of-life services
• Suspend your own beliefs and values about assisted dying, and not judge them
• Raise the issue of advance care planning to give the patient a sense of control
• Acknowledge the limits of your knowledge and confidence, where necessary, and involve others who have overall responsibility and more experience
• Be clear about the legal position, if asked directly about assisted dying.

It is important to assess the mental state of the patient, including whether they have mental capacity and if they are suffering from depression, which would contribute to a sense of hopelessness (➋ see Depression, pp. 581–2). If you have concerns that a patient has active suicidal ideas, you should involve senior colleagues and, where necessary, the patient's GP (➋ see Suicide and suicidal ideas, p. 583). Discussions of dying and assisted suicide can be very stressful and emotive, so it is important to take time to think about the situation, reflect on the experience, and discuss it with colleagues.

Reflection point
• Can you recall any situations you have encountered in your practice that raised ethical questions for you about assisted suicide?
• How did you deal with them at the time, and is there anything you would do differently now, having had time to reflect on them?

Further reading

British Medical Association, Resuscitation Council (UK), Royal College of Nursing (2014). *Decisions Relating to Cardiopulmonary Resuscitation*, 3rd ed. Available at: ➶ https://www.resus.org.uk/dnacpr/decisions-relating-to-cpr/

General Medical Council (2010). *Treatment and Care Towards the End of Life: Good Practice in Decision Making*. Available at: ➶ http://www.gmc-uk.org/guidance

Ho A. Relational autonomy or undue pressure? Family's role in medical decision-making. *Scand J Caring Sci* 2008;22:128–35.

Hudson P, Hudson R, Philip J, Boughey M, Kelly B, Hertogh C. Legalizing physician-assisted suicide and/or euthanasia: pragmatic implications. *Palliat Support Care* 2015;13:1507.

Jack A. Which way now for the Cancer Drugs Fund? *BMJ* 2014;349:g5524.

Mental Capacity Act 2005. Available at: ℘ https://www.gov.uk/government/collections/mental-capacity-act-making-decisions

Moulton B, King JS. Aligning ethics with medical decision-making: the quest for informed patient choice. *J Law Med Ethics* 2010;38:85–97.

Mullick A, Martin J, Sallnow L. An introduction to advance care planning in practice. *BMJ* 2013;347:f6064.

NHS National End of Life Care Programme (2011). *Capacity, Care Planning and Advance Care Planning in Life Limiting Illness. A Guide for Health and Social Care Staff.* Available at: ℘ https://www.ncpc.org.uk/sites/default/files/ACP_Booklet_June_2011.pdf

Royal College of Nursing. *When Someone Asks for Your Assistance to Die. RCN Guidance on Responding to a Request to Hasten Death.* London: Royal College of Nursing; 2011.

References

4 Beauchamp T, Childress J. *Principles of Biomedical Ethics*, 7th ed. New York, NY: Oxford University Press; 2013.

5 Sokol DK. Update on the UK law on consent. *BMJ* 2015;350:h1481.

Clinical Management of Cancer

Chapter 14

Diagnosis and staging

Diagnosis, classification, and staging of cancer

Early diagnosis still offers the best opportunity for cure or extended survival for many types of cancer. Therefore, fast and accurate diagnosis is essential to ensure the most effective and appropriate approach to managing cancer. Over the last decade, in the UK, there has been emphasis on promoting the early diagnosis of cancer via various cancer access targets, with patients seen within 2 weeks of referral and commencing treatment within 62 days if cancer is identified.

Cancer classification

Classifying cancers into specific histology (grade) and extent of spread (stage) allows for prognostic information and planning of appropriate treatment, as well as comparison of treatment results, e.g. survival, cure, and QoL, within countries and worldwide. For specific types of tumour, biological factors might also be used to classify tumours (e.g. tumour receptor status in breast cancer) (➲ see Cancer biology, p. 32 for classification of the main tissue types).

Cancer diagnosis

The chosen approach depends on the presenting signs and symptoms, clinical performance status (see Table 14.1), the anticipated goal of treatment, the availability of equipment, and the patient's and their family's own expectations and wishes. It is essential to consider how an individual will cope with going through a whole host of invasive tests and also whether or not it would be worthwhile.

There are no single tests specific and sensitive enough to determine the exact diagnosis of an individual cancer. Therefore, a range of tests, both invasive and non-invasive, need to be carried out before an individual patient can have an accurate diagnosis.

Advances in diagnosis

Improved computed tomography (CT) and MRI scanning, the introduction of positron emission tomography (PET) scans, and use of US-guided biopsies have all led to more accurate diagnosis and staging of many cancers. This has led to more effective targeting of treatments, e.g. reducing futile surgery in both lung and rectal cancer. More accurate diagnosis of cancer at a cellular and genetic level has improved staging and treatment planning. For example, the expression of specific gene products is now used to predict responses to treatment, and in the future, it is likely that biological markers will elucidate whether a drug is working on the target. As time progresses, it is very likely that the diagnostic phase will involve a detailed genetic screen, with new cancer treatments increasingly targeted at specific genes. This approach has become known as 'personalized medicine', although some elements of a more personalized approach to diagnosis have been in place for some years (e.g. HER-2 status in breast cancer).

Areas that need to be explored during the diagnostic process are covered on the following pages under the following headings:
- Patient history
- Presenting signs and symptoms
- Laboratory studies
- Surgical/specialist viewing
- Radiological imaging.
- Staging and grading.

Diagnosis: multidisciplinary evaluation

Many members of the health-care team will be involved. Diagnosis can be a point for potential delays, which can impact on overall survival and cause high levels of anxiety. Effective coordination of the MDT is essential to ensure an efficient and well-supported patient journey through this difficult time. Patient pathways have been designed for many cancers to reduce diagnostic and treatment delay.

Nurses are heavily involved in this process. Nurses will support the patient with information and symptom management. Specialist nurses may coordinate the MDT and evaluate the patient pathway. Some nurse specialists may also be involved in performing diagnostic tests, such as digital rectal examination and cystoscopy, or in telling patients their diagnosis (➜ see Role of the cancer nurse in giving significant news, p. 115). Increasingly, nurses are involved in the diagnostic pathway, with many specialist nurses now undertaking courses in medical assessment.

Table 14.1 Clinical performance status

Performance status (PS) is an attempt to quantify cancer patients' general well-being. This measure is often used to determine whether they can receive chemotherapy whether dose adjustment is necessary and as a measure for the required intensity of palliative care. Clinical trials often include performance status as one of the criteria patients must meet for joining.

The main scales are the WHO/Eastern Cooperative Oncology Group (ECOG) scales summarized below. Other scores such as the Karnofsky score after Dr David Karnofsky are also in use. This runs from 100% 'perfect' health to 0% death in intervals of 10%.

Grade	WHO/ECOG performance status scores
0	Fully active, able to carry on all pre-disease performance without restriction
1	Restricted in physically strenuous activity, but ambulatory and able to carry out work of a light or sedentary nature, e.g. light housework, office work
2	Ambulatory and capable of all self-care, but unable to carry out any work activities. Up and about for >50% of waking hours
3	Capable of only limited self-care, confined to bed or chair for >50% of waking hours
4	Completely disabled. Cannot carry out any self-care. Totally confined to bed or chair
5	Dead

Further reading

Tobias J, Hochauser D. Staging of tumours. In: Tobias J, Hochauser D (eds). *Cancer and Its Management*, 7th ed. Oxford: Blackwell; 2015. p. 44.

Vogel WH. Diagnostic evaluation, classification and staging. In: Yarbro CH, Wujcik D, Gobel BHM (eds). *Cancer Nursing: Principles and Practice*, 7th ed. Massachusetts: Jones and Bartlett; 2010. pp. 166–99.

Patient assessment

Patient history

Past medical history, family history, risk factors, and physical examination are all an essential part of diagnosis. A thorough history needs to be taken, including the duration and speed of onset or any progression, and general and specific symptoms. Cancer can take years to progress, so signs/symptoms may have been there for many years.

The patient's own expectations, beliefs, physical, social, spiritual, and emotional needs all need to be assessed and discussed, alongside any risk factors associated with lifestyle. This may take time and should be a part of an ongoing assessment process (➲ see Introduction to assessment, pp. 462–3).

Presenting signs and symptoms

Screening has increased the number of non-palpable cancers identified at diagnosis. However, more typically, other signs and symptoms of disease take the individual into the health-care system. For common presenting symptoms, see Box 14.1.

Knowledge of the common presenting signs/symptoms of each cancer gives health-care professionals a benchmark against which to screen patients. In the UK, the Department of Health has produced referral guidelines for all cancers. These highlight patient signs and symptoms that should be referred urgently to cancer specialists.[1]

Laboratory studies

These include tests such as full blood count (FBC), liver and renal function tests, blood chemistry, urinalysis, faecal occult bloods, and specific tumour markers (➲ see Tumour markers, p. 179).

Tumour markers

These are hormones, enzymes, or antigens produced by tumours or by tissue stimulated by tumours. They vary in sensitivity and specificity. Many tumour markers are highly sensitive, i.e. they are generally identifiable if the tumour is there. However, they are often not very specific, i.e. they are often present when the disease is absent, but other non-malignant causes account for the marker's presence. This reduces their use as a diagnostic test. However, some can be useful in assessing response to treatment (see Table 14.2).

Box 14.1 Common presenting symptoms

- Weight loss
- Persistent pain
- Unexplained fever
- Unusual bleeding or discharge
- A sore which does not heal
- Change in bladder and bowel habits

- Fatigue
- Painless lump
- Obvious change in wart or mole
- Persistent cough/hoarseness
- Indigestion/difficulty in swallowing

Table 14.2 Some commonly used tumour markers

Marker	Indications	Uses
Carcinoembryonic antigen (CEA)	Breast, colorectal, lung	Monitoring patients with known disease
Prostate-specific antigen (PSA)	Prostate cancer, benign prostate enlargement	Initial screening, response to treatment, recurrence
Human chorionic gonadotrophin (HCG)	Germ cell tumours (testicular, some ovarian), pregnancy	Diagnosis, prognostic indicators
Alpha-fetoprotein (AFP)	Germ cell tumours, liver, cancer, pregnancy	Diagnosis, monitoring, response to treatment
CA-125	Ovarian, colorectal, gastric cancers	Monitoring response to treatment
CA19-9	Oesophageal, pancreatic, colorectal	Diagnosis, monitoring response to treatment

Table 14.3 Common diagnostic tests and indications

Diagnostic test	Common indications
Core or fine-needle aspirate	Breast or thyroid cancer
Excision biopsies	May be used for malignant melanoma, other skin cancers, and some breast cancers
Endoscopy (± biopsy)	Lung, gastrointestinal (GI), genitourinary (GU) cancers
Laparoscopy	Lymphoma, GI, urological, gynaecological cancers
Liver biopsy	Liver metastases of uncertain origin, primary hepatic tumours
Bone marrow aspirate	Haematological cancers or suspected spread to bone marrow
Colposcopy	Cervical and vaginal cancers

Surgical evaluation

This is where the cancer is looked at macroscopically and a biopsy may also be taken. Obtaining an accurate tissue sample is essential in establishing a cancer diagnosis. Different cancers in the same organ may require very different treatment approaches, e.g. small cell and non-small cell lung cancer.

Other tests that are also carried out include paracentesis or lumbar puncture (see Table 14.3).

References

1 National Institute for Health and Care Excellence (2015). *Suspected Cancer: Recognition and Referral*. NICE guideline [NG12]. Available at: ℘ https://www.nice.org.uk/guidance/ng12

Radiological imaging

Imaging aims to demonstrate the anatomy of a particular area of the body and detect any abnormalities. It is used within oncology to provide a detailed understanding of primary tumours, their likely routes of spread, and their response to treatment.

Main imaging modalities

(See Table 14.4.)
- Plain X-rays
- Fluoroscopy
- CT
- MRI
- Nuclear medicine (NM) and US
- PET.

These modalities can be used either alone or in combination to produce an image that can be interpreted.

The dose of radiation received from radiological imaging should be kept to a minimum (➔ see Radiation protection, p. 196). US and MRI are the preferred imaging modalities, where possible, as neither uses ionizing radiation.

It is important to select the correct imaging tool for the examination required, based on the efficiency of detecting lesions and the least risk and discomfort to the patient. Cost will also be a factor.
- MRI and CT are particularly effective at imaging soft tissue abnormalities and for imaging bony structures.
- A combination of imaging tools can sometimes give the health-care professional a clearer understanding of any abnormalities present. In some cases, it is now possible to fuse different types of images together.

Diagnosing different cancer sites

Several different modalities may be used to assist in accurately diagnosing and staging a specific cancer. The actual diagnostic and imaging modalities used for individual cancers are listed within each cancer site section.

Contrast media

Contrast media are substances that are used in conjunction with some imaging modalities, to help visualize anatomical structures. For example, when imaging the urinary system, the introduction of a contrast agent enables the radiographer to visualize the kidneys more easily and can track the flow of urine through the system. An allergic reaction can occur when a contrast medium is used. Emergency drug therapy must therefore be readily available to treat reactions (➔ see Anaphylaxis, pp. 633–4).

In an ideal situation, a patient would be transferred to the imaging department for their investigation; however, it is possible for some imaging to be carried out on the ward. Mobile X-ray units and portable US equipment can be used at the bedside.

Note: it is important that appropriate radiation protection procedures are followed when mobile X-ray units are used (➔ see Radiation protection, p. 196).

Table 14.4 Types of imaging and specific indications

Imaging modality	Clinical indication
Plain X-ray Use of X-rays to produce an image on film or digitally	Chest, e.g. lung lesions/pleural effusions/infection Abdomen, e.g. blockages Skeletal system, e.g. bony abnormalities such as metastatic disease
Fluoroscopy Continuous use of low-dose X-rays to produce a dynamic image	GI tract abnormalities. Often contrast media, such as barium, are used to outline the GI tract Arteriography Has been superseded by CT-guided biopsy/US-guided biopsy
CT scan Use of X-rays to produce transverse sections of the head and body. The X-ray tube rotates around the patient	Any region of the body can be scanned. Can be used for diagnosis, staging, and radiotherapy planning
MRI scan Images produced by applying a pulse of strong magnetic energy to tissue. The energy released is processed into high-quality images	CNS, musculoskeletal, cardiac, breast, abdomen, and pelvis Not useful for lung imaging. Some patients unable to have MRI, as the magnetic field may displace any metallic implants or foreign bodies
Nuclear medicine Use of radioisotopes injected or inhaled into the body, imaged using a gamma camera. Typically shows abnormal physiology of the body, rather than anatomical detail, e.g. bone scan	Skeletal: bone metastases Thyroid: focal nodules Respiratory: pulmonary embolus
PET scans PET and its fusions with other imaging modalities helps health-care professionals to see not only the blood flow and metabolism of the tumour, but also the anatomical location in the fused image	It offers improved accuracy in staging several cancers, including non-small cell lung, upper GI, lymphomas, and recurrent bowel cancers. It has reduced the futile thoracotomy rate in non-small cell lung from about 40% to about 20%
US High-frequency sound waves are used. Different tissues transmit different sound waves that are converted into an electrical current and subsequent image. Bone and air are poor conductors of sound. Fluid is a good conductor	Abdomen: liver, gall bladder, pancreas, kidneys, testes Breast and ovary: distinguish between solid and cystic mass Thorax: confirms pleural effusions and plural masses

Staging and grading cancer

Grading

This is a method of classifying tumour cells, based on cellular differentiation or resemblance to their normal cell of origin, in terms of behaviour, structure, and maturity (see Table 14.5).

Grading can be very important, indicating the potential for spread or the likely rate of growth of a particular tumour.

- High-grade tumours tend to be fast-growing and more 'aggressive' and are more likely to spread quickly.
- Low-grade tumours tend to be slower-growing and less likely to spread quickly.

Examples of grading systems include the Gleason system used to grade prostate cancer and the Fuhrman system used for kidney cancer.

Staging

Staging is a classification system based on the anatomical spread of a cancer. The most commonly used system is tumour node metastasis (TNM). This was set up by the Union for International Cancer Control (UICC) nearly 50 years ago and has been regularly updated. Stage classifications have been determined for most cancer sites by the American Joint Committee of Cancer.[2] TNM assesses:

- T: size of the primary tumour
- N: absence or presence of regional lymph nodes
- M: absence or presence of distant metastases.

Information from each part are combined together to determine the stage of the cancer. Most cancers are then staged from stage I to IV, though there may be further subdivisions, e.g. into stage IIIa and IIIb. The stage should be given at diagnosis, if possible, but often changes after surgery as a more accurate picture of the extent of disease emerges (see Table 14.6).

Limitations

There are limitations with the TNM system. It is not always sensitive enough to accurately determine prognosis or treatment. It is also not useful in several cancers. For example, it cannot be used for haematological cancers. Leukaemias are classified according to cell type and differentiation. Acute leukaemias are further subdivided by the French–American–British (FAB) classification. Hodgkin's and non-Hodgkin lymphomas are classified by cell type and then through a system based on the areas or region of lymph node involvement plus the presence or absence of 'b' symptoms.[3]

Other staging systems sometime run alongside TNM, e.g. Duke's (colorectal cancer) and Clark's (malignant melanoma). In CNS tumours, the system is based on the biological behaviour of the tumour (grade), size, and location. A higher grade is more malignant. N is not used, as the brain is not supplied with lymphatic drainage.

Other prognostic factors

As cancer biology and genetics become more fully understood, the range of prognostic factors becomes more complex. Oestrogen and progesterone

Table 14.5 Cancer grading

Grade	Differentiation	Appearance
Grade 1 (low grade)	Well differentiated	Mature cells—resembling normal tissue
Grade 2	Moderately differentiated	Cells with some level of immaturity
Grade 3	Poorly differentiated	Little resemblance to normal tissue
Grade 4 (high grade)	Undifferentiated	No resemblance to normal tissue

Table 14.6 General TNM definitions

	Stage designation	Definition
T	Primary tumour	Size or depth of primary tumour
	Tx	Cannot be assessed
	T0	No evidence of primary tumour
	Tis	Carcinoma *in situ*
	T1–T4	Increasing size or depth of primary tumour
N	Regional lymph node spread	Extent and location of lymph node involvement
	Nx	Cannot be assessed
	N0	No regional lymph node involvement
	N1–N3	Increasing number and size of involved regional lymph nodes
M	Metastasis	Absence or presence of distant metastases
	Mx	Cannot be assessed
	M0	No distant spread
	M1	Distant metastatic disease present

receptors, Her-2/Neu, and vascular endothelial growth factor (VEGF) are examples of cell surface receptors that are important prognostic factors and which also now offer specific targeted therapy options.

Further reading

National Institute for Health and Care Excellence (2015). *Suspected Cancer: Recognition and Referral.* NICE guideline [NG12]. Available at: ℘ https://www.nice.org.uk/guidance/ng12

References

2 Amin M, Edge S, Greene F, *et al.* (eds). *The AJCC Cancer Staging Manual*, 8th ed. New York, NY: Springer International Publishing; 2017.

3 Hoffbrand A, Moss P. *Essential Haematology*, 6th ed. Oxford: Blackwell Science; 2011.

Surgery and cancer

Cancer surgery

Despite developments in radiotherapy, chemotherapy, and other drug therapies in the last two decades, surgery remains a major treatment modality. A treatment plan containing a surgical approach offers the best hope of a cure for many patients with many different types of tumour.

Surgery can still be used as a single treatment, e.g. removing a very small breast cancer lump or colonic polyps. However, it is now more usually combined with other treatments such as radiotherapy or chemotherapy (see Box 15.1).

Surgery is used in a number of different ways in managing cancer:
- Diagnosis, e.g. tissue biopsy of a primary tumour
- Staging, e.g. lymph node sampling
- Tumour excision: primary cancer or metastatic disease with intention to cure, e.g. colorectal cancer with single liver metastases
- Palliative surgery
- Supportive procedure, e.g. central venous catheters (CVCs), PEG tubes
- Reconstructive surgery (➔ see Reconstructive surgery, p. 190)
- Stoma formation (see ➔ Care of the patient with a stoma, p. 328).

Principles

Effective surgical removal of a tumour relies on a key number of principles.

Accurate staging

If the tumour has metastasized from the original site, has become too large to be removed, or involves, or is adjacent to, vital structures, then surgery alone may not be successful. Accurate staging prior to surgical intervention can also prevent futile surgery on widespread disease. In some diseases where there are single or small numbers of metastases, these can also be removed surgically, with some survival benefit, e.g. removal of liver metastases in colorectal cancers.

Good excision margins

If a tumour can be removed completely, with a buffer of unaffected tissue around the excised tumour, then surgery is likely to be more successful.

Box 15.1 Multiple treatment modalities

Breast cancer is a good example of the multimodality treatment of cancer. A woman with breast cancer may typically have the following treatment pathway:
1. Surgical removal of the primary disease and sampling of lymph nodes.
2. Radiotherapy to the affected breast, to reduce the risk of local relapse.
3. Adjuvant combined chemotherapy treatment to reduce distant metastatic recurrence (some women with a large tumour or small breast may have chemotherapy prior to surgery—neo-adjuvant).
4. Endocrine therapy (if oestrogen or progesterone receptor positive) to reduce recurrence.

A clear margin will generally be more successful in reducing relapse; however, this may increase the surgical morbidity for the patient, i.e. more extensive and potentially damaging surgery. Assessment of surgical margins will vary on a case-to-case basis and often forms part of the discussion at MDT meetings.

Comorbidities

If the patient is fit and well and able to tolerate surgery, then a surgical plan is more likely to be successful.

Quality of life (cost/benefit)

If surgical treatment is liable to seriously affect the ability of an individual to function in society and drastically reduce their QoL, then the option of surgery needs to be considered within the MDT setting and through discussion with the patient.

Adjuvant and neo-adjuvant treatments

Chemotherapy and radiotherapy can be employed prior to surgery. This is termed neo-adjuvant treatment and is normally employed to reduce the size of a tumour to make excision easier or the margins more accessible (see Chemotherapy regimens, p. 209). More commonly, adjuvant treatments are utilized following surgery and are used to prevent the tumour from spreading via micrometastases. The primary tumour site and lymph nodes can be irradiated to reduce the risk of local metastases, and chemotherapy can be given to treat systemically to eradicate any existing micrometastases. In some cases, it is appropriate to utilize both neo-adjuvant treatments prior to surgery and adjuvant treatments post-surgery. For example, downstaging chemoradiation can be used to shrink a tumour, making it more amenable to surgery; further chemotherapy could be employed post-operatively to reduce the possibility of recurrence.

Developments in surgery

↑ knowledge of cancer biology, improved surgical techniques, and technological advances in imaging equipment have all combined to improve patient outcomes in a number of settings. Breast cancer surgery has become less mutilating, with more use of breast-conserving surgery. In rectal surgery, total mesorectal excision (TME) has improved survival rates and QoL for a number of patients. There has also been an ↑ use of less invasive surgery, using endoscopic/laparoscopic approaches, both for staging and disease excision.

With surgery becoming more specialized in the UK, many types of surgery are increasingly carried out exclusively in regional specialist centres. The aim is for surgeons to have sufficient expertise in their particular cancer surgery. This can have other impacts on patients and their families, with many having further to travel for treatment.

Further reading

Bartlett DL, Thirunavikarusu P, Neal MD (eds). *Surgical Oncology: Fundamentals, Evidence-based Approaches and New Technology*. New Delhi: Jaypee Brothers Medical Publishers; 2011.
McLatchie G, Borley N, Chikwe J. *Oxford Handbook of Clinical Surgery*, 4th ed. Oxford: Oxford University Press; 2013.

Preparing patients for cancer surgery

Prior to patients undergoing surgery, there are a number of important issues that need to be addressed.

Staging

Prior to a full surgical assessment, it is vital that the MDT are aware of the size, position, and pathology of the tumour and the presence of any local or distant metastatic spread. This is normally evaluated by radiological methods. It is now possible to assess tumours with a high degree of accuracy due to the availability of very sensitive diagnostic imaging techniques such as MRI and PET scanning (➔ see Diagnosis, classification, and staging of cancer, p. 176).

Lymph node assessment

An important aspect of any staging investigation is to determine whether cancer may have spread to lymph nodes. This is important as it may be possible to remove lymph nodes during surgery, and adjuvant treatment (e.g. radiotherapy) can be employed to treat any affected nodes. A relatively new technique used to assess the spread of cancer to lymph nodes is sentinel lymph node biopsy.

Sentinel node biopsy

This technique is increasingly employed in order to accurately assess the spread of cancer to surrounding lymph nodes. It has proven particularly useful in treating melanoma and, more commonly, breast cancer. The tumour site is infused (normally by injection) with a radiological marker and/or a blue dye. Time is allowed for the marker to diffuse to the first, or 'sentinel', lymph node. This equates to the first node to which cancer cells would diffuse to. Once identified, this node is then removed and examined for the presence of cancer cells. If it is clear, then it is almost certain that other nodes will not have been affected and will need not be removed. If the sentinel node is positive, then this node and other nodes further up the chain are removed.

   The technique allows surgeons to preserve lymph nodes, wherever possible, and spares patients the possible side effects of lymph node removal such as lymphoedema (➔ see Diagnosis, classification, and staging of cancer, pp. 176–8 for more information on staging systems).

Preoperative assessment

A good preoperative assessment is vital. It determines whether an individual is able to tolerate surgery both physically and psychosocially. It will also help determine if a patient will tolerate any long-term side effects from the surgery itself, and therefore the overall viability of a surgical approach. It is useful to have a wide-ranging spectrum of assessments if surgery is likely to be complex and have long-term side effects. For example, an anaesthetist, a specialist nurse, and a dietician may assess a patient's physical condition, and a psychologist may assess the patient's ability to adapt to major surgery. The individual's social situation may also have to be considered and may be highly relevant, e.g. an elderly frail person who lives alone being assessed for the formation of a permanent ileostomy.

Multidisciplinary team discussion

In situations where complex surgery may be required, it is important that any decisions made at an MDT meeting are based on the assessments of the whole MDT. It is also important that the decisions made are fully discussed with the patient. Details of the proposed treatment plan should be disseminated to all the clinicians caring for the patient. This ensures a consistent approach.

Information giving

Once a proposed treatment plan has been formulated, then it is vital that information is passed on to the patient and family prior to consent being sought for the operation. A valuable role in supporting the patient and their family through this process will be that of the CNS or key worker. The information that an individual and their family requires in order to make decisions about surgery needs to be tailored according to their own specific needs (➔ see Patient and family involvement in decision-making, p. 120).

Consent for surgery

Although the issue of consent is important when considering any cancer treatment, it has particular relevance in surgery, since surgery often results in major, and sometimes permanent, changes to an individual's body image, functional ability, and QoL.

The consent procedure should ideally address issues around treatment intent (whether curative or palliative), the need for further adjuvant treatments, and the benefits of any surgery weighed up against any possible long-term side effects and other risks.

Perioperative care of patients

There are a number of perioperative risks associated with surgery, which require careful management to minimize risks. Cancer surgery sometimes requires large excisions around other complex physiological structures to remove tumours that may also be highly vascular. Tumours can also alter blood chemistry and disrupt the clotting cascade. A patient's nutrition may also be poor, and many cancer patients have major comorbidities such as cardiorespiratory limitation. This can increase the number of perioperative complications and reduce effective recovery and wound healing.

These risks and their management have been summarized (see Table 15.1).

Palliative surgery

As well as being a curative treatment, surgery can be used to palliate symptoms or reduce discomfort. A full discussion with the patient about the realistic risks and benefits is essential. The clinicians need to be mindful that the patient may decline palliative surgery and should openly discuss other possible palliative support. Some of the areas where surgery can be used in a palliative way are:

- Removal of a tumour which is causing pain or psychological distress, i.e. a fungating lesion (➔ see Chapter 51, Skin and mucosal alterations).
- Relieving an obstructive process in the intestinal tract, e.g. stenting an oesophageal lesion or removing a tumour causing a bowel obstruction.
- Decompressing the spinal cord (➔ see Metastatic spinal cord compression, p. 641).
- Providing haemostasis in a tumour that is causing high levels of blood loss.
- Managing airway obstruction by forming a tracheostomy.
- Debulking a large tumour, even when not all the tumour can be removed, e.g. in ovarian cancer, this can both prolong survival and improve symptoms such as pain.

Reconstructive surgery

Surgery can also be used to restore form and function, following excision of a tumour. Good examples of this are:

- Breast reconstruction following mastectomy (➔ see Breast reconstruction, pp. 305–7).
- Facial and oral reconstruction following surgery for H&N cancers.
- Skin grafting following removal of lesions.
- Surgery which allows or facilitates the use of prostheses.

This form of surgery has developed rapidly over the last two decades, with vascular microsurgery being employed to utilize 'free flaps' (moving tissue, complete with its own vascular network, from another site in the body) to repair deficits left by tumour excision. This has led to improvements in breast reconstruction, reducing the long-term impact on body image. Developments in flap repair of the tongue or mandible has improved long-term function for many patients.

Table 15.1 Perioperative risks and their management

Risk	Management
Nutrition	• Refer to dietician preoperatively for full nutritional assessment • Maximize calorie intake preoperatively • Assess for tube-feeding or parenteral nutrition throughout perioperative period • Monitor weight and protein levels regularly
Wound healing	• Monitor and maintain adequate oxygen perfusion • Assess cardiac and pulmonary function preoperatively—administer oxygen, as required • Ensure adequate nutrition (see 'Nutrition' above) • Reduce risks of infection (see 'Infection' below)
Bleeding/ deep vein thrombosis (DVT)	• Correct blood chemistry preoperatively where possible • Utilize anti-embolus aids • Help the patient to get back to normal levels of mobility as quickly as possible post-operatively • Regular post-operative observations • Observe wound site regularly post-operatively • Monitor any blood loss carefully
Infection	• Good hygiene and technique throughout the perioperative period • Administer preoperative and post-operative antibiotic regimens • Thorough and regular post-operative observations • Observe wound site regularly for signs of infection
Pain	• Detailed preoperative pain assessment and education • Manage post-operative pain with infusional analgesics, which should preferably be 'patient-controlled' • Regular assessments of pain • Ensure that the period of transition between acute post-operative pain and longer-term post-operative pain is well managed • Manage the patient's anxiety effectively (see 'Anxiety' below)
Anxiety	• Give good and clear information throughout the operative period • Information should be given regularly and be in response to the patient's needs • Involve specialist teams where pain is not adequately controlled

Psychological effects of surgery

Despite reconstructive surgery being more widely available and accessible, not all surgical side effects can be resolved and many patients suffer from short- and long-term effects of cancer surgery. These can range from shorter-term side effects, such as wound infections and seroma formation (collections of fluid post-breast surgery) to long-term body image alteration such as loss of a breast or facial disfigurement. Even short-term problems or slight changes in appearance and function can have a profound effect on an individual's body image, causing a loss of confidence and a range of psychosocial difficulties from sexual problems to social withdrawal. The greater the post-operative changes, the greater the difficulties are likely to be (⊕ see Body image, p. 607).

Enhanced Recovery Schemes

Much of the physiological stress placed on the body by major abdominal surgery can be reduced by optimizing perioperative care. The Enhanced Recovery Scheme, developed by Henrik Kehlet in Denmark, results in reduced length of stay in hospital, reduced morbidity, and faster overall recovery.

The technique applies a number of key principles:
- To avoid deviation from normal function, e.g. no bowel prep or periods of 'nil by mouth', instead to maximize carbohydrate intake preoperatively
- To avoid long periods of patients resting in bed and to promote early mobilization
- Good fluid balance, e.g. to ensure patients are neither dehydrated nor hypotensive, but also to avoid fluid overload
- To avoid unnecessary drains
- To avoid hypothermia preoperatively
- Patient able to return home with support as soon as possible.

In 2012. a working party in the UK, including the then National Cancer Director, made a statement confirming that enhanced recovery should be adopted as standard practice across the UK and work is proceeding to make this a reality.

Further reading

NHS Improving Quality. Enhanced Recovery *Care Pathway: A Better Journey for Patients Seven Days a Week and a Better Deal for the NHS*. London: Department of Health; 2013.

Chapter 16

Radiotherapy

Principles and uses

Radiotherapy works by destroying cells within the body. It is delivered in as uniform a dose as possible to an accurately defined target to minimize physiological and psychological consequences for the patient. The aim is to kill the tumour cells, whilst minimizing the dose to normal structures.

When radiation is directed at tumour cells, it damages vital structures such as the cells' DNA or enzymes. Cells are generally more vulnerable to the lethal effects of radiation when they are dividing; therefore, the rate of cell division within a tumour will have an impact on its response to that treatment. Cells may also repair themselves. Cancer cells are generally less effective at repairing themselves than cells in normal tissue. This, in part, accounts for the ability of radiotherapy treatment to destroy a cancer, whilst enabling normal tissues repair (➋ see The 4 'Rs' of radiotherapy, p. 195).

Radiosensitivity

Different types of tissues and organs have different tolerances to radiation. Lymphoid tissue, haematopoietic tissue, ovaries, testes, and lenses of the eye are the most sensitive, requiring a smaller dose to cause lethal damage. The lung, liver, gut, and skin are moderately sensitive. Muscle, bone, and connective tissue are the least sensitive. The tolerance of normal tissues to radiation is one of the main dose-limiting factors of radiotherapy. For example, doses to the spinal cord will need to be considered when treating a H&N cancer.

Use of radiotherapy

~ 40% of patients with cancer will have radiotherapy as a treatment at some point in their disease. Radiotherapy can be employed as:

- **Primary treatment:** for some diseases, e.g. skin, prostate, and H&N cancers and Hodgkin disease, radiotherapy can be the primary treatment
- **Adjuvant treatment:** more commonly, radiotherapy is given as an adjuvant with surgery and/or chemotherapy, e.g. breast and H&N cancers, to cure or control a cancer
- **Palliative treatment:** palliative radiotherapy is used frequently to manage a range of symptoms in many cancers. These symptoms include spinal cord compression, pain, haemorrhage, and fungating wounds.

Fractionation

The amount of times a dose of radiation is delivered is known as the number of fractions. The number of fractions will vary, depending on whether the patient is having radical or palliative treatment and the area being treated. The ideal fractionation allows normal tissue to recover, whilst maximizing damage to cancer cells.

- **Radical (curative intent):** a high dose of radiation divided into small fractions, delivered daily over several weeks, to eliminate a tumour and minimize side effects, but remaining within the tolerance of normal tissues
- **Palliative:** a smaller amount of radiation given in a short number of fractions over a shorter time span with few acute side effects.

Chemo-irradiation

Concurrent chemotherapy and radiation treatment (particularly with radiation-sensitizing drugs) is increasingly used as a radical treatment modality in a number of cancers, including oesophageal, H&N, and cervical (➔ see Concurrent chemo-irradiation, pp. 209–10). The use of two concurrent treatment modalities increases cure and cancer control rates, but at the expense of more short-term side effects.

The 4 'Rs' of radiotherapy

There are four main principles that influence the biological response of a tumour and normal tissue, and these help guide the planning of radiotherapy treatment.

Repair

Radiation has two main damaging effects—direct breaks to DNA and indirect effects where it interacts with water molecules and oxygen to create free radicals. Free radicals are highly reactive molecules, which can oxidize and damage DNA synthesis. Most cells do not die immediately but instead die after several divisions, due to damaged DNA and cell mechanisms such as apoptosis (➔ see Cancer biology, p. 32). The ability of cells to repair this damage will impact on the effectiveness of radiotherapy as a treatment. Fractionating the dose aims to take advantage of the ability of normal tissue to repair itself more effectively than the cancer.

Repopulation

During radiotherapy, tumour cells not destroyed by the treatment begin to grow to replace the damaged cells. Some fast-growing cancers show accelerated growth. Reducing the overall treatment time of radical treatments and ensuring that there are no delays in treatment schedules are important. In tumours with fast growth, some patients may have >1 treatment a day. This is known as hyper-fractionation, which has been used in both H&N cancer and lung cancer.

Reoxygenation

Oxygen has an important role to play in the effectiveness of radiotherapy. The more oxygenated the tumour cells are when irradiated, the more effective the radiation is at destroying DNA. Many tumours have areas of reduced oxygen (hypoxia) due to poor vascularity. This makes them more resistant to radiation damage. Ways of improving oxygenation include ensuring patients are not anaemic [having a haemoglobin (Hb) level of above 12g/dL] and the development of drugs that can sensitize hypoxic cells. Fractionating radiotherapy increases the chance of killing cells that have already survived one treatment, as with each fraction, the tumour becomes less hypoxic and more oxygenated.

Redistribution

Cells that are initially destroyed by radiotherapy will have been dividing (in the cell cycle). Over time, cells moving from G_0 into the cell cycle replace these cells (➔ see Cancer biology, p. 32). Therefore, fractionating radiotherapy allows a greater chance of damaging cells at a sensitive stage of the cell cycle (particularly mitosis—M phase).

Treatment modalities

External beam radiotherapy

The main treatment machines used today are called external beam megavoltage linear accelerators. These produce extremely accurate, high-energy beams that are able to destroy cells. The unit of radiation dose is known as a gray (Gy). This is the amount of energy that is absorbed per unit mass, so 1Gy = 1J/kg.

Proton beam treatment

Proton therapy is a type of radiotherapy that utilizes positively charged particles (protons), instead of high-energy X-rays. These protons are produced from a particle accelerator and then focused into a beam, which can be focused on the tumour in the same way as the more traditional external beam radiotherapy. The advantage of using this modality is that protons deliver the dose of radiotherapy at the end of their range of penetration, allowing radiation doses to be concentrated at a more specific level, thus allowing more control of treatment when near other sensitive structures. Because of the high cost of delivering proton therapy and the uncertain benefit currently, protons are only commissioned by the NHS to treat a limited range of tumour types in the UK. In addition, the treatment of ocular tumours by specialist low-dose proton therapy machines is also commissioned. As research continues and proton therapy develops, it is possible that the application of protons in radiotherapy may increase.

Unsealed sources

These can be administered directly via either oral or IV routes. They are used to treat specific cancers, such as thyroid cancer where radioactive iodine is given orally and is taken up by the thyroid gland.

Brachytherapy (sealed source)

Radiotherapy can also be delivered via a radioactive source placed inside a body cavity or directly into a tumour (see Table 16.1).

Radiation protection

Radiation is potentially dangerous. It can cause cancer, although the chance of this being caused by diagnostic X-rays is small, due to the low dose used.

In order for radiotherapy treatment to be safe, the maximum 'tolerance' dose should not be exceeded, as above this dose, there is an ↑ chance of permanent damage to tissues. Radiotherapy must only be used when there is potential benefit for the patient.

The Ionising Radiation (Medical Exposure) Regulations (IRMER) 2000 specifies responsibilities for staff and employers using radiation on patients. It sets training requirements, and it requires justification of exposures for individuals. The employer has to provide a safe framework for staff to work with, including lists of trained staff and written procedures.

Table 16.1 Radiotherapy: main treatment modalities

Superficial and orthovoltage	Uses low-energy X-rays to treat superficial skin lesions such as basal cell carcinomas (BCCs) and SCCs
Megavoltage (external beam)	For deeper structures in the body. Uses a range of X-ray energies produced from an external electrical source. Patients may require complex planning of treatment, using a range of imaging modalities, to help localize the tumour. This is usually performed using a CT or MRI scanner (➔ see Treatment planning, and delivery, p. 198)
Electrons	For skin lesions and scars. Particularly useful for treating skin lesions and areas overlying bony structures, as the energy of the beam is lost rapidly upon interaction with tissues, producing a high dose close to the skin surface
Unsealed source	Radioactive isotopes administered IV or orally, e.g. iodine-131, which is used orally to treat thyroid cancer. Iodine-131 is taken up selectively by the thyroid gland
Brachytherapy	Treatment using a radioactive source element, such as irridium-192 or caesium-137, that is placed inside a body cavity, e.g. the cervix or use of radioactive wires, needles, or seeds that can be inserted directly into a tumour, e.g. tongue, breast, penis, and prostate (➔ see Treatment planning, and delivery, p. 198)

Radiation protection issues

- All personnel employed in a radiotherapy department must wear a radiation dose monitor, usually at waist level. Those staff who may come into contact with a patient who could be radioactive (e.g. radioactive iodine patients, brachytherapy patients, patients having a radioisotope scan) may wear additional monitors, e.g. on their fingers. Some may be monitored more regularly.
- All staff should avoid prolonged contact with patients who are radioactive, but it is advisable for staff who are pregnant or breastfeeding to avoid contact completely.
- Radiation protection equipment (e.g. mobile, thick lead screens) should be used when nursing patients who are radioactive. The intensity of radiation decreases with distance, and so the further you are away from the source of radiation, the safer you are.
- All radioactive waste should be disposed of in accordance with the local rules governing each oncology ward or department.
- Once a patient who has been radioactive leaves the ward, the area should be monitored, using a Geiger counter, to ensure no residual radioactivity is present.
- Patients leaving hospital following treatment with unsealed sources, such as iodine-131, should take some precautions during the first week at home. This may involve using personal sets of crockery and cutlery. Washing cutlery and crockery with soap and hot water will remove contamination. If patients use a dishwasher, they do not need to keep utensils and crockery separate.
- Patients should try to use a separate toilet area; if this is not possible, flush the toilet twice after use. It is important to keep the toilet area clean.

Treatment planning and delivery

Treatment planning

Radical radiotherapy

Planning generally happens in two stages: localization and verification.

1a. Localization: planning imaging

- CT/MRI-CT fusion/PET-CT fusion and US can all be used to aid in locating a tumour for radiotherapy planning. External markings, such as permanent body tattoos, can be placed onto the patient's skin as reference points to aid in the planning of treatment. These will be clearly visible on the scan(s). Newer techniques of skin mapping with IR beam localization can now allow 'tattoo-less' planning.

1b. Localization: computer planning

- The digital planning image is loaded into a planning computer where treatment can be modelled and adjusted to produce the maximum dose to the tumour, whilst minimizing the dose to surrounding normal tissues and organs. The treatment fields are defined, based on these principles, and any structures requiring shielding are identified (e.g. spinal cord or the lens of the eye). The prescribed dose is calculated and checked to ensure accuracy. The process is known as virtual simulation, as both the patient and the treatment beam data are modelled virtually within the computer program to produce the treatment plan, without the patient being called back repeatedly as the treatment is modelled and improved/adjusted.

2. Verification

- The treatment is verified on day 1 of the course of treatment by taking verification images in the treatment unit (linear accelerator). These may be two-dimensional images comparable to a plain X-ray, a three-dimensional dataset comparable to a CT scan, or a four-dimensional dataset using real-time imaging, such as breathing motion, to track the movement of a tumour during treatment. These images are assessed by a radiographer who has undertaken additional training to be competent in undertaking this task. Verification images are taken regularly (up to daily with each treatment) during the course of treatment to ensure that the treatment volume is still being treated as planned and there have been no changes due to patient weight loss or gain or changes in tumour size.

Treatment delivery

Megavoltage treatment delivery (external beam)

- Information from the treatment planning stage is used to position the patient on the treatment couch. Laser lights and the field light in the machine are used to line up with the marks and permanent body marks drawn on the patient. Whilst the treatment is delivered, staff leave the treatment room due to the high level of radiation.

Note: in many solid tumours, patients may have a second phase of treatment that focuses more specifically on the tumour, known as a boost. This requires a further planning session during treatment.

Proton treatment

The planning process in proton therapy is broadly similar to that employed in conventional external beam therapy, but the manner in which the beams are produced differs and treatment verification utilizes specialist equipment.

Brachytherapy/radioisotope/interstitial treatment delivery

Treatments can last several hours or even days.
- The patient will be required to remain in a specially designed room for the duration of their treatment.
- Nursing staff are responsible for checking that the treatment is being delivered. This may involve checking to make sure the source of radiation has not moved out of place or checking for machine failure. Any changes must be reported to a named staff member within the radiotherapy team responsible for brachytherapy.
- Any nursing procedures that need to be carried out must be done as quickly and efficiently as possible and utilize any radiation protection equipment as appropriate (➲ see Radiation protection, pp. 196–7). Nursing staff must wear radiation monitors if they are involved in patient care.

Advances and new technology in radiation therapy

Radiotherapy treatment
- Three-dimensional conformal treatment: this involves shaping the beam to 'fit' the shape of the tumour, using individual leaves of lead in the head of the machine. This aims to minimize the amount of normal tissue in the treatment field.

Intensity-modulated radiotherapy

A number of different techniques can be used to allow better shaping (conforming) of a treatment to match more closely the three-dimensional shape of the tumour. This takes into account any inconsistency within the tumour volume and improves the beam shape and profile. Intensity-modulated radiotherapy (IMRT) may involve a larger number of treatment fields or modulate a number of different beam characteristics at the same time (such as field size and shape and the beam dose rate). This enables the dose to the tumour to be escalated, whilst often reducing the dose to surrounding normal tissues, and thus reducing side effects. This reduction in side effects can enable patients to continue with day-to-day life during treatment and may allow escalation of the treatment dose to increase tumour cure rates. IMRT is now the standard mode of delivery for many clinical applications.

Stereotactic ablative radiotherapy (SABR)

This technique is currently used to treat smaller tumours in the brain or lung. In some cases, this treatment can be as effective as primary surgery in treating tumours.

Management of radiotherapy treatment and its side effects

Undertaking a course of radiotherapy can be an emotionally and physically demanding time for patients and their families. It may last several weeks plus the initial planning time, requiring daily travel, often over a long distance. Radiotherapy treatment may occur after or alongside other treatments, adding to the potential for debilitating side effects.

Many patients have fears of radiotherapy and its side effects. They may also have misunderstandings about the nature of the treatment. Media coverage of nuclear accidents and weapons raises concerns about radioactive fallout and dangers of getting other cancers or being a danger to others, e.g. 'will I be radioactive?' Initial assessment needs to:

- Clarify the individual's beliefs and concerns about radiotherapy treatment
- Explain the actual treatment process, potential side effects, and management of these.

After treatment is completed, patients may still face acute and long-term side effects (➜ see Community support, pp. 202–3).

Side effects

Radiotherapy side effects occur because of radiation damage to the cells. As the radiation cannot distinguish between normal and cancerous cells, it is inevitable that some normal cells will be damaged. This may lead to the patient experiencing radiation side effects, but some of these sides effects can be minimized by the use of modern treatment techniques such as IMRT. Side effects are generally localized to the area being treated (see Table 16.2). However, the main systemic side effect is fatigue (➜ see Chapter 42, Cancer-related fatigue).

Acute and long-term side effects

Side effects occur at different stages of the treatment, depending on the amount of treatment being delivered and the duration of the course of treatment. Side effects can be acute or long-term. Acute side effects can continue to worsen after treatment has been completed for up to 2–3 weeks. Most acute side effects will disappear a few weeks after treatment has been completed, though some may take longer and continue, becoming long-term. Symptom management is therefore a key element of continuing care and follow-up.

Understanding the tolerance dose of radiation treatment that a normal tissue or organ can withstand and advances in treatment planning and delivery greatly reduce the risk of long-term side effects occurring.

Multidisciplinary team

The management of radiotherapy side effects can involve many healthcare professionals, including: oncologists and their medical teams, oncology nurses, including CNS, therapeutic radiographers, radiotherapy physicists, dieticians, speech and language therapists, occupational therapists, physiotherapists, psychologists, counsellors, GPs, and other community healthcare professionals.

Table 16.2 Side effects of radiotherapy

Area treated	Acute side effects	Long-term side effects
Brain/CNS (including spinal cord)	Raised intracranial pressure (ICP), headache, nausea, blurred vision, unsteady gait, tiredness, dysphasia	Neurological defects, including neuroendocrine abnormalities, rarely cognitive dysfunction, spinal cord myelopathy, and rarely CNS necrosis
H&N	Pain, dysphagia, mucositis, xerostomia, fungal infection, weight loss, skin reaction	Pain, bone necrosis, dysphagia, xerostomia, skin changes
Breast (including axilla)	Pain, skin reaction, tiredness	Brachial plexopathy, skin telangiectasia and pigment changes (rare with modern linear accelerators), lymphoedema, rib and sternal necrosis (rare), lung fibrosis, psychosocial problems
Thorax	Breathlessness, pain, dysphagia, weight loss, tiredness	Pneumonitis and lung fibrosis, pericardial complications
GI tract (including oesophagus, small and large bowel)	Nausea, vomiting, pain, diarrhoea, weight loss, tiredness	Oesophagus: dysphagia, oesophageal ulceration/perforation (rare)
		Small bowel: rarely malabsorption syndromes, hypermotility, long-term diarrhoea, pain, ulceration, fistulae, perforation, ischaemia, bleeding
		Large bowel: rarely colitis, stricture, bowel obstruction, ulceration, fistulae, perforation, ischaemia, tenesmus, bleeding
Pelvis (including bladder/prostate, gynaecological)	Pain, difficulty in micturition, frequency, nocturia and urgency, cystitis, haematuria, proctitis, diarrhoea, tiredness	Bleeding, scarring, vaginal stenosis and dryness, fibrosis, cystitis, urinary incontinence, erectile dysfunction, urethral dysfunction, large bowel complications

Note: for detailed management of the main side effects listed in the Table 16.2, ➔ see Section 7, Symptom management.

Skin toxicity

The basal layer of the epidermis is sensitive to radiation because of its high proliferation rate. Radiotherapy treatment temporarily reduces cell division within the basal layer, therefore preventing normal repopulation. Skin toxicity occurs when the rate of repopulation of the basal cell layers cannot match the rate of cell loss caused by the treatment.

- The dose of radiation needed to induce a skin reaction depends on the amount of dose delivered with each fraction, the duration of the course of treatment, and the energy of treatment dose used.
- The degree of skin reaction will vary, depending on the area of the body being treated. Common areas that experience acute skin reactions include the breast, H&N, groin, and particularly areas where there are skinfolds. For radical treatments, skin reactions tend to occur within 2–3 weeks into a course of treatment and will heal within a few weeks of completion of radiotherapy.
- The evidence base for managing skin reactions remains limited, and practice remains variable. However, many radiotherapy departments now follow the skincare clinical guidelines developed by the Society and College of Radiographers and updated in 2011 (see Table 16.3).

Community support

When patients finish their radiotherapy treatment, many are still experiencing the physical side effects of the treatment. However, many can also experience emotional, social, financial, and spiritual difficulties. This is not only due to the effects of treatment, but also the process of returning to 'normal'.

Assessing the need for follow-up and community support is an important part of supporting the patient post-treatment. Patients should receive advice and information on the support services that are available to them. There should be a coordinated care package for each patient that should include the contact details of their cancer nurse specialist and other important members of the MDT.

The department/ward must work in partnership with primary care staff to ensure the patient's needs are met following completion of radiotherapy treatment. Communication between the radiotherapy centre/ward and primary care should be initiated early on, and protocols should be in place that ensures any post-radiotherapy problems are dealt with promptly. Understanding and awareness of the roles and contribution hospital and community health-care professionals have will help ensure a collaborative approach to care post-radiotherapy is achieved.

Table 16.3 Intervention guidelines

Skin reaction	Intervention
No visible skin reaction	• Continue with own skincare moisturizing regime • Assess weekly
Faint or dull erythema (mild tightening of the skin or itching)	• Advise patient to frequently apply a moisturizer to soothe • Assess weekly
Bright erythema and dry desquamation (sore, itchy, tight skin)	• Advise patient to apply moisturizer to soothe • Steroid creams should only be used following medical advice from the radiotherapy department. These creams should not be used on broken skin • If the skin breaks, patients should be advised to discontinue the cream and ask for further advice • Assess daily
Patchy moist desquamation (yellow or green exudate; soreness with oedema)	• Use appropriate dressing • Do NOT use gentian violet • Moisturizer can still be applied to other parts of the field • Assess daily
Confluent moist desquamation (yellow/pale green exudate; soreness with oedema)	• Use suitable dressings for the amount of exudates. Do not use adhesive dressings • Do NOT use gentian violet • Take a swab if there are any signs of infection • Seek advice from a tissue viability nurse • Assess daily

Reproduced from *Summary of Interventions for Acute Radiotherapy-Induced Skin Reactions in Cancer Patients: A Clinical Guideline College of Radiographers 2011* with permission from the Society and College of Radiographers.

Further reading

Barker HE, Paget JT, Khan AA, Harrington KJ. The tumour microenvironment after radiotherapy: mechanisms of resistance and recurrence. *Nat Rev Cancer* 2015;15:409–25.

Bhide SA, Nutting C. Recent advances in radiotherapy. *BMC Med* 2010;8:25.

Department of Health. *Ionising Radiation (Medical Exposure) Regulations 2000, Statutory Instrument No. 1059*. London: HMSO; 2000.

Faithfull S, Wells M. *Supportive Care in Radiotherapy*. Edinburgh: Churchill Livingstone; 2003.

Haas ML. Radiation therapy: toxicities and management. In: Yarbro CH, Frogge MH, Goodman M (eds). *Cancer Nursing: Principles and Practice*, 7th ed. Sudbury, MA: Jones and Bartlett; 2010. pp. 313–49.

Harris R (2011). *Summary of Interventions for Acute Radiotherapy-Induced Skin Reactions in Cancer Patients: A Clinical Guideline Recommended for Use by The Society and College of Radiographers*. Available at: ℘ https://www.sor.org/learning/document-library/summary-interventions-acute-radiotherapy-induced-skin-reactions-cancer-patients-clinical-guideline

Systemic anti-cancer therapy

Introduction to systemic anti-cancer therapy

The term systemic anti-cancer therapy (SACT) is now currently employed widely within the UK and elsewhere to describe medication which is administered systemically via a range of routes (oral, SC, IV), in order to treat cancers.

The term has developed to replace the generic description 'chemotherapy' over the last 5 years, in response to the rapidly increasing number of agents which could be described as biological, immuno-, or targeted therapies.

The term SACT is also the chosen description employed by UK health services (e.g. NHS England) when referring to cytotoxic, biological, and hormonal therapies as a group of treatments.

With this in mind, the overarching SACT chapter contains three large sections on cytotoxic chemotherapy, biological and targeted therapies, and hormonal therapies.

Cytotoxic chemotherapy: principles and uses

The term 'cytotoxic chemotherapy' is used here to differentiate between broad-spectrum cytotoxic agents affecting the cell cycle and targeted and immunotherapy and hormone therapies. Cytotoxic chemotherapy can be used with curative or palliative intent, either alone or in conjunction with other treatment modalities. Cytotoxic drugs disrupt cell division and replication, with rapidly proliferating cells being most susceptible to their action. As cytotoxic drugs are unable to distinguish between cancer cells and normal cells, rapidly proliferating cells of the bone marrow, GI tract, reproductive system, and hair follicles are particularly vulnerable to their effects, resulting in many of the common side effects of chemotherapy. Normal cells have a greater capacity for repair and renewal than cancer cells. Despite the more recently developed biological therapies having a more sophisticated selective approach, with the capability to target specific tissues and processes within tumour cells, it seems likely that cytotoxic chemotherapy will remain part of the armoury used to treat cancer for some years to come.

Cancer cell growth

Chemotherapy aims to reduce the number of actively dividing cells in a tumour, thereby reducing the growth potential. Smaller tumours tend to have a faster growth rate, are likely to have more actively dividing cells, and are therefore more sensitive to chemotherapy. Examples would be germ cell tumours and small cell cancer.

Effects of cytotoxic drugs on the cell cycle

Cytotoxic drugs have the greatest effect on actively dividing cells. Many cytotoxic drugs act on specific phases of the cell cycle, e.g. S phase (cell cycle-specific drugs), whilst others act on cells in any phase of the cell cycle (cell cycle-non-specific drugs). Drugs acting on a specific phase of the cycle will only affect cells that are in that phase at the time of administration. Cell cycle-non-specific drugs affect both cells that are actively cycling and quiescent cells. Multiple courses of chemotherapy are required to affect cells entering different phases of the cell cycle at different times. Examples of cell cycle-specific and cell cycle-non-specific drugs are shown in Table 17.1.

Classification of drugs

Cytotoxic drugs have differing modes of action, which are not yet fully understood. Most disrupt cell reproduction either by damaging DNA or by affecting mitosis and are categorized according to their mode of action (see Table 17.2).

Table **17.1** Examples of cell cycle-specific and cell cycle-non-specific drugs

Cell cycle-specific drugs	Cell cycle-non-specific drugs
Cytosine arabinoside, fluorouracil (5FU), gemcitabine, methotrexate (S phase)	Chlorambucil, doxorubicin, procarbazine, cisplatin, cyclophosphamide, ifosfamide, melphalan
Bleomycin, etoposide, irinotecan, topotecan (G2 phase)	
Vincristine, vinorelbine, docetaxel, paclitaxel (M phase)	
L-asparaginase (G1 phase)	

Table **17.2** Classification of cytotoxic drugs

Classification	Mode of action	Examples
Antimetabolites	Replace or compete with naturally occurring purines, pyridamines, or folates necessary for synthesis of nucleic acids	Methotrexate, cytosine arabinoside, 5FU, gemcitabine, 6-thioguanine, capecitabine, fludarabine
Anthracyclines (cytotoxic antibiotics)	Inhibit synthesis of ribonucleic acid (RNA) and DNA by different mechanisms, e.g. breaks and cross-links in strands of DNA, intercalation of base pairs	Doxorubicin, epirubicin, idarubicin, mitoxantrone
Alkylating agents (plus platinum agents)	Cause breaks and cross-links in strands of DNA	Chlorambucil, cyclophosphamide, ifosfamide, melphalan, dacarbazine, busulfan, cisplatin, carboplatin, carmustine, lomustine, procarbazine
Mitotic inhibitors: vinca alkaloids	Inhibit mitosis by binding to tubulin, an essential component of the mitotic spindle	Vincristine, vinblastine, vindesine, vinorelbine
Taxanes	Cause mitotic arrest by binding to microtubules	Paclitaxel, docetaxel
Topoisomerase inhibitors	Inhibit topoisomerase enzymes necessary for DNA replication. Cause single-strand breaks in DNA strands	Etoposide, topotecan, irinotecan (drugs from other categories, e.g. doxorubicin, mitoxantrone, are also topoisomerase inhibitors)

Chemotherapy regimens

Different cytotoxic drugs with proven efficacy against a particular cancer are combined in different chemotherapy regimens. Other agents with anti-cancer activity, e.g. hormonal and biological therapies, may also be included in these regimens. The dose and combination of drugs aim to achieve the maximum therapeutic effect with acceptable toxicity levels. A fine balance exists between the therapeutic dose of a cytotoxic drug and a lethal dose.

Combination chemotherapy

Combinations of drugs are used to overcome problems associated with single-agent drug resistance. Most chemotherapy regimens include a combination of cell cycle-specific and non-specific drugs to increase malignant cell destruction. Drugs with different, but complementary, actions and efficacy are combined. Drug toxicities should differ or occur at different times, so that maximum tolerated doses of drugs can be administered without severe toxicity.

Scheduling and sequencing of drugs

The order in which drugs are given can either affect their efficacy or cause ↑ toxicity, e.g. clearance of paclitaxel is significantly ↓ if it is administered after cisplatin, leading to ↑ myelosuppression.[1] Other drugs are synergistic, enhancing each other's effect, e.g. cisplatin and etoposide.

Intervals between pulses of chemotherapy

The time interval between pulses of chemotherapy is important; too short and normal cells will not have recovered, resulting in ↑ toxicity; too long and cancer cells may regrow between treatments. The interval between pulses is the period of time required for the most sensitive normal cells (usually the bone marrow) to recover. Most chemotherapy regimens are therefore repeated every 3–4 weeks. However, this is dependent on the toxicity of the drugs used.

Modes of use

Chemotherapy can be used in different ways and with different intent.
- **Curative**: chemotherapy is used as first-line treatment to cure a number of cancers, particularly haematological and lymphatic cancers.
- **Adjuvant**: following surgery, to remove the primary tumour, adjuvant chemotherapy is used as a means of destroying micrometastases.
- **Neo-adjuvant**: neo-adjuvant chemotherapy is used before surgery to:
  - Reduce the size of the primary tumour (possibly making it more amenable to surgery)
  - Reduce metastatic potential
  - Measure tumour response to chemotherapy.

It is used to treat various cancers, including H&N, bladder, cervical, non-small cell lung (NSCLC), and early breast cancers. Clinical trials continue to investigate the effectiveness of neo-adjuvant chemotherapy for different cancers.

Concurrent chemo-irradiation

Chemotherapy is administered concurrently with radiotherapy to increase the effectiveness of radiotherapy, whilst reducing the potential for metastatic disease. Certain cytotoxic drugs, e.g. cisplatin, 5FU, and gemcitabine, are known to have radio-sensitizing properties, increasing the sensitivity of cancer cells to radiotherapy and increasing therapeutic potential. The use of concurrent radiotherapy has been investigated for various cancers, including colorectal, cervical, oesophageal, laryngeal, pancreatic, cervical, NSCLC, and stomach.

The optimal dose, schedule, and combination of drugs to use concurrently with radiotherapy have yet to be established. Ongoing clinical trials are investigating the effects on both survival and toxicity profiles. Concurrent therapy may increase treatment toxicities, e.g. haematological and GI in cervical cancer, neutropenia and acute oesophagitis in NSCLC, and severe mucositis in H&N cancer.

High-dose therapy

High-dose therapy involves increasing the dose of cytotoxic drugs to a point where they are lethal to the normal bone marrow. Bone marrow then has to be replaced by haematopoietic stem cell transplant (HSCT). High-dose therapy and HSCT are used mainly for haematological and lymphoid cancers (➔ see Chapter 18, High-dose therapy (autologous transplant)).

Palliative

Palliative chemotherapy is used to control symptoms, improve quality of life, and treat oncological emergencies, e.g. superior vena cava syndrome. There may be no survival benefit associated with palliative chemotherapy, and treatment toxicities may impact on QoL. Therefore, the costs of chemotherapy need to be balanced against the survival benefit and compared to the cost of best supportive care.

References

1 Wilkes G, Barton-Burke M. *The 2015 Oncology Nursing Drug Handbook*. Sudbury, MA: Jones and Bartlett Publishing; 2015.

Chemotherapy: safe handling

Cytotoxic drugs are known to be teratogenic, mutagenic, and carcinogenic and therefore are potentially hazardous to patients, staff, and the environment. Exposure can occur through ingestion, inhalation, and absorption through the skin. Exposure can occur at all stages of preparation, administration, and disposal of drugs, most notably when reconstituting or mixing drugs, connecting and disconnecting IV tubing, and disposing of used equipment and patient excreta.[2]

It is vital that health-care professionals involved in the preparation, administration, and disposal of cytotoxic drugs and waste adopt safe handling procedures to protect themselves and others from the potential health risks associated with exposure.

Legal requirements
The preparation, administration, and disposal of cytotoxic drugs and waste must comply with the relevant legislation:
- Medicines Act (1968 and 2012).
- Environmental Protection Act (1990).
- Management of Health and Safety at Work Regulations (1999).
- Control of Substances Hazardous to Health (COSHH) Regulations (2002).

Pregnant workers
The EEC Council Directive 92/85/EEC (EEC, 1992) identifies cytotoxic drugs as potentially hazardous to pregnant workers. Employers have a duty to assess the risk to health and decide what measures should be taken. Pregnant workers can choose not to be involved in activities involving exposure to cytotoxic drugs.

Measures to reduce exposure to cytotoxic drugs
The evidence supporting safe handling practices is incomplete. However, various guidelines exist, based on the available evidence and expert opinion.

Preparation
Cytotoxic drugs should be reconstituted by appropriately trained personnel, wearing personal protective equipment, under aseptic conditions in a biological safety cabinet or an isolator within a pharmacy department. Cytotoxic drugs should only be reconstituted outside pharmacy departments in exceptional circumstances.

Transport and storage
Cytotoxic drugs should be transported and received in patient areas by staff trained in safe handling and safe storage procedures. Cytotoxic drugs should be securely stored in appropriate conditions in a clearly marked location, separate to other medicines.

Personal protective equipment
Gloves should be worn at all times when handling cytotoxic drugs and excreta. No gloves are completely impermeable to cytotoxic drugs. Permeability of gloves increases with time, and gloves should be changed on a regular basis to reduce the potential for exposure.

Eye and respiratory protection is advised when there is a risk of splashing or if the risk of generating an aerosol exists.[3,4] Aprons and gowns can protect clothing and subsequent skin exposure. A COSHH risk assessment should be undertaken for each handling activity to assess whether a gown or plastic apron offers the most protection.

Administration

Drugs should be supplied ready for administration and not require any further mixing or reconstitution. Oral preparations should not be handled. Tablets should not be crushed, and capsules should not be opened. A recent Cochrane Review (2018) illustrated that there was not enough good quality evidence to support the use of 'closed systems' in reducing exposure to staff administering chemotherapy.

Disposal of waste

Gloves and aprons should be worn when disposing of used IV equipment, excreta, blood, and body fluids. Contaminated needles, syringes, and IV giving sets should be disposed of intact. All waste should be placed in clinical waste bags and clearly marked cytotoxic. Patient excreta may contain traces of cytotoxic drugs for up to 72 hours following administration.

Spillage

Procedures should be in place for preventing and dealing with spillage. Spillage kits should be available in all areas where cytotoxic drugs are administered. Any spillage should be dealt with promptly. A warning sign should be in place to indicate the spill and prevent exposure and contamination, measures taken to contain the spill, and protective clothing worn. Contaminated materials should be clearly labelled and packaged for disposal. Porters and laundry staff should be aware of procedures for handling and disposing of contaminated materials.

Copious amounts of soap and water should be used for skin contact. Eyes should be flooded with water or an isotonic eye wash solution for at least 5 minutes, and medical advice obtained.[3] Spillage of a large amount of cytotoxic drug incurring exposure to people should be reported to RIDDOR[5] (Reporting Injuries, Diseases, and Dangerous Occurrences Regulations 2013).

Cleaning

Drug residue may be left on work surfaces in drug administration areas. All staff involved in cleaning areas where cytotoxic chemotherapy is administered should have training in minimizing exposure. Procedures for minimizing exposure should also be in place.[4]

References

2 Health and Safety Executive (2003). *Safe Handling of Cytotoxic Drugs. HSE Information Sheet.* Available at: ℘ http://www.hse.gov.uk/healthservices/safe-use-cytotoxic-drugs.htm

3 Royal College of Nursing. *Clinical Practice Guidelines: The Administration of Cytotoxic Chemotherapy. Recommendations.* London: Royal College of Nursing; 1998.

4 Scottish Executive Health Department (2005). *Guidance for the Safe Use of Cytotoxic Chemotherapy.* Available at: ℘ https://www.sehd.scot.nhs.uk/mels/HDL2005_29.pdf

5 Health and Safety Executive (2013). *Reporting Accidents and Incidents at Work: A Brief Guide to the Reporting of Injuries, Diseases and Dangerous Occurrences Regulations 2013 (RIDDOR).* Available at: ℘ http://www.hse.gov.uk/pubns/indg453.pdf

6 Close-system drug-transfer devices plus safe handling of hazardous drugs versus safe handling alone for reducing exposure to infusional hazardous drugs in health-care staff, Cochrane Worg Group, 27th March 2018.

Chemotherapy: safe administration

Cytotoxic drugs can have severe and potentially fatal consequences if administered incorrectly. Prevention of errors and patient safety are of paramount importance, and policies and procedures relating to cytotoxic drug administration should be adhered to at all times. All practitioners involved in chemotherapy administration must have undertaken specific education and training, be knowledgeable about the drugs they are administering and their side effects, and have demonstrated competence in their role.

- Patient consent should always be obtained and documented before the administration of chemotherapy.
- Cytotoxic chemotherapy should be administered during normal working hours, in a specifically designated area.
- Administration should not be rushed, and care should be taken to avoid distraction during administration.
- Practitioners should be aware of emergency situations which may occur during and following administration of cytotoxic drugs, e.g. allergic reactions, anaphylaxis, and extravasation, and be competent in managing them.
- Resuscitation equipment, emergency drugs, and extravasation kits should be available in all areas where cytotoxic drugs are administered.

Before administering drugs, practitioners should be familiar with the individual patient's:

- Blood count and general physical condition. Neutropenia or thrombocytopenia may mean that chemotherapy is delayed. Abnormal liver or renal function may require dose modification
- Allergy history
- Any contraindications to chemotherapy administration
- Any drugs they are taking (including non-prescription drugs) and any possible interactions
- Recommended dose range and maximum dose of drugs
- Route of administration
- Potential adverse reactions
- Short- and long-term side effects
- Route of excretion
- Compatibility of any drugs or IV fluids to be administered in conjunction with cytotoxic drugs.

Note: the *British National Formulary* and specific drug information sheets should always be consulted before drugs are administered.

Chemotherapy guidelines for safe practice

The *Manual of Cancer Standards* (England and Wales)[6] and *Guidance for the Safe Use of Cytotoxic Chemotherapy* (Scotland)[7] set clear guidelines for the administration and handling of chemotherapy. Local trusts are able to adapt these to their own local circumstances where appropriate.

All staff must follow their local Trust guidelines on administration and handling of cytotoxic chemotherapy at all times. These guidelines must be available in any area where cytotoxic drugs are administered.

References

6   Department of Health. *Manual of Cancer Standards*. London: Department of Health; 2004.
7   Scottish Executive Health Department (2005). *Guidance for the Safe Use of Cytotoxic Chemotherapy*. Available at: ℜ https://www.sehd.scot.nhs.uk/mels/HDL2005_29.pdf

Chemotherapy: routes of administration

Cytotoxic drugs can be administered by a number of different routes. The route of administration is chosen to achieve maximum cancer cell death by optimizing the bioavailability and exposure of cancer cells to drugs, thereby improving efficacy.

Main routes of chemotherapy administration

- Intravenous (IV)
- Intrathecal (IT)
- Intracavity, e.g. intravesical, intraperitoneal
- Subcutaneous (SC)
- Intramuscular (IM)
- Intra-arterial
- Topical
- Oral

Intravenous

The IV route remains the most commonly used route for the administration of cytotoxic drugs.[8] It is the most reliable route, as the drug is delivered systemically. Drugs can be delivered through a variety of venous access devices (VADs).

Venous access devices

The choice of device depends upon the condition of the patient's veins, the drugs to be administered, and the length of treatment. For those having lengthy courses of treatment, a central VAD (CVAD) should be considered. Choosing the right VAD for the treatment to be administered is important in reducing potential complications. Prevention of infection is vital, and strict asepsis is required, irrespective of the choice of VAD. Extravasation and subsequent tissue damage are major potential problems with the IV route (see Table 17.3).

Peripheral cannulation

Careful placement of any peripheral VAD is required, and nurses administering chemotherapy need to be skilled in cannulation. Individuals with cancer may have veins difficult to cannulate.

- Patients may have experienced previous problems with venous access and should always be asked if they have a preferred choice of arm for cannulation.

Table 17.3 Venous access devices

Type of cannula	Use
Peripheral cannula	Short-term use
Mid-line cannula	Medium term use (2–4 weeks)
Peripheral IV central catheter	Can be used for several months
CVAD (e.g. Groshong and Hickman catheters)	Long-term use
Implantable port (e.g. Port-a-cath)	Long-term use

- Limbs affected by lymphoedema, dermatitis, cellulitis, skin grafts, previous fractures, stroke, arteriovenous fistulae, or wounds should be avoided. The forearm is the cannulation site of first choice. Joints such as the antecubital fossa and wrist should be avoided, as there is a greater chance of dislodging the cannula.
- If the first cannulation attempt is unsuccessful, a subsequent one should be proximal to the first.
- The smallest gauge of cannulae should be used and be firmly secured.
- Pre-existing IV lines should be avoided for chemotherapy administration, wherever possible.

Administration

Drugs may be administered by direct bolus injection, by bolus injection into the side arm of a fast-running infusion of 0.9% normal saline, or by infusion. The choice of method depends upon the pharmacological properties of the drug (e.g. whether it is a vesicant or requires dilution, stability, osmolarity, and pH of the drug) and the type of VAD used. Any prescribed pre-hydration fluids or anti-emetics should be given before chemotherapy is commenced.

Before any drug is administered, the patency of the VAD should be assessed by withdrawing blood and then flushing with 0.9% sodium chloride. If a peripheral cannula is being used, the site should be closely observed throughout the infusion for signs of tissue infiltration or extravasation, e.g. resistance, swelling, pain or discomfort, redness, or signs of leakage. Cannula dressings should allow clear visibility of the insertion site and surrounding area. Cannulae should be flushed between drugs and after completion of drug administration with a compatible fluid.

Note: sodium chloride is not compatible with all drugs.

Intrathecal

Many cytotoxic drugs are unable to cross the blood–brain barrier, and the IT route is used in the treatment of acute lymphocytic leukaemia and some lymphomas. Cytotoxic drugs are injected into the cerebrospinal fluid, usually into the subarachnoid space, via a lumbar puncture, but drugs can also be injected into a ventricular space. Only certain drugs can be safely administered IT: methotrexate, cytosine arabinoside, and thiotepa.

Box 17.1 highlights the key recommendations for prescribing, issuing, dispensing, transport, storage, and administration of IT chemotherapy.[9]

Fatal vinca alkaloid administration

Around 55 patients worldwide, some in the UK, have died or been paralysed due to erroneous IT injection of vinca alkaloids (usually vincristine) causing severe or fatal neurotoxicity. Strict guidelines for everyone involved in IT administration of cytotoxic drugs have now been implemented.

Full details of guidance for IT administration can be found at ℘ http://webarchive.nationalar http:/www.dh.gov.uk/prod_consum_dh/groups/dh_digitalassets/documents/digitalasset/dh_086844.pdf

The implications of these guidelines for Scotland[8] are outlined at ℘ https://www.scot.nhs.uk/publications/

Box 17.1 Intrathecal chemotherapy guidelines
- A written local protocol must be in place.
- A register of named people trained and authorized to prescribe, dispense, issue, check, or administer IT chemotherapy must be kept, and only those on the register can undertake these procedures.
- Those on the register must have specific education and an annual review of competence.
- Drugs should be transported by the administering doctor or designated pharmacist.
- IT drugs should be stored in a dedicated lockable container or refrigerator.
- IT drugs should be administered after IV drugs.
- IT drugs should only be issued following written confirmation that IV chemotherapy drugs have been administered.
- A specific area should be designated for IT administration.
- All IV vinca alkaloids should be clearly labelled. Avoid negative labelling.

From Department of Health. HSC 2008/001. (2008). *Updated National Guidance on the Safe Administration of intrathecal chemotherapy*. London: DH © Crown Copyright, reproduced under the Open Government License v.4.0.

Intra-cavity

Cytotoxic drugs are instilled into body cavities such as the bladder (intravesical) and peritoneum. Malignant cells are therefore exposed directly to the drug, maximizing effectiveness.

Intravesical

Intravesical chemotherapy is used, following surgery to treat bladder cancer (➲ see Cancer of the bladder and ureter, pp. 369–71). Patients are catheterized, residual urine in the bladder drained, and the cytotoxic drug instilled slowly. The drug is retained for 2 hours either by clamping the catheter or by removing it and asking the patient not to pass urine for 2 hours. Patients should be encouraged to change position every 15 minutes from back to front and from side to side, so that all of the bladder mucosa is exposed to the cytotoxic drug. Drugs most commonly used are mitomycin and doxorubicin.

Most drugs can irritate the bladder, inducing chemical cystitis, and a high fluid intake is recommended after the drug has been voided. Urinary frequency, urgency, and burning when passing urine may be common following intravesical chemotherapy. Contact dermatitis may be experienced, particularly with mitomycin, and this can be avoided by thorough washing of the hands and genitals immediately after instillation and subsequent voiding of urine. Sexually active patients should protect their partners from exposure to cytotoxic drugs by wearing a condom.

Few systemic side effects are experienced with mitomycin and doxorubicin, although allergic reactions have been reported with doxorubicin.

Intraperitoneal

The peritoneal cavity can act as a sanctuary site for tumour cells, and cytotoxic drugs may be instilled to treat malignant ascites and control tumour growth. Intraperitoneal chemotherapy has been used primarily for treating ovarian cancer. Cytotoxic drugs can be delivered by a temporary suprapubic catheter, a Tenckhoff external catheter, or an implantable port. Drugs are usually diluted in 2L of fluid, warmed, and instilled by gravity.

Complications include catheter-related complications, abdominal pain, fatigue, haematological effects, metabolic abnormalities, and neuropathy. Respiratory distress, abdominal discomfort, and diarrhoea may also be experienced due to ↑ abdominal pressure. Infection is a further common problem, and temperature should be monitored.

Subcutaneous and intramuscular routes

Few cytotoxic drugs are administered by these routes because of the potential for tissue damage, bleeding, discomfort, and fibrosis. Drug absorption is also slow via these routes. However, more of the biological therapies are now administered SC.

Cytotoxic drugs administered by these routes include methotrexate (for some indications), asparaginase, and cytosine arabinoside.

The smallest needle size should be used and sites rotated to prevent side effects. For IM administration, a large muscle and the Z track technique should be used to avoid leakage of the drug into the skin. Platelet counts should always be checked before administration to reduce the possibility of bruising and bleeding.

Intra-arterial

A high concentration of cytotoxic drug is delivered directly to the tumour by the artery that provides tumour blood supply. The concentration of the drug to the tumour is ↑, whilst systemic circulation is ↓, thus reducing the occurrence of side effects. An example of this technique in action would be 'TACE' (trans-arterial chemo-embolization). This is a minimally invasive technique used in specialist centres to treat primary liver cancers whereby chemotherapy is introduced into the liver via the hepatic artery; other smaller vessels within the liver are deliberately occluded. Using this methodology, high doses of chemotherapy can be delivered directly into primary liver cancers.

Topical

Topical cytotoxic drugs may be used for skin lesions such as SCC and T-cell lymphoma; 5% 5FU cream is most commonly used. With repeated applications, tissue necrosis and sloughing of dead tissue occur. Normal tissue surrounding the lesion should be protected. Systemic effects are uncommon, although slight nausea may occur.

References

8 Scottish Executive Health Department (2004). *Safe Administration of Intrathecal Cytotoxic Chemotherapy* [issued under NHS HDL (2004) 30, 2 June 2004]. Available at: ℘ http://www.sehd.scot.nhs.uk/mels/HDL2004_30.pdf

9 Department of Health. *HSC 2008/001. Updated National Guidance on the Safe Administration of Intrathecal Chemotherapy.* London: Department of London; 2008.

Oral chemotherapy

The role of oral chemotherapy has markedly ↑ with the introduction of capecitabine in metastatic colorectal and breast cancers, and oral vinorelbine in lung and breast cancers. Other examples of drugs given orally include etoposide, chlorambucil, and procarbazine. Many chemotherapy and biological agents in development are also oral, so this trend towards oral therapy is likely to continue.

Advantages of oral chemotherapy

There are many potential advantages:
• Most patients prefer it
• Reduction of complications due to IV lines and pumps, e.g. spillage, infection, extravasation
• Shorter treatment time/reduction in patient–staff contact can free up nursing time for other service activities
• Improved QoL
• Improved side effect profile
• Cost-effectiveness
• Allows for easier modernization of chemotherapy pathways, e.g. nurse-led clinics, nurse prescribing of chemotherapy, and telephone assessment.

Potential risks

However, there are a number of important issues when managing individuals receiving oral chemotherapy:
• Patients and health-care professionals may think that oral chemotherapy is less serious or less dangerous than IV therapy.
• Patients have ↑ responsibility for administering their chemotherapy, as well as monitoring and responding appropriately to adverse events.
• Patient compliance is difficult to assess. Patients need information about the importance of strict adherence to the prescribed drug regimen, the correct dosage, what to do if they miss a dose, and what to do if they have any side effects.

As a general rule, the benefits from oral chemotherapy outweigh the risks. This is reflected in the recommendation from NHS England, which promotes 'maximizing the use of oral medications' as a way of reducing in-patient visits in chemotherapy.[10]

In 2008, in the UK, the National Patient Safety Agency (NPSA) published an alert outlining the large number of dosing errors associated with oral cytotoxic agents resulting in three deaths and several hundreds of incidents. The NPSA recommended that chemotherapy should be 'initiated by a cancer specialist and non-specialists who prescribe, dispense, or administer ongoing oral anti-cancer medication should have ready access to written protocols and treatment plans, including guidance on monitoring and treatment of toxicity'.

Note: it is essential to assess whether patients are able to safely manage an oral chemotherapy regime. Issues to consider include reading ability, manipulative abilities of elderly/frail patients, memory/concentration, and support at home from family or other professionals.

- Patients have less contact time with staff. Patient education time may therefore be quite short, e.g. all initial vital information may need to be given at a one-off visit prior to treatment. Educational strategies and patient information material need to be well designed and evaluated.
- Oral drugs can have varied metabolism between patients; therefore, dose modification and interruptions are a normal and essential part of therapy in response to any adverse events, i.e. hand and foot syndrome (HFS), diarrhoea, nausea and vomiting, and mucositis. Absorption of oral drugs may also be affected by food, GI problems, e.g. nausea and vomiting or diarrhoea, and concurrent medications. In the presence of any of these factors, patients may experience ↑ toxicity or a lower dose of the drug than prescribed. These issues all serve to highlight the need for good patient education in order to maintain patient safety and compliance.[11]

Patient compliance and education

To ensure that patients are safe in self-administering oral chemotherapy at home, effective patient education is essential. Pre-chemotherapy assessment clinics, dedicated oral chemotherapy clinics, and nurse-led follow-up (outpatient or telephone contact) are examples of developments that can support this process. Clear communication channels between primary and secondary care need to be developed. Well-designed information packs, treatment guides, and patient diaries will all help.

Patients may not wish to report adverse events if they think that dose reduction or interruption will reduce the efficacy of the drug. It is essential to inform patients that dose reductions of up to 50% and short interruptions in treatment will not reduce the efficacy of their treatment.

Essential aspects of patient information and education include:
- Correct dosage and administration schedule
- Accurate and clear information about how to recognize, grade, and manage common side effects
- Who to report to if any concerns
- The role of dose reduction and interruptions.

Further reading

(Whole journal issue dedicated to issues of oral chemotherapy) *Eur J Oncol Nurs* 2004;**8**(Suppl 1).

References

10 2013/14 NHS standard contract for cancer: chemotherapy (adult) – NHS England NHS England /B15/S/a. Available at: ℘ https://www.england.nhs.uk/wp-content/uploads/2013/06/b15-cancr-chemoth.pdf

11 Wood L. A review on adherence management in patients on oral cancer therapies. *Eur J Oncol Nurs* 2012;16:432–8.

Chemotherapy: administering vesicants and extravasation

Vesicant drugs have the potential to cause tissue damage and necrosis if extravasated. Extravasation is defined as infiltration of a drug into the subcutaneous tissues. The amount of damage usually correlates directly with the amount of drug infused. Damage may not be apparent immediately, and it may be 1 or 2 days before evidence of progressive tissue damage occurs.[12] Damage can continue for several weeks after extravasation (see Table 17.4). In severe cases, extravasation can result in loss of function or amputation. Surgical debridement or skin grafting may also be required. Prevention of extravasation is paramount when administering vesicant drugs. Extravasation is most frequently associated with peripheral cannulae but can also occur with the use of CVADs.

In 2012, the European Society of Medical Oncology (ESMO), together with the European Oncology Nursing Society (EONS), classified drugs into three groups to help develop a grading system for extravasation risk (see Table 17.5).

Table 17.4 Extravasation risk factors and prevention

Risk factors	Prevention
Previous chemotherapy as veins are often fragile and difficult to cannulate	Avoid small veins
	Avoid veins adjacent to tendons, nerves, or arteries
	Avoid sites distal to recent venepuncture or cannulation attempts
	Winged steel devices, such as 'butterfly' needles, should not be used, as they can easily dislodge and puncture vein walls
	Flexible cannula should be used
Previous radiotherapy	Avoid previously irradiated areas
Circulatory impairment, e.g. lymphoedema, peripheral vascular disease, Raynaud's disease, and comorbidity, e.g. diabetes, superior vena cava syndrome	Administer vesicants first when vein integrity is greatest, to reduce the risk of extravasation[13]
	Administer bolus slowly into a fast-running infusion
	Check infusion flow quality and cannula site regularly throughout infusion
	Never rush drug administration
	Never use infusion devices and pumps for vesicant drugs
	Use a peripherally inserted central catheter (PICC) or central catheter for slow infusion of high-risk drugs
No return blood flow from CVAD	Do not administer vesicant drugs before the patency of CVAD is evaluated
Needle dislodgement with implanted ports	Monitor needle placement with continuous infusion of vesicants, particularly during movement, which increases the risk of dislodgement

Table 17.5 Classification of chemotherapy drugs according to their ability to cause local damage after extravasation (ESMO-EONS guidelines)

Vesicants	Irritants	Non-vesicants
DNA-binding compounds	*Alkylating agents:*	Arsenic trioxide
	Carmustine	Asparaginase
Alkylating agents:	Ifosfamide	Bleomycin
Mechloretamine	Streptozocin	Bortezomib
Bendamustine*	Dacarbazine	Cladribine
Anthracyclines	Melphalan	Cytarabine
Doxorubicin	*Anthracyclines (others):*	Etoposide phosphate
Daunorubicin	Liposomal doxorubicin	Gemcitabine
Epirubicin	Liposomal daunorubicin	Fludarabine
Idarubicin	Mitoxantrone	Interferons
Others (antibiotics):	*Topoisomerase II inhibitors:*	Interleukin-2
Dactinomycin	Etoposide	Methotrexate
Mitomycin	Teniposide	Monoclonal antibodies
Mitoxantrone*	*Antimetabolites:*	Pemetrexed
Non-DNA-binding compounds	Fluorouracil	Raltitrexed
	Platin salts	Temsirolimus
Vinka alkaloids:	Carboplatin	Thiotepa
Vincristine	Cisplatin	Cyclophosphamide
Vinblastine	Oxaliplatin*	
Vindesine	*Topoisomerase I inhibitors:*	
Vinorelbine	Irinotecan	
Taxanes:	Topotecan	
Docetaxel*	*Others:*	
Paclitaxel	Ixabepilone	
Others:		
Trabectedin		

* Single case reports describe both irritant and vesicant properties.

Reprinted from Perez-Fidalgo J et al (2012) – Management of chemotherapy extravasation: ESMO-EONS Clinical Practice Guidelines. *Annals of Oncology* 23 (Supplement 7): vii167–vii173 with permission from Oxford University Press.

Nurses administering chemotherapy should be knowledgeable about the vesicant properties of the drugs they are administering, observe the vein regularly during the administration procedure, recognize the signs and symptoms of extravasation, and be competent in managing such an emergency, should it occur. Prompt recognition and management are imperative.

References

12 Bertelli G. Prevention and management of extravasation of cytotoxic drugs. *Drug Saf* 1995;12:245–55.

13 Perez-Fidalgo J, Garcia Fabregat L, Cervantes A, Margulies A, Vidall C, Roila C; ESMO Guidelines Working Group. Management of chemotherapy extravasation: ESMO-EONS clinical practice guidelines. *Ann Oncol* 2012;23(Suppl 7):vii167–73.

Chemotherapy: recognizing extravasation

Signs of extravasation may initially be slight, and neither nurses nor patients may notice them (see Table 17.6). Patients should be asked to report any feelings of pain, burning, or discomfort, as they may quickly recognize if an injection feels different to previous experiences. Initially, it may be difficult to differentiate between an extravasation and other reactions.

Patient reports of pain, burning, or discomfort are particularly important for CVADs. Extravasation may not be immediately apparent. Signs and symptoms include:

- Difficulty withdrawing blood from CVADs
- Shoulder pain—may be described as dull, aching, burning, or stinging sensation
- Supraclavicular, chest wall, or lower back pain can occur with extravasation from an implantable port
- Pyrexia
- Erythema, warmth, and tenderness of chest wall or around port site
- Pain and swelling along catheter tunnel or around port site.

Managing extravasation

Management of extravasation is controversial. Local protocols and procedures should be followed. Table 17.7 outlines generally accepted principles in the management of extravasation.

Table 17.6 Signs and symptoms of extravasation

Signs and symptoms	Other reaction complicating diagnosis
Erythema, discoloration, swelling, leakage, or a change in skin temperature	Flare reactions, common with drugs such as doxorubicin and epirubicin, often present as a red streak along the vein, blotchy skin, urticarial reactions, and pruritus. Flare reactions are temporary and subside within 30–90 minutes
Burning, stinging, and pain	Venospasm may also result in pain on administration. Usually described as dull ache. Stinging and pain may occur with flare reaction
↑ resistance to syringe or slowing of infusion rate	Patient position and kinking of administration set may also cause ↑ resistance
Lack of blood return	Can be misleading. The act of withdrawing blood can pull the cannula back into the vein, and blood can be withdrawn. On recommencing administration, extravasation occurs through the hole in the vessel wall, exacerbating the injury
	Vessel wall puncture can occur during venepuncture; the cannula remains in the vein, and blood is returned, but drugs can leak through the puncture hole into surrounding tissues

Table 17.7 Management of extravasation

Management	Rationale
Stop infusion immediately	Prevent further extravasation
Leave the cannula in place	Allows aspiration of the drug and administration of antidote
Inform a doctor experienced in the management of extravasation injuries	Management of extravasation is controversial; an experienced person should always advise on management
Mark the affected area with a pen	Extravasated area is clearly marked
Aspirate as much of the drug as possible from the cannula. SC injection of 0.9% sodium chloride may help to dilute the drug	Remove the drug from tissues, although it is recognized that little may be obtained
Remove the cannula	Causes vasoconstriction and reduced local uptake of the drug
For all drugs other than vinca alkaloids, the principle of 'localize and neutralize' is used. Ice packs should be applied regularly for 24–48 hours	
Topical dimethylsulfoxide (DMSO) may be applied	Has been found to be particularly successful in the treatment of anthracline extravasation
For anthracycline extravasation, then administration of dexrazoxane should be considered	Has been found to be effective in reducing tissue damage if regime commences no later than 6 hours after extravasation occurred
For vinca alkaloid extravasation, administer SC hyaluronidase 1500U as an antidote. Apply warm	The principle of 'spread and dilute' is used for vinca alkaloid extravasation
Elevate the limb following application of warm or cold packs	To remove extravasated material whilst preserving the overlying skin
Some authorities advocate flushing the infiltrated area with 0.9% sodium chloride, using multiple stab incisions in the subcutaneous tissue around the extravasated area	
Accurately document the extravasation incident	

Chemotherapy: side effects and complications

See Table 17.8 for common side effects and complications of chemotherapy. Management of side effects and patient care are discussed in subsequent chapters.

Table 17.8 Short- to medium-term side effects and complications

Short- to medium-term side effects	
GI	Skin and nails
• Nausea and vomiting (can be delayed with some drugs, e.g. cisplatin) • Mucositis • Constipation • Diarrhoea • Anorexia • Taste changes • Metallic taste (e.g. cyclophosphamide)	• Alopecia • Plantar–palmar erythrodysesthesia (HFS) • Rash • Erythema • Hyperpigmentation • Radiation recall • Ridging of nails and Bowman's lines • Nail loss
Bone marrow	General side effects
Myelosuppression, neutropenia, thrombocytopenia, anaemia May be prolonged or delayed with some drugs, e.g. carmustine, lomustine, melphalan, mitomycin	Fatigue Flu-like symptoms Fluid retention and oedema (docetaxel, paclitaxel)
Reproductive system	Cardiac
Amenorrhoea/early menopause Infertility (particularly alkylating agents)	Tachycardia and other rhythm disturbances Hypertension (mainly anthracyclines)
Neurological	Renal and bladder
Peripheral neuropathy Autonomic neuropathy Cranial nerve neuropathy Ocular nerve toxicities	Hyperuricaemia Coloured urine (doxorubicin, epirubicin, mitoxantrone) Haemorrhagic cystitis (cyclophosphamide, ifosfamide)

Complications
• Hypersensitivity reactions and anaphylaxis   • Tumour lysis syndrome   • Sepsis   • Pulmonary toxicity (e.g. pulmonary fibrosis with bleomycin, busulfan, chlorambucil, carmustine)   • Cardiomyopathy (anthracyclines)   • Neurotoxicity   • Ototoxicity (tinnitus and hearing loss with cisplatin)   • Nephrotoxicity   • Hepatotoxicity (asparaginase, amsacrine, carmustine, cisplatin, chlorambucil, dacarbazine, methotrexate); hepatic veno-occlusive disease (busulfan)   • Secondary cancers   • Cognitive dysfunction

Chemotherapy closer to home

Use of chemotherapy in the home and non-traditional environments such as mobile chemotherapy units or local clinics is likely to expand in the future. This is linked to changes in the way health care is delivered, with an increasing move to care closer to patients' homes and an increasing number of oral and SC anti-cancer therapies available (➔ see Oral chemotherapy, pp. 219–20). Nurses caring for patients in these environments need to be knowledgeable about the drugs the patient is receiving, potential side effects, safe handling, and who to contact if they need advice or support.

Before administration is commenced, it is vital that policies and procedures are developed for all aspects of cytotoxic drug administration, including management of side effects and emergency situations, e.g. spillage, extravasation, and hypersensitivity reactions. Safe handling guidelines and regulations should be adhered to at all times.

Considerations when administering chemotherapy in non-traditional environments

- Drugs should be transported in a robust and tamper- and leak-proof container, clearly marked cytotoxic.
- Drugs should be stored in correct conditions and kept out of the reach of children and pets.
- Clear information on safely handling oral chemotherapy, e.g. handwashing, not crushing tablets.
- Disposal methods for cytotoxic drugs and waste should be clearly established.
- All necessary equipment should be available before drug administration, including spillage and extravasation kits for IV chemotherapy.
- Administration and checking procedures should be adhered to.
- Clear communication pathways should be established between primary and secondary care and the teams delivering the chemotherapy.

Further reading

Department of Health. *National Guidelines on the Safe Administration of Intrathecal Chemotherapy*. London: Department of Health; 2001.

Health and Safety Executive (2013). *Reporting Accidents and Incidents at Work: A Brief Guide to the Reporting of Injuries, Diseases and Dangerous Occurrences Regulations 2013 (RIDDOR)*. Available at: ➘ http://www.hse.gov.uk/pubns/indg453.pdf.

Skeel RT, Khleif S. *Handbook of Cancer Chemotherapy*, 8th ed. Philadelphia, PA: Lippincott, Williams, and Wilkins; 2011.

Introduction to targeted and biological therapies

In recent years, we have developed a greater understanding of the tumour microenvironment and the role of the immune system in the development of cancer. Our increasing knowledge of the mechanisms of cell division, and more recently the complexity of cell signalling pathways, has led to an explosion in the number of new targeted and biological therapies moving into clinical trial and standard use.

The number of potential targets for anti-cancer treatments continues to grow, and the hope is that this will continue to enable future development of anti-cancer therapies.

This chapter will cover the main principles of commonly used targeted and biological therapies and highlight some of the more commonly used agents. However, due to the regular changes in treatment guidelines, it is essential that the reader consults current NICE guidelines to ensure that they are properly up-to-date with current practice (ᔑ http://www.nice. org.uk/Guidance).

Further reading

Keeping tabs on MABs. The latest on monoclonal antibodies. *Br J Nurs* 2015;24(16), Suppl 1.
Semin Oncol 2012;39:243–366 (Note: whole journal volume focusing on cancer vaccine development).
Zeron-Medina J, Ochoa de Olza M, Brana I, *et al*. The personalization of therapy: molecular profiling technologies and their application. *Semin Oncol* 2015;42:775–87.

Small molecule inhibitors

An ↑ knowledge of the mechanism of cell growth, in particular signal transduction pathways and signal amplification, has led to a number of new protein targets for new small molecules. These inhibit the functions of proteins in growth signalling pathways.

Tyrosine kinase inhibitors

Tyrosine kinase (TK) is an enzyme that has a key function as an on/off switch in growth factor signalling pathways. The two main classes are:
- Cell surface receptors with TK activity, e.g. epidermal growth factor (EGF) receptor, human epidermal growth factor receptor 2 (HER-2)
- Intracellular growth factor signalling proteins, active in the receptor signalling pathway, e.g. c-Abl.

There are a number of anti-cancer drugs that inhibit TK activity in growth signalling pathways, including:
- EGFR signalling pathway, e.g. erlotinib
- HER-2/Neu signalling pathway, e.g. lapatinib
- VEGF pathway, e.g. sorafenib.

Some other drugs have a broad-spectrum inhibition of >1 pathway, e.g. sunitinib.

Commonly used drugs

Imatinib

Oral medication used for both chronic myeloid leukaemia (CML) and GI stromal tumours (GISTs); targets the mutant form of the Abl protein encoded by the *Bcr–Abl* fusion gene.

In metastatic GISTs, it has provided an effective treatment where previously there were no therapeutic options. It produces response rates of around 50%, with 2-year survival of >70%.

Common side effects include:
- Oedema/effusions
- Nausea
- Diarrhoea
- Rash
- Myelosuppression.

Gefitinib

Oral medication which targets the EGFR pathway. Used as first-line treatment in patients with locally advanced or metastatic NSCLC, with a positive *EGFR* mutation.

Common side effects include:
- Diffuse acneiform rash
- Diarrhoea
- Fatigue.

Erlotinib

Also targets the EGFR pathway. Encouraging results in:

- NSCLC: in patients with locally advanced or metastatic NSCLC, with a positive *EGFR* mutation
- Pancreatic cancer: used in clinical trials in combination with gemcitabine.

Common side effects include:

- Diffuse, often distressing acneiform rash
- Diarrhoea
- Fatigue.

Sunitinib

Inhibits the VEGF receptor but also affects closely related pathways. Reduces cell proliferation and also has an anti-angiogenesis effect. Main use is in advanced renal cell carcinoma (RCC). Also used in pancreatic neuro-endocrine tumours (NETs) and GIST tumours resistant to imatinib.

Common side effects include:

- Fatigue
- Diarrhoea
- Skin toxicity—dry, cracked, yellowing
- Hypertension.

Everolimus

Oral medication which targets the mammalian target of rapamycin (mTOR) pathway. Inhibits cell division. Main use in metastatic RCC. Also used in pancreatic NETs.

Common side effects include:

- Skin rash
- Stomatitis
- Fatigue
- Risk of infection.

Side effect management

The ↑ use of tyrosine kinase inhibitors (TKIs) has seen a related increase in the number of patients presenting with rash, HFS, and diarrhoea. Diarrhoea should be managed as with other causes (➔ see Diarrhoea, pp. 502–5). Appropriate dose reduction and/or interruption is an important aspect of toxicity management, with oral medications. It is important that nurses make themselves aware of the individual drug protocols and grading of treatment toxicities, as they may be a first contact point for these patients, who will often be managing their medication from home.

Dose modification

Despite side effects, many patients will struggle with advice to reduce or stop medication, when they see it as their main chance to treat their cancer effectively. Assessing and supporting compliance with correct dosing is an essential part of the cancer nurse's role for these patients.

Tyrosine kinase inhibitors: skin toxicity

- Ensure that patients are reviewed regularly and have any skin toxicities graded. Many problems may be reduced by avoiding hot showers, reducing sun exposure, and wearing loose-fitting clothing.
- In mild rash, ensure topical treatments are available—urea-containing lotions, fragrance-free moisturizers. Can use topical steroid cream, e.g. hydrocortisone 1%.
- For HFS, give patients advice regarding the need to moisturize the hands and feet (including the use of urea-based creams) and to avoid rubbing (e.g. ill-fitting shoes). Patients need monitoring for superimposed infections and may need antibiotic support and possible dermatological referral.
- If toxicities reach grade 3, then the anti-cancer drug should be interrupted till improvement to grade 1 and can be restarted at a reduced level.

Note: other side effects, e.g. fatigue, risk of infection, are covered in the appropriate chapters under those headings.

Immunotherapy

The principle of immunotherapy is the administration of antibodies to the patient with cancer, enabling their immune response to attack cancer cells within their body.

Immune checkpoint inhibitors

This cell surface receptor has a key role in downregulating the immune system, suppressing T-cell activity. It keeps T-cells from attacking other cells by attaching to programmed death-ligand 1 (PD-L1). This is a protein which is found on some normal cells but is often found in large numbers on cancer cells, helping them to evade immune attack. Monoclonal antibodies that target either programmed cell death protein 1 (PD-1) or PD-L1 can block this binding and boost the immune response against cancer cells. These drugs have shown a great deal of promise in treating a number of cancers.

PD-1 inhibitors

For example:
- Pembrolizumab (Keytruda®)
- Nivolumab (Opdivo®).

These have shown efficacy in treating several types of cancer, including melanoma of the skin and NSCLC. Trials are also being undertaken in a number of other cancers.

PD-L1 inhibitors

For example:
- Atezolizumab (Tecentriq®).

Used to treat bladder cancer and NSCLC.

CTLA-4 inhibitors

CTLA-4 is another protein on some T-cells that acts as a type of 'off switch' to keep the immune system in check. CTLA-4 inhibitors target this protein to prevent it from working, therefore boosting the immune response against cancer cells.
- Ipilimumab (Yervoy®) has shown excellent efficacy in treating metastatic melanoma.

Side effects

A key issue is the ↑ risks of severe immune-mediated inflammation of the lungs, colon, liver, or kidneys and the endocrine system, which can be fatal. Detailed and regular assessment of respiratory function, diarrhoea, and liver function tests (LFTs) is essential, as well as assessment of possible endocrine disorders. Patients will need intensive courses of corticosteroids if symptoms occur.

Cytokines

Cytokines are soluble proteins, which have biological activity on several tissues, mainly on those originating from the haematopoietic and immune systems. Cytokines can both inhibit and promote tumour growth. The main cytokines that have therapeutic activity in cancer are:
- Interferons
- Haematopoietic growth factors.

Interleukins and TNF have also been used experimentally in some advanced cancers.

Interferons

Several types of interferon are produced by the immune system in response to viral infections. Interferon alfa is the interferon used to treat a range of cancers (see Box 17.2), though, in most cases, its first-line use has been replaced by the development of newer targeted therapies.

Interferons have the following anti-tumour activity:

- They interfere with, or directly stop, tumour cell growth.
- They affect the expression of oncogenes.
- They enhance the cytotoxic activity of natural killer cells, macrophages, and T-cells. They reduce the amount of blood vessels around the tumour.
- They promote tumour cells to change to less aggressive cells.

The main **side effects** of interferons are: flu-like symptoms (>90%), anorexia, fatigue, ↑ LFTs, rashes, GI complaints, lethargy, depression, and thrombocytopenia. Flu-like symptoms can be treated with prophylactic paracetamol. Patients usually begin to tolerate the side effects of interferons after prolonged administration. The side effects are reversible once treatment stops. Slow-release (pegylated) versions of interferons are now commercially available, allowing less frequent administration than normal interferons.

Interleukins

Interleukins are cytokines produced by several immune system cells. They have an important role in mediating many immune responses. Interleukin-2 has been clinically evaluated in several advanced cancers (see Box 17.2).

It is limited in clinical practice by its toxicity profile. The main **side effects** are: flu-like symptoms, capillary leak syndrome, severe hypotension, angina, arrhythmias, respiratory distress, somnolence, anaemia, thrombocytopenia, and multi-organ failure.

Box 17.2 Cancers treated by cytokines

Interferon-α

- Hairy cell leukaemia
- Multiple myeloma
- Cutaneous T-cell lymphoma
- Malignant melanoma

- CML
- RCC
- KS
- Carcinoid tumours

Interleukin-2

- RCC
- Trials in melanoma

TNF

- Trials in melanoma and sarcoma

Tumour necrosis factor

TNF is a mediator of the inflammatory response. It is still an experimental treatment. The clinical use of TNF is limited by severe side effects, including acute fever, anaemia, thrombocytopenia, liver, renal, and CNS toxicity. Prospective randomized controlled trials in melanoma and sarcoma have had disappointing results.

Haematopoietic growth factors

Haematopoietic growth factors are cytokines that have a role in controlling the formation and development of blood cells. Recombinant DNA technology has enabled the synthetic production of naturally occurring growth factors for use in clinical practice. They are primarily used to reduce the impact of bone marrow suppression caused by anti-cancer therapy. There are three main growth factors used in cancer care:
- Erythropoietin (EPO)
- Granulocyte colony-stimulating factor (G-CSF)
- Granulocyte-macrophage colony-stimulating factor (GM-CSF).

Erythropoietin

EPO has a role in stimulating red blood cell production. In the cancer setting, it is used to manage anaemia caused by chemotherapy (➔ see Erythropoietin, p. 488).

Granulocyte colony-stimulating factor

G-CSF is a cytokine that regulates proliferation and differentiation of a range of haematopoietic cells. G-CSF:
- Can reduce the risk of neutropenia, febrile neutropenia, and infection in patients receiving myelosuppressive anti-cancer drugs
- Is used with treatment where there is a high risk of febrile neutropenia, e.g. high-dose chemotherapy, blood and stem cell transplant settings. It is also used to maintain the dose and schedule of drugs in standard chemotherapy regimes, e.g. testicular cancer, breast cancer
- Is recommended by current European guidance as primary prophylaxis if the risk of febrile neutropenia is ≥20%
- As secondary prophylaxis, following an episode of febrile neutropenia, is an alternative option to dose reduction in the adjuvant setting
- Is also used in mobilizing stem cells for stem cell harvest
- Has a short half-life and requires regular SC injections for each treatment. Pegylated G-CSF (pegfilgrastim) has an ↑ half-life, and only one injection is required in each course of chemotherapy.

Granulocyte-macrophage colony-stimulating factor

GM-CSF increases the number of neutrophils and monocytes. It also stimulates dendritic cells to divide, which help the immune system to recognize and attack cancer cells.

It is currently being used in trials to boost the numbers of dendritic cells and also in cancer vaccine trials.

Bacille Calmette–Guérin (BCG)

Activates macrophages, T- and B-lymphocytes, and natural killer cells. Also induces local response via interleukins.

Its main use in cancer treatment is in treatment of superficial bladder cancer (◆ see Cancer of the bladder and ureter, pp. 369–71).

Intravesical instillation for superficial bladder cancer

- 38% reduction of recurrence in Ta and T1 bladder cancer. Main treatment for bladder carcinoma *in situ*. Complete response rate of >70%.
- Side effects: dysuria, haematuria, mild fever, urinary frequency. Rarely sepsis.

Monoclonal antibodies

Monoclonal antibody therapy is a therapeutic modality that has become mainstream in the treatment of a number of cancers, e.g. breast, melanoma, lung, gastric, ovarian, colorectal, haematological, often combined with more conventional chemotherapy agents.

All cells have protein markers on their surface, known as antigens. Monoclonal antibodies are designed in the laboratory to recognize particular protein markers on the surface of some cancer cells or other cells such as T-cells (e.g. PD-1 or CTLA-4). The monoclonal antibody then 'locks' on to this protein.

Monoclonal antibodies have several mechanisms of action by which they destroy or prevent the replication of malignant cells, such as:

- Triggering the immune system to attack cancer cells, e.g. rituximab, ofatumumab
- Blocking molecules that stop the immune system from working (checkpoint inhibitors), e.g. ipilimumab, nivolumab, pembrolizumab
- Blocking signals from telling cancer cells to divide, e.g. cetuximab, bevacizumab
- Carrying toxic therapy to specific cell targets by combining radionuclides, cytotoxic drugs, or cell toxins with the antibody, known as 'conjugated' monoclonal antibodies, e.g. brentuximab, ibritumomab.

Staff safety issues

Monoclonal antibodies are not infective, but as they are proteins, there is a theoretical risk of operator sensitization to non-human monoclonal antibodies on repeated exposure. However, there is little evidence to suggest this is a problem in practice. Ideally, the manipulation of monoclonal antibody preparations should be undertaken in pharmacy aseptic facilities, to ensure operator protection from contamination and patient protection from cross-contamination.

- Vials should not be shaken to avoid prolonged foaming.
- It is important not to create aerosols when removing content from the vial.
- On addition of the vial's contents to an infusion bag, gently invert the bag to mix. Do not shake.

Hypersensitivity reactions

The most common side effects of monoclonal antibodies are infusion-related, including flu-like symptoms and a cytokine release syndrome. This is generally observed with the first or second dose, and the probability of it occurring increases in patients with a large tumour burden or pulmonary insufficiency. The symptoms of this sort of reaction normally appear 1 or 2 hours after the infusion and range from very mild to a severe and/or fatal anaphylactic reaction (→ see Anaphylaxis, pp. 633–4). It can also be associated with features of tumour lysis syndrome (TLS) (→ see Tumour lysis syndrome, pp. 649–50). The risk of such reactions means that these drugs should be administered in areas where resuscitation equipment is available.

Rapid infusion protocols

Protocols exist in many areas for rapid infusion of a number of monoclonal antibodies, when patients have tolerated licensed rates without any signs of reaction.

There are several examples of monoclonal antibodies, which have become standard treatments for some cancers.

Trastuzumab

Trastuzumab is a humanized monoclonal antibody used to treat breast cancer patients whose tumours overexpress the HER-2 protein. The HER-2 protein is overexpressed in 20–30% of breast cancers and is a poor prognostic factor. Trastuzumab targets the HER-2 protein. Immunohistochemistry assays are required to assess whether patients are overexpressing the HER-2 protein. There is a standard scoring system (0, +1, +2, or +3). Patients with a HER-2 score of +3 are eligible for treatment with trastuzumab.

Established treatment:
- Combined with adjuvant chemotherapy in early HER 2 +ve breast cancer
- In metastatic HER-2 +ve breast cancer (➲ see Adjuvant treatment of early breast cancer, p. 299; ➲ see Management of metastatic breast cancer, pp. 303–4)
- Combined with chemotherapy in metastatic gastric/gastro-oesophageal junction (GOJ) cancer.

Trastuzumab works by:
- Downregulating HER-2 receptors
- Inhibiting growth signalling pathways
- Engaging natural killer cells of the immune system to attack the tumour
- Inducing cell lysis
- Enhancing chemotherapy cytotoxicity.

Side effects:
- Cardiotoxicity—patients' cardiac function must be monitored [echocardiography or MUGA (multigated acquisition) scanning at baseline and then at 3-monthly intervals during treatment]
- Fever or chills—can be prevented with prophylactic paracetamol
- Hypersensitivity reactions; can be delayed onset (➲ see Allergic reactions in oncology, p. 633).

Rituximab (Mabthera®)

Rituximab is used for CD20-positive B-cell NHL, in combination with chemotherapy (usually CHOP). Rituximab binds the antigen CD20 on the cell surface, which is found in high levels on B-cell malignancies, e.g. NHL. This causes cell lysis.

Main therapeutic use:
- NHL: with or without CHOP chemotherapy (➲ see Non-Hodgkin lymphoma, Treatment, pp. 412–13)
- Chronic lymphocytic leukaemia: combined with chemotherapy (see ➲ Chronic lymphocytic leukaemia, pp. 405–7).

Side effects:
- Infusion-related side effects of rituximab usually occur during the first infusion and include fever, chills, and hypersensitivity reactions (➔ see Hypersensitivity reactions, p. 633).
- Patients should be pre-medicated with paracetamol and chlorphenamine to minimize these side effects.
- Patients at higher risk of this side effect include those with a high tumour burden, pulmonary insufficiency, or tumour infiltration. These patients will also need to be treated with allopurinol or rasburicase to reduce their risk of TLS (➔ see Tumour lysis syndrome, pp. 649–50).
- Rituximab should be used with caution in patients receiving cardiotoxic chemotherapy or in those with cardiovascular disease.

Bevacizumab (Avastin®)

Bevacizumab is a recombinant human monoclonal antibody against the extracellular VEGF. VEGF is produced and secreted by most malignant cells, as it is required for the formation of blood vessels. Its established uses include:
- Metastatic colorectal cancer (➔ see Chapter 24, Colorectal cancer)
- Metastatic breast cancer (➔ see Management of metastatic breast cancer, pp. 303–4)
- Epithelial ovarian, Fallopian tube, or primary peritoneal cancer (➔ see Gynaecological cancers, pp. 385–7).

Serious side effects:
- GI perforation, delayed wound healing
- Infections
- Thrombosis and haemorrhage.

Cetuximab (Erbitux®)

Cetuximab is a monoclonal antibody against the epidermal growth factor receptor (EGFR), causing inhibition of the EGFR signalling pathway. Its main clinical roles are in:
- EGFR-expressing KRAS wild-type metastatic colorectal cancer (➔ see Chemotherapy in advanced colorectal cancer, pp. 326–7)
- Locally advanced, recurrent, or metastatic SCC of H&N (➔ see Head and neck cancer, pp. 418–19).

Main side effects:
- Hypersensitivity reactions (~3%)
- Acneiform rash
- Sore mouth
- Diarrhoea
- Common side effects of TKIs.

Management of common side effects of monoclonal antibodies

Chills and rigors

These begin after around 30 minutes and can last for up to 90 minutes. Pre-medication with paracetamol and chlorphenamine. Provide warmth (hot water bottles, blankets) and reassurance (can be very frightening for both the patient and carers).

Fever and sweating

Occur after chills, often with headache, tachycardia, and hypotension. Pre-medication with paracetamol. Encourage ↑ fluid and food intake.

Diarrhoea

The increasing use of checkpoint inhibitors has ↑ the incidence of potentially life-threatening colitis-induced diarrhoea in patients receiving them (➜ see Chapter 40, Altered bowel function). If colitis is suspected, then immediate treatment should be established with high-dose steroids.

Note: other side effects are covered in the appropriate chapters under those headings.

Biosimilars

In 2017, the first biosimilar monoclonal antibodies was introduced into the UK: biosimilar rituximab for haematological malignancies and biosimilar trastuzumab for breast cancers. It is expected that many more biosimilar MABs will be introduced into clinical practice in the next decade. Nurses will have a key role in informing and reassuring patients about possible changes to their treatment.

Tumour vaccines

Tumour vaccines are a form of biological therapy used to prevent the development of virus-induced cancers and treat non-virus induced cancers.

Virally induced tumours

- A HPV vaccination programme is now in place in the UK to target HPV strains 16 and 18, which are responsible for over 70% of cervical cancer.
- Hepatitis B vaccine is a widely used vaccine against hepatocellular carcinoma (HCC).
- Tumour vaccines are also in development for EBV, which is closely linked to the development of Burkitt's lymphoma and NHL.

Non-virally induced tumours

- Vaccines are also in development for cancers that are not caused by a virus. Tumour cells or extracts of tumour cells can be used as cancer vaccines to enhance an immune response to the relevant tumours.
- Tumour vaccines using tumour-associated antigens are also being developed. These vaccines work by stimulating the immune system to recognize and destroy specific cancer cells.

Talimogene laherparepvec

This is a genetically modified herpesvirus, indicated for the local treatment of unresectable skin and nodal lesions in patients with recurrent melanoma. It is given as a direct intralesional injection. It directly replicates in the lesion and may also stimulate an immune response.

- Main side effects: fatigue, chills, fever, and nausea.

Vaccines are undoubtedly one of the most interesting and exciting areas in the genesis of new cancer therapies. Treatments are in development, targeting breast, colon, bladder, and lung cancers and melanoma.

Future advances

There will be a continuing increase in the knowledge of cancer and related biology, plus technological advances, which allow more accurate and quicker mapping of genes and more accurate diagnosis and delivery of drugs. These may lead to treatments tailored and stratified by individual tumour biology.

Further vaccines to prevent cancer or reduce risk may be just over the horizon. However, it is always difficult to predict the future. Gene therapy was hailed as the new breakthrough over 20 years ago and has yet to make a major impact. Yet few people foresaw the introduction of a tablet—imatinib—with few side effects that would fundamentally change the outlook for individuals with CML.

Nursing issues

Information support

The rapid development of new cancer drugs has a number of implications for cancer nurses at all levels. Nurses working in chemotherapy units have a range of new drugs to get to understand and inform patients about. Many new medications are tablets. These give patients ↑ autonomy when managing their medication. However, they also require highly skilled information giving and support for patients regarding the safety aspects of each particular medication and their safe dosing and storage. Many centres have set up oral chemotherapy clinics to support patients in managing their medication at home, including accurate reporting of side effects and assistance with dose modification or interruption.

Hormonal therapy: background

Some tumour growth is stimulated by one of the body's hormones. These cancers can respond to hormonal therapy; they include breast, prostate, endometrium, renal cell, ovary, testis, and thyroid cancers. The best evidence of this relates to the sex steroid hormones progesterone and oestrogen in breast and endometrial cancers and androgens in prostate cancer.

Breast and prostate cancer treatment accounts for the vast majority of hormonal therapy that is administered, and these are the main focus of this section. More detail of specific disease treatments are found within the relevant chapters (➲ see Chapter 22, Breast cancer; ➲ Gynaecological cancers, pp. 385–7; ➲ Prostate cancer, pp. 57–8).

The aim of hormonal therapy is to inhibit the production of the hormone influencing cancer growth or to block the effect of the hormone on the target organ. By inhibiting the action of the hormone, tumour cell growth can be slowed down or the tumour volume can be shrunk. These treatments can often prolong survival for many years. However, hormone-sensitive tumours can become resistant to hormonal therapy if the treatment fails to reduce the levels of hormones below the level needed for tumour cell growth.

Knowledge of how hormones or hormone antagonists act on cancer cells is the basis of hormone manipulation in cancer treatment. When a hormone enters a cell, it binds to a receptor. This receptor–hormone complex, in turn, stimulates the action of the hormone in the cell nucleus.

The strategies for hormonal therapy modifying tumour growth are:
* To reduce the overall amount of the stimulating hormone in the body
* To prevent the hormone from binding to a cell receptor by:
  * Competitive inhibition of the receptor site
  * Reduction in receptor numbers
* To block the hormone–receptor complex from activating the cell nucleus.

Key hormone targets in cancer therapy

Tumour type	Hormone to be blocked by treatment
Breast	Oestrogen
Endometrium	Oestrogen
Prostate	Testosterone

Oestrogen production

In pre-menopausal women, the ovaries are the source of 90% of oestrogen production. This is regulated by the hypothalamus and the pituitary gland. If oestrogen levels are low, the hypothalamus releases luteinizing hormone-releasing hormone (LHRH), also known as gonadotrophin hormone-releasing hormone (GHRH). This stimulates the release of the gonadotrophic hormones luteinizing hormone (LH) and follicle-stimulating hormone (FSH) by the pituitary. These stimulate the ovaries to produce oestrogen. Many tissues, including breast tissue, have specific receptors, which will be stimulated by oestrogen.

Around 10% of oestrogen is produced in subcutaneous fatty tissue under the control of the adrenal glands. This continues after the menopause. The androgens that the adrenal gland produces are converted to oestrogen by the enzyme aromatase.

Testosterone production

Testosterone, an androgen hormone, is produced by the testes. A small amount is also produced by steroids released from the adrenal glands. Like ovarian production of oestrogen, it is under pituitary control, via LHRH and LH. Prostate tissue is dependent on androgens, mainly testosterone, for growth and function. Androgen receptors are found in the nucleus of prostate cells.

Hormonal therapy in prostate cancer aims to reduce testosterone production (LHRH analogues) or block the androgen receptors (anti-androgens). In recent years, two powerful anti-androgens have been developed for administration where other hormonal therapies and cytotoxic chemotherapy have proven ineffective. Enzalutamide and abiraterone acetate are currently used in metastatic, castrate-resistant (does not respond, or stops responding, to standard hormonal therapies) disease, but research is ongoing into their use in earlier-stage prostate cancer.

Treatment decision-making

There are now several different options involving hormonal therapy for the treatment of breast and prostate cancers. However, hormonal therapy does have both short- and long-term effects, which can have far reaching implications for the QoL, particularly in terms of sexual functioning, for both men and women, and in menopausal symptoms in pre-menopausal women. Patients need accurate and timely information and support to aid them in making decisions about the appropriate treatment approach, as in some cases, patients are asked to make a choice between extended longevity and QoL[13] (→ see Aromatase inhibitors and breast cancer, p. 300, → Prostate cancer, Hormonal therapy alone, p. 374).

Main hormone drugs

The mechanism of action, efficacy, and side effect profile for each medication is taken into account when deciding on the best hormonal therapy for a patient. In some cancers, notably breast cancer, it is possible to assess which hormone receptors are present in tumours. This ensures that the patient receives the most appropriate hormonal treatment for the characteristics of their cancer.

The main classes of hormonal treatments used in cancer include oestrogens, progestogens, and hormone antagonists. (See Table 17.9 which shows examples of drugs in each of these classes and their use in treating different tumour types.)

Table 17.9 Commonly used hormonal therapies

Drug class	Mode of action	Tumour type	Drug
ER antagonist	Block ERs	**Breast:** used as adjuvant in early breast cancer to reduce recurrence post-surgery. Can also be used as a neo-adjuvant, pre-surgery to shrink a tumour	• Tamoxifen
Aromatase inhibitors	Inhibit the conversion of androgens to oestrogens peripherally. This stops the stimulation of oestrogen-dependent tumours	**Breast:** used first, second, or third line in post-menopausal breast cancer (➔ see Chapter 22, Breast cancer)	• Anastrozole • Exemestane • Letrozole • Fulvestrant • Toremifene
Progestogens	Directly reduce adrenal and ovarian sex hormones and indirectly reduce pituitary gonadotrophin levels. Anti-oestrogen	Endometrium, breast, prostate	• Medroxyprogesterone acetate • Megestrol acetate
LHRH agonists	Treatment causes downregulation of the pituitary, preventing LH release and causing a fall in serum testosterone levels in men and serum oestradiol levels in women	**Prostate:** used in a range of situations (➔ see Prostate cancer, pp. 385–7) **Breast:** adjuvant treatment for pre-menopausal women with early disease. Also used in metastatic disease in pre-menopausal women. Initial treatment can cause a flare in symptoms by temporarily increasing hormone levels. Men can be treated with anti-androgens given immediately prior to, and for the first few weeks of, treatment. In women, these effects are managed symptomatically	• Buserelin • Goserelin • Leuprorelin • Triptorelin

(Continued)

Table 17.9 (Contd.)

Drug class	Mode of action	Tumour type	Drug
Anti-androgens	Block testicular and adrenal androgens	**Prostate**: used alone or in combination with LHRH agonists	• Bicalutamide • Cyproterone acetate • Flutamide • Enzalutamide • Abiraterone acetate
Oestrogens	Oppose the action of androgens. This suppresses the growth of androgen-dependent prostate cancer	Prostate	• Diethylstilbestrol • Ethinylestradiol

* More specific treatment information can be seen in ⊕ Breast cancer and ⊕ Prostate cancer.

Hormone testing in breast cancers

As part of the normal pathology assay of breast tumours, all are tested for sensitivity to hormones. This is normally expressed as the degree of oestrogen receptor (ER) or progesterone receptor (PR) positivity. The Allred scale is used, giving a score out of a maximum of 8 (e.g. ER 7/8 and PR 7/8 for a tumour with a high number of both ERs and PRs). These scores are used to guide the provision of hormonal therapies.

References

13 Baumgart J, Nilsson K, Stavreus-Evers A, Kallak T, Sundström Poromaa I. Sexual dysfunction in women on adjuvant endocrine therapy after breast cancer. *Menopause* 2013;20:162–8.

Hormonal therapy: assessment and management of side effects

As with any drug therapy, hormonal therapy can have side effects. Patients need to be assessed regularly for their response to treatment and any side effects they may be experiencing. The main side effects of the drugs are shown in Table 17.10.

The risks and benefits of treatment must be assessed if patients experience severe side effects. It is sometimes beneficial for patients to be prescribed another drug in the same class if they are experiencing severe side effects.

Management of menopausal symptoms

These can be severe and are generally worst in women who are initially premenopausal. Women with breast cancer are also currently advised not to take HRT, so they are more likely to suffer from these symptoms.

Problems include:

• Disruptions to the menstrual cycle, amenorrhoea
• Hot flushes, night sweats (can be severe)
• Difficulty sleeping, fatigue, depression
• Joint pain, headaches
• Vaginal dryness, painful intercourse
• Psychological impact: ageing, body image, loss of fertility.

Patients need detailed and honest information about the whole potential impact of the menopause. An in-depth assessment is useful to plan with each individual what aspects of the menopause, if any, are major issues for her. A management package of pharmacological and non-pharmacological measures can then be planned.

Hot flushes (also occur with men having LHRH treatment)

Can range from frequent and severe to mild. They can be very disruptive, may be accompanied by drenching sweats, and can occur many times a day. They are generally more severe in those having cancer treatments, rather than natural menopause.

Pharmacological approaches

• Use of HRT is generally considered unsafe, due to oestrogen and the risk of breast cancer. However, there is controversy about whether HRT increases cancer recurrence.
• Gabapentin, selective serotonin reuptake inhibitors (SSRIs), e.g. venlafaxine or paroxetine, clonidine. Many women find the side effect profile problematic (see *British National Formulary* for further information).

Self-help/behavioural measures

Many women will employ a range of self-help measures:[14]

• Behavioural modification, e.g. loose-fitting layers of thin, absorbent clothes (cotton)
• Keeping diaries to identify patterns of flushing and exacerbating factors

Table 17.10 Common side effects of hormonal therapy

Drug	Common side effects
Tamoxifen	↑ risk of endometrial cancer, DVT and stroke, mood swings, cataracts, hot flushes, fatigue, irregular menstrual cycles, vaginal discharge or bleeding, vaginal skin irritation, rashes, GI disturbances, headache, visual disturbances
Anti-androgens	Loss of libido, impotence, damaged liver function, steroidal effects, hypertension, fluid retention, seizures
Aromatase inhibitors	Hot flushes, osteoporosis, joint pains, drowsiness, fatigue, lethargy, rash, vaginal dryness, pain on intercourse
Progestogens	Nausea, fluid retention, weight gain, tremors, sweating, muscular cramps, Cushingoid features
LHRH analogues	Women: tumour flare, joint pains, loss of libido, fatigue Men: loss of libido, impotence, tumour flare, gynaecomastia
Oestrogens	Sodium retention with oedema, thromboembolism, jaundice, nausea, impotence, gynaecomastia (men)

- Complementary therapies, e.g. evening primrose oil, black cohosh (limited evidence of effectiveness)
- Cognitive strategies that have been effective include relaxation techniques. These may also improve other side effects and feelings of control in general[15] (➲ see Progressive muscle relaxation, p. 588).

Osteoporosis

- Dietary advice regarding ↑ calcium, exercise; improved fitness and muscle strength, monitoring for bone density. Dietary and exercise advice should also consider issues of weight gain

Body image
(➲ See Body image, p. 607.)

Sexual health issues
(➲ See Sexuality and cancer, p. 606.)

Further reading

Tobias J, Hochhauser D. *Cancer and its Management*, 7th ed. Oxford: Blackwell; 2014.

National Institute for Health and Care Excellence (2018). *Early and Locally Advanced Breast Cancer Overview* (section on adjuvant endocrine treatments). Available at: ℛ https://pathways.nice.org.uk/pathways/early-and-locally-advanced-breast-cancer

References

14 Fenlon D. Endocrine therapies. In: Corner J, Bailey C (eds). *Cancer Nursing: Care in Context*, 2nd ed. Oxford: Blackwell Press; 2008. pp. 262–79.

15 Fenlon D. A randomized controlled trial of relaxation training to reduce hot flashes in women with primary breast cancer. *J Pain Symptom Manage* 2008;35:397.

High-dose therapy (autologous transplant)

Principles and uses of high-dose therapy

Many haematological cancers are treated more effectively by higher doses of chemotherapy and radiotherapy than by lower doses. Continuing to escalate the dose given might theoretically increase the cure rate. However, the dose-limiting factor is the toxicity to normal tissues. The first tissue to be seriously affected is the bone marrow. Bone marrow suppression results in:

- Neutropenia—with ↑ risk of infection, particularly by bacteria and fungi
- Anaemia—with resulting dependence on red cell transfusions
- Thrombocytopenia (low platelets)—with ↑ risk of bleeding and dependence on platelet concentrate transfusions.

High-dose therapy (HDT) with autologous stem cell support has been developed to overcome the problem posed by bone marrow toxicity. High doses of chemotherapy and/or radiotherapy are administered, followed by infusion of haematopoietic (blood-forming) stem cells. These have been previously collected from the patient and stored, in order to speed the recovery of the bone marrow and to minimize the risk of resulting marrow suppression. HDT is used routinely in a number of situations (see Table 18.1).

Note: HDT should, in theory, improve survival for patients with solid tumours. However, results from clinical trials of HDT in solid tumours have been extremely disappointing.[1]

Stem cell priming, collection, and storage

Prior to the HDT procedure, stem cells from the patient must be collected and stored. The most common way of collecting stem cells is peripheral blood stem cell (PBSC) collection.

Stem cell priming

Three approaches are used to increase the number of haematopoietic blood cells circulating in the peripheral blood of the patient (stem cell priming):

1. Chemotherapy is administered to the patient. The number of circulating stem cells increases, as the bone marrow recovers from the suppression caused by the chemotherapy. About 10% of patients require admission for neutropenic fever as a result of the conditioning chemotherapy.
2. Growth factor (G-CSF) is administered. This appears to encourage the haematopoietic stem cells in the marrow to dislodge and enter the peripheral circulation. G-CSF is very safe and well tolerated, although it may produce bone pain, which is usually responsive to simple analgesia.
3. Plerixafor is occasionally required to further encourage movement of haematopoietic stem cells from the marrow to enter the peripheral circulation. Its main side effects are nausea and diarrhoea. It is typically given the evening before a stem cell harvest and is often used as a 'rescue' therapy for patients who are struggling to harvest stem cells via more standard methods.

Table 18.1 Indications and outcome for HDT with autologous stem cell support (placing)

Indication	Intended outcome of HDT
Myeloma (frontline therapy)	Increases survival by ~1 year
Relapsed Hodgkin lymphoma responsive to chemotherapy	Potentially curative
Relapsed high-grade NHL responsive to chemotherapy	Potentially curative
Relapsed low-grade NHL responsive to chemotherapy	Induces prolonged remission (unlikely to cure)

Data sourced from BSBMT Indications for BMT, Version Oct 2013. ℬ http://bsbmt.org/wp-content/uploads/2013/10/BSBMT-Indications-Table-Updated-October-20131.pdf

Stem cell collection is usually scheduled for 8–10 days after the initial conditioning chemotherapy is given. A predictive count blood test can be used to determine the number of immature blood cells circulating in the bloodstream, and therefore the best time to collect.

Stem cell collection

PBSC collection is achieved by an apheresis procedure. Blood from the patient is passed through an apheresis machine, which separates out stem cells in a centrifuge. The machine is programmed to collect white blood cells with a molecule on the surface called CD34. This marks out immature blood cells, and some of these cells will be haematopoietic stem cells. These are separated from the rest of the blood, and the remainder of the blood is returned to the patient.

To collect sufficient cells, the patient typically needs to spend 3–4 hours per day on the machine, for up to 2 or 3 consecutive days. The most common complication is citrate toxicity, which occurs because citrate is used in the machine tubing to prevent the blood from clotting. This can reduce blood calcium, which is managed by taking oral calcium. Other complications include reduced platelet count and venous damage.

Special rigid lines or large-bore peripheral cannulae are required for apheresis, due to the high rate of blood withdrawal and return.

Bone marrow harvest is a less common way of collecting stem cells directly from the patient. This involves a general anaesthetic and multiple punctures of the posterior portion of the iliac crest, with a bone marrow aspirate needle. The main side effects are post-operative pain, anaemia requiring a blood transfusion, and complications of the anaesthetic.

Note:

Further detail on haematopoietic stem cell mobilization and apheresis can be found in the European Group for Blood and Marrow Transplantation (EBMT) publication *A Practical Guide for Nurses and Other Allied Health Care Professionals. European Group for Blood and Marrow Transplantation* (➔ see Further reading, p. 255).

Stem cell storage

Stem cells are stored in liquid nitrogen. A chemical called DMSO is added to the cells before freezing, as a preservative to protect them from the freezing process. Stem cells can be stored for as long as is needed, although if they have been stored for many years, a check on their viability should be performed before they are re-infused into the patient.

References

1 Pedrazzoli P, Ledermann JA, Lotz J-P, *et al.*; European Group for Blood and Marrow Transplantation (EBMT) Solid Tumors Working Party. High dose chemotherapy with autologous hematopoietic stem cell support for solid tumors other than breast cancer in adults. *Ann Oncol* 2006;17:1479–88.

Conditioning

Chemotherapy and/or radiotherapy administered prior to stem cell infusion is called conditioning chemotherapy. The role of conditioning therapy in autologous transplantation is simply to kill the cancer. The type of chemotherapy depends upon the condition being treated. Regimens commonly used in the UK are outlined in Table 18.2.

Note: by convention, the day of stem cell infusion is termed day zero (D0), and therefore, conditioning therapies are administered on day −5, −4, etc.

Stem cell administration

On the day of stem cell infusion (D0), the frozen bags containing the cells are brought to the ward. They are placed in a water bath to thaw them to 37°C, prior to being administered to the patient. The usual means of infusion is via a CVC, although a peripheral cannula can also be used.

The most common complication of a stem cell infusion is an allergic-type reaction to DMSO. The patient may complain of an itch or a wheeze or they may develop an urticarial rash. Before the stem cells are given, the patient receives a pre-med of chlorphenamine 4mg orally or 10mg IV and hydrocortisone 100mg IV. In severe cases, anaphylaxis may occur with severe bronchospasm, tachycardia, and hypotension.

The patient is carefully and frequently monitored during and shortly after the stem cell infusion, which is carried out according to local ward protocols. A mild reaction may be treated with:

• Slowing the infusion.
• Hydrocortisone 100mg IV.

A more severe reaction should be treated as an anaphylactic episode (➜ see Anaphylaxis, pp. 633–4).

Patients are also pre- and post-hydrated to counter the dehydrating effects of DMSO. Urine output is carefully monitored throughout. Nausea and sometimes vomiting are also side effects of DMSO; this should be managed preventatively with anti-emetics. The number of bags of stem cells given depends upon the dose of stem cells per bag. This is highly variable and depends upon how well the stem cells were mobilized during the harvest. If many bags are given, the patient may develop headache, lethargy, and possible renal or liver impairment as a result of DMSO toxicity.

Table 18.2 Common conditioning regimens in the UK

Name of regimen	Drugs administered	Condition
BEAM	Bleomycin Etoposide Cytarabine (Ara-C) Melphalan	Relapsed Hodgkin lymphoma Relapsed high- or low-grade NHL
High-dose melphalan	Melphalan	Myeloma
Cy/TBI	High-dose cyclophosphamide Total body irradiation	Lymphoblastic lymphoma

Nursing issues of high-dose therapy

Patients who have had HDT are prone to similar side effects to those who have had standard chemotherapy regimes. However, these are often more severe and prolonged, and patients may face a range of concurrent side effects. The specific side effects are dependent on the drug regimens.

Bone marrow suppression

- Neutropenia: the more prolonged the neutropenia, the greater the risk of severe and overwhelming infection, with patients at risk of septic shock and becoming extremely unwell very quickly (➔ see Treatment of neutropenic sepsis, p. 481). Continued immunosuppression post-transplant can increase the risk of fungal infections and *Pneumocystis jiroveci* pneumonia (PJP). Prophylactic administration of co-trimoxazole is used in this setting to reduce the risk of PJP. Patients are often supported with G-CSF to ensure rapid maturation of newly forming neutrophils (➔ see *Granulocyte colony- stimulating factor*, p. 233). This can reduce neutropenia from near 21 days to around 10–14 days. Patients need to be informed about signs and symptoms of longer-term infections, as well as the need to immediately contact their GP or the haematology centre about any potential signs of infection.
- Nursing assessment includes: daily weight, regular observations, and observation for any signs and symptoms of infection, including daily line site dressings.
- Anaemia and thrombocytopenia: ➔ see Chapter 37, Bone marrow suppression.

Mucositis

This can be severe. Patients may require opioids to relieve pain, and IV fluid support due to inability to take oral fluids. Nutritional support is normally in the form of supplements. Patients can require NG feeding to support them during this stage of the transplant (➔ see Oral mucositis and related problems, pp. 617–19).

Diarrhoea

Often develops at the same time as oral mucositis. This should be actively managed with fluid support—IV fluids, if necessary, to prevent dehydration. Once infection is excluded, then can use loperamide and codeine to reduce output (➔ see Diarrhoea, pp. 502–5).

Alteration in taste

This often occurs because of the high dose of the drugs used and because of mucositis. It can be a troubling symptom and can take many months to resolve.

Veno-occlusive disease

This is a serious, but uncommon, liver condition (➔ see Chapter 19, Allogeneic haematopoietic stem cell transplantation).

Late side effects

Late side effects of HDT are also regimen-dependent. For those receiving radiotherapy, cataracts and long-term infertility are common. Cataracts are unusual in chemotherapy-only regimens. The risk of infertility is more variable in chemotherapy-only regimens. It is more common in older women (➔ see Sexuality and cancer, p. 606).

Patients receiving HDT can require intensive nursing support, involving:

- Administering IV fluids, a range of antimicrobial agents, and nutritional support
- Regular vital signs and blood count monitoring, and daily weights
- Administering blood and platelet support
- Managing infection risk and severe pain from mucositis
- Limiting the psychological effects of isolation and boredom, and separation from family
- Psychological support for both the patient and family facing a life-threatening illness and a rigorous treatment regimen. For some, this may be their first hospital experience or their first experience away from their usual haematology centre.

Such intensive nursing is rewarding but can also be extremely stressful. Nurses in such areas should have access to support networks such as clinical supervision.

Further reading

Browne M, Cutler T. *Haematology Nursing*. Chichester: Wiley-Blackwell; 2012.

European Group for Blood and Marrow transplantation. *Haematopoietic Stem Cell Mobilisation and Apheresis: A Practical Guide for Nurses and Other Allied Health Care Professionals*. Available at: ℅ http://www.iwmf.com/sites/default/files/docs/documents/autologous_stem_cell_collection.pdf

Hoffbrand AV, Moss PAH. *Essential Haematology*, 6th ed. Oxford: Blackwell Science; 2011.

Singer CRJ, Baglin T. *Oxford Handbook of Clinical Haematology* (Oxford Medical Handbooks). Oxford: Oxford University Press; 2009.

Allogeneic haematopoietic stem cell transplantation

Principles of allogeneic transplant

An allogeneic stem cell transplant is where the source of haematopoietic (blood-forming) stem cells is from someone other than the patient. There are a number of reasons why an allogeneic stem cell transplant may be useful:

• It enables high doses of chemotherapy to be given, whilst minimizing the time spent with low blood counts, due to bone marrow suppression. The high doses of chemotherapy are given to increase the chance of eradicating the underlying cancer.
• Autologous stem cells (➔ see Chapter 18 High-dose therapy (autologous transplant)) used in people with haematological malignancies may well be contaminated with cancer cells. An allogeneic source of stem cells prevents this.
• The main benefit is thought to be due to the graft-versus-malignancy (GvM) effect (➔ see Graft-versus-malignancy, p. 258).

Graft-versus-malignancy

Haematopoietic stem cells produce all of the cellular components of blood, including lymphocytes. Lymphocytes are designed to recognize anything that is not of the host (i.e. non-self) and to attack it. Lymphocytes made from a stem cell that is not from the patient (i.e. derived from an allogeneic donor) will recognize the patient as non-self. This has the beneficial effect of seeing the patient's cancer cells as non-self and attacking them—the so-called GvM effect. On the other hand, lymphocytes will also recognize the patient's normal tissues as non-self and attack them. This causes the potentially serious side effect of allogeneic stem cell transplantation called graft-versus-host disease (GvHD) (see Fig. 19.1) (➔ see Graft-versus-host disease, p. 261)

Uses of allogeneic transplant

The main indications for allogeneic stem cell transplantation are:
• Poor-risk acute myeloid leukaemia (AML) in first remission
• Relapsed AML in second remission
• Poor-risk (especially Philadelphia chromosome-positive) acute lymphoblastic leukaemia in first remission
• Aplastic anaemia.

Less common indications include myelodysplasia, relapsed high- or low-grade NHL, Hodgkin lymphoma, myeloma, and myelofibrosis.

Donor source

There are two main sources of donor:
• Matched sibling (brother or sister): this is normally the preferred type of donor. Matching is done using the human leucocyte antigen (HLA) system (see Box 19.1)
• Matched unrelated donor (MUD)—also known as voluntary unrelated donor (VUD). The complication rate is higher using this sort of donor.

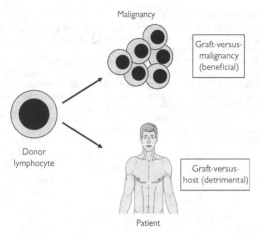

Malignancy

Graft-versus-
malignancy
(beneficial)

Donor
lymphocyte

Graft-versus-
host (detrimental)

Patient

Fig. 19.1 Mechanism of graft-versus-malignancy and graft-versus-host effect.

Box 19.1 Human leucocyte antigen matching

- In order to minimize the complications of a transplant, the donor should be a reasonable HLA match with the patient. HLA is the name given to a number of genes producing molecules involved in the immune recognition process.
- A mismatch in a number of the HLA genes may result in rejection of the transplant or more severe GvHD. For a sibling, the chance of being an HLA match is 1 in 4. If a patient does not have a sibling match, then the chance of finding an unrelated donor depends largely on the ethnic origin of the patient.
- Ethnic minority patients often have great difficulty in finding a match due to the relatively low number of donors from a similar group (and therefore of a similar genetic make-up) on the transplant registers.

Occasionally, stem cells can be obtained from the umbilical cord of a newborn baby, and rarely an identical twin is used as a donor (syngenic transplant). These are an exact HLA match. Though this reduces some of the risks of transplant, such as rejection and GvHD, there is a loss of GvM effect.

Note: a sibling donor is usually preferred over an MUD, as even though both donors may be fully matched, a sibling donor is more likely to be matched for other important genes, which are not currently tested for.

Stem cell collection

Collection of stem cells from a donor is similar to that used for the collection of autologous stem cells from a patient (➲ see Chapter 18, High-dose therapy (autologous transplant)).

The main difference is that priming only involves the use of growth factor injections, and no chemotherapy is used. Most commonly, collection is through PBSC harvest. However, direct bone marrow harvest from the donor's iliac crests can also be used as a source. Donors should be informed and counselled about the different options to support them coming to a decision. Some concerns have been raised over the potential long-term effects of using G-CSF in a healthy donor, but there is currently no good evidence to support these.

Complications of allogeneic transplant

This section will deal with complications specific to allogeneic stem cell transplantation. High-dose chemotherapy and radiotherapy used in the conditioning process also have their own associated complications (➔ see Chapter 18 High-dose therapy (autologous transplant)).

Graft-versus-host disease

GvHD is caused by donor T-lymphocytes recognizing and attacking the recipient's normal tissues. If this occurs within 100 days of the transplant, it is called acute GvHD; if it persists or develops after 100 days, it is called chronic GvHD. Whilst a small amount of GVHD is thought to be a positive development, enhancing the GvM effect, extensive GVHD can be a life-threatening complication.

Predisposing factors include:
- HLA-mismatched transplant
- Cytomegalovirus (CMV)-seropositive patient
- Increasing age of the patient and donor
- Sex-mismatched transplant.

Clinical features

Acute GvHD frequently involves:
- Skin—erythema which may progress to blistering and desquamation
- Gut—diarrhoea which may progress to abdominal pain, ileus formation, and perforation
- Liver—mild alteration in LFTs, jaundice which may progress to fulminant hepatic failure.

Chronic GvHD may affect any organ. It may result in thickened, fibrotic skin, a sore and dry mouth, dry vagina, photosensitive or dry eyes, hepatitis, and lung involvement with obliterative bronchiolitis.

Prevention

A number of measures are taken to reduce the risk of GvHD:
- Donor selection: a good HLA match reduces the risk of GvHD (see Box 19.1)
- Immunosuppression—various immunosuppressive agents which dampen down T-lymphocyte activity are used, e.g. ciclosporin
- Low-dose methotrexate is often used in the early post-transplant period to prevent GvHD
- T-cell depletion of the transplant—although this is effective in reducing GvHD, it is also thought to reduce the GvM effect, leading to higher rates of relapse.

Management

Severe, acute GvHD requires intensive medical and nursing input.
- Accurate measurement of stool volumes should be attempted, as this determines the severity of gut GvHD and guides treatment. Attention is required to the skin around the anus, as this may become excoriated and a site for infection. Strict fluid balance and fluid replacement. Gut biopsy may be indicated.
- Regular fluid balance assessment, including daily or twice-daily weight.

- Careful attention to pressure areas.
- Regular temperature, pulse, blood pressure, respiratory rate, saturations.
- Daily urea and electrolytes, magnesium, calcium, and phosphate, with replacement of depleted electrolytes.
- Patients with GvHD are profoundly immunosuppressed, so that frequent septic screens are needed (blood cultures, CMV, urine cultures, CXR, stool cultures).
- Symptomatic treatment involves:
  - Diarrhoea: loperamide and possibly octreotide. Barrier creams to prevent excoriation, Sudocrem® or Metanium® with olive oil to clean. Ensure ciclosporin and other drugs are given IV, so as to ensure absorption
  - Liver failure: avoidance of sedatives, monitoring of electrolytes and blood glucose. Reviewing of all IV drugs, so as to reduce toxicity on the liver
  - Pain: paracetamol initially, but opioids are often necessary. Involvement of the acute pain team or palliative care team may be indicated if difficult to manage
  - Skin: pressure area care needs to be managed extremely carefully, with regular turning and special mattresses essential. Daily bath/wash with use of emollients to dry affected skin.
- Specific treatment involves:
  - Continuing GvHD prophylaxis, usually with ciclosporin or tacrolimus. Ciclosporin levels are monitored frequently to ensure correct dosing and minimize toxicity
  - IV high-dose steroids (methylprednisolone).

Note: if the GvHD is steroid-resistant, the outlook is extremely poor, with a very high mortality rate. Other immunosuppressant options exist but have limited success rates.

GvHD nursing

Nursing a patient with severe GvHD is extremely complex and stressful. The symptoms are difficult to manage. The effect on the patient's body image and self-esteem can be dramatic. In the worst-case scenario, a patient may have a combination of skin desquamation, severe liver failure, and continuous uncontrollable diarrhoea. They may be confused and in severe pain. Intensive physical and psychological support is required for both the patient and their family. These patients need at least one-to-one nursing care, possibly even more at times. Involvement of palliative care specialists can support effective symptom management and work with the emotional distress of the family and other carers.

Veno-occlusive disease

Hepatic VOD is due to the obstruction of small blood vessels within the liver, which causes damage to the surrounding liver cells. It usually occurs due to chemotherapy and/or radiotherapy given during an allogeneic stem cell transplant. Increasing age, previous hepatic disease or dysfunction, and prior intensive chemotherapy are risk factors for developing VOD. Although approximately half of all cases resolve, the mortality rate can be over 90% in severe cases.

Clinical features
The following typically occur within 21 days of the transplant:
- Enlarged liver
- Ascites
- Weight gain of >5% from baseline
- Raised bilirubin.

Prevention
A continuous infusion of low-dose unfractionated heparin can be used during the transplant period to reduce the risk of VOD.

Treatment
- Supportive care:
  - Ascites: low-salt diet, avoid saline infusions, cautious use of loop diuretics such as furosemide
  - Confusion (hepatic encephalopathy): avoid sedatives and opiate analgesia; correct known causative factors such as constipation, electrolyte imbalance, and infection
  - Avoid drugs which damage the liver, and ensure ciclosporin level is not too high as the kidneys are at risk of damage.
- Specific treatment:
  - IV defibrotide infusion.

VOD nursing
- Meticulous skin hygiene, with daily bath/wash to remove build-up of waste products. Use of emollients can help manage itch due to bilirubin build-up.
- Continuous assessment of fluid balance and abdominal girth and weight is essential. It allows assessment of the distribution of the patient's body fluids, guiding appropriate therapy.
- Patients can be confused, requiring psychological support and maintenance of a safe environment. They may also develop respiratory symptoms due to hepatosplenomegaly and pleural effusion. If liver damage is severe, then pain management can be problematic and may require support from the specialist palliative care team.

Cytomegalovirus reactivation and disease
CMV is a common infection in children and young adults. After an acute infection, the virus persists in the body without causing disease (a state called latency). If that person then becomes profoundly immunosuppressed, the virus can reactivate. They may be initially asymptomatic (see Fig. 19.2), but continued reactivation leads to CMV disease, which can be very serious.

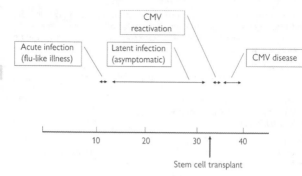

Fig. 19.2 Stages of CMV infection in a patient who has an allogeneic stem cell transplant aged 32.

In the past, CMV disease was a major killer of stem cell transplant patients, but with improved detection of reactivation before it can cause disease, along with treatment at this stage (called pre-emptive treatment), death from CMV disease is now thankfully rare.

CMV management
The patient and their donor are tested for CMV immunoglobulin prior to the transplant. If the patient or donor are CMV-positive, then the patient is tested regularly for CMV reactivation. If two consecutive tests are positive, then treatment with ganciclovir is commenced. Foscarnet is used for ganciclovir-resistant cases.

Prevention of CMV
* Aciclovir prophylaxis is often given to transplant patients where the donor or the recipient is seropositive.
* If the patient and donor are CMV-seronegative, patients receive CMV-negative blood products before and after the transplant.

Note: the risk of transmission of the virus in leucodepleted blood products (which are now routinely used) is very low, and in an emergency, CMV-unscreened products can be used.

CMV disease
CMV may manifest in a variety of ways, but it most commonly causes colitis (with bloody diarrhoea) or pneumonitis (with cough and breathlessness). Treatment is as for CMV reactivation, i.e. ganciclovir and foscarnet for ganciclovir-resistant cases. IV immunoglobulin can also be used.

Other infections
Stem cell transplant patients are susceptible to a wide variety of infections, due to profound immunosuppression. The most common are bacterial, causing line infections, pneumonias, UTIs, and septicaemia.

Table 19.1 Relatively common infections in allogeneic stem cell transplant patients

Infection	Clinical problem	Treatment
Invasive fungal infection, e.g. Aspergillus	Pneumonia (common), abscesses, e.g. liver, brain	Antifungals, e.g. amphotericin, voriconazole, caspofungin
PJP	Pneumonia (may cause pneumothorax)	High-dose co-trimoxazole
Respiratory syncytial virus (RSV)	Pneumonitis	Nebulized ribavirin

The exact treatment depends on the type of infection and the time elapsed since the transplant. A patient who has recently had a transplant should be treated urgently with broad-spectrum antibiotics, even if they are not neutropenic, as they remain profoundly immunosuppressed (see Table 19.1).

Interstitial pneumonia syndrome

Interstitial pneumonia syndrome (IPS) may occur anytime, from a few days to several months after treatment when the patient has returned home. High-dose chemotherapy/radiotherapy can directly damage the cells of the lungs. A dry, non-productive cough or shortness of breath are both early manifestations of IPS. Any patient experiencing these symptoms after HDT should be seen by a haematology doctor immediately, since this can be a fatal complication. It is essential that patients, carers, and their GPs are fully informed about this risk.

Long-term survival

Allogeneic stem cell transplantation is a high-risk procedure. The mortality rate from the procedure varies greatly, according to:

- Age
- General fitness, performance status, and comorbidities of the patient
- Disease being transplanted
- Remission status at time of transplant
- Type of transplant (sibling versus MUD)
- CMV status of the donor and recipient.

For conventional transplantation in a young person, the usual mortality rate of the procedure is in the region of 15–20% for a matched sibling transplant.

Reduced-intensity conditioning transplants

The high mortality rate of a conventional transplant means that it is only suitable for patients up to their mid 40s. This is due to the intensity of the conditioning chemotherapy, which typically involves high-dose cyclophosphamide and often total body irradiation.

In an attempt to reduce the mortality rate and extend the age limit, reduced-intensity conditioning (RIC) transplants have been developed. These use more gentle conditioning regimens, with the aim of preventing graft rejection by the patient.

Once the transplant has engrafted, more reliance is placed on the GvM effect to eradicate any residual disease. Various protocols have been developed, with more or less intense conditioning regimens. In the UK, a typical conditioning regimen involves fludarabine and melphalan or cyclophosphamide with or without alemtuzumab to deplete T-cells.

RIC transplants are increasing in popularity. The indications are as for conventional transplantation (→ see Uses of allogeneic transplant, p. 258), but the age and fitness of the patient are less of a consideration. RIC is now commonly performed in patients into their mid to late 60s. The mortality rate is around 10%. The development of RIC has led to renewed interest in treating solid tumours such as RCC with high-dose chemotherapy. This is currently still under evaluation.

Donor lymphocyte infusions

In the event of a relapse after an allogeneic stem cell transplant, one treatment option available is donor lymphocyte infusions (DLIs). Lymphocytes are collected from the original donor—this usually requires just one additional apheresis session (with no priming required).

The lymphocytes are then infused into the patient at a given dose, according to the patient's weight. The T-lymphocytes in the infusion then recognize the patient's cancer cells as non-self and attack them.

The lymphocytes themselves would normally be rejected by the patient, but they are not, due to the previous stem cell transplant. The main disadvantage of DLIs is that they can induce GvHD.

Further reading

Browne M, Cutler T. *Haematology Nursing*. Chichester: Wiley-Blackwell; 2012.

Hoffbrand AV, Moss PAH. *Essential Haematology*, 6th ed. Oxford: Blackwell Science; 2011.

Singer CRJ, Baglin T. *Oxford Handbook of Clinical Haematology* (Oxford Medical Handbooks). Oxford: Oxford University Press; 2009.

Chapter 20

Clinical trials

Clinical trials in the cancer setting

Research governance and research guidelines in a clinical setting

Historically, medical experiments were conducted with only the ethics and morality of individual researchers and some local agreements guiding the conduct of the study. However, following the horrific medical experiments conducted during World War II, there has been international and national guidelines and legislation developed to regulate trial conduct.

These are now specified in the **International Conference of Harmonisation Tripartite Guidelines for Good Clinical Practice** (ICHGCP), which sets out responsibilities for researchers and underpins current research practice. It is a requirement that researchers in the UK are trained in ICHGCP.

They are also embedded in European legislation through the **EU Clinical Trials Directive 2001**—which aims to allow agents trialled and licensed in one European country to be adopted in another, without further research being required.

Ethics approval

Before a clinical trial can proceed within the UK, it needs to have approvals from properly constituted independent ethics committees (independent of both the researchers whose work they are reviewing and those who pay for the research). Until a research ethics committee approves a clinical trial, researchers cannot ask any participants to join it.

Ethics committees that review clinical trials in the NHS are part of the Health Research Authority's National Research Ethics Service (NRES). The committees will ensure that the dignity, rights, safety, and well-being of participants are key considerations when granting approval for a clinical trial.

Medicines and Health Care Products Regulatory Authority

Where medicinal products are involved in a clinical trial, approval for use of the product must be sought from the Medicines and Health Care Products Regulatory Authority (MHRA). Following review of the preclinical and clinical data, if the product is deemed to be safe, then clinical trial authorization will be granted.

Research and development department

This is needed where clinical trials involve NHS staff, patients, data, or equipment. Where their Trust is involved in a clinical trial, the Chief Executive needs to grant approval.

In order to gain approval from the regulatory bodies, clinical trials must have undergone expert independent scientific review. All research staff participating in clinical trial activity must be qualified by education, training, or experience and must have appropriate supervision, support, and training. The training needs of research staff are not clearly described; however, in practice, biannual evidence of ICHGCP training is considered acceptable in many hospital settings.

Since 2005, the Research Governance Framework (RGF) has outlined the responsibilities of the main people and organizations involved in health and social care research. In the UK, the Health Research Authority takes responsibility for issuing advice and guidance on research in England. From March 2016, the new 'UK Policy Framework for Health and Social Care' replaces the RGF.

Among the many responsibilities of the clinical trial sponsor is the role of the monitor [monitors visiting trial sites are often referred to as Clinical Research Associates [CRAs]). This involves checking that the data being collected are accurate, which will positively impact on the quality of the results and subsequent analysis of trial data. The sponsor must ensure that any suspected unexpected serious adverse reactions (SUSARs) are reported promptly, promoting safety for trial participants.

Further information on the conduct of clinical trials can be found at the NHS Health Research Authority website, available at: ℘ http://www.hra.nhs.uk/

Phases of clinical trials

The initial phase of all new drug development is the preclinical stage where new agents, or combinations, are investigated by performing pharmacological, pharmacokinetic, and toxicology testing in animal and *in vitro* models. Once an agent, or a combination, has been found to be of potential benefit, it is moved from the laboratory to clinical testing.

Clinical trials are then conducted using human volunteers. In most cancer treatment trials, patients with cancer are most likely to be the participants in the trial, rather than the more common use of healthy volunteers. This is due to the toxic nature of many of the agents being tested. The trials are conducted in three phases.

Phase I: is it safe?

This is the first use in humans, and in cancer, treatments are usually offered to patients for whom there is no other available treatment. The primary aim is to determine the maximum tolerated dose.

They may be offered to patients with a variety of tumour types. The exceptions to this are trials of gene therapies and vaccines which are specifically designed for individual tumour types and therefore will only be tested on patients with an appropriate diagnosis.

The dose of the drug is ↑ in stages until the toxicity is considered unacceptable. Three to six patients are treated at each dose level, and the level is only ↑ once the toxicity has been assessed at the lower dose and it is considered safe to increase. Pharmacokinetic and pharmacodynamic testing is conducted as part of the phase I trial, which will determine the potential treatment schedules for further trials.

Phase II: does it work?

The aims are to assess the activity of the drug in designated tumour types and the toxicity at a given dose and treatment schedule. These trials are normally offered to patients with metastatic disease, and activity is measured by assessing tumour response. Multiple studies of the same drug may be conducted in different tumour types at the same time. The number of patients participating in each phase II study varies but often start recruiting up to 25, then may increase if found to be effective.

Phase III: is it better than what is already being used?

This is the first time a new agent, or combination, will be directly compared with either the current standard treatment, or placebo where no standard treatment exists. This comparison takes the form of a randomized controlled trial. QoL is also normally assessed during this type of trial, as there may be little difference in terms of efficacy, but significant differences in terms of tolerability and impact on patient well-being.

In addition, some drugs are followed up in phase IV or post-marketing studies. Phase IV trials in cancer treatments are uncommon, as many of the phase III trials have an endpoint of evaluating survival and therefore follow patients up for life, rendering the phase IV trial superfluous.

Nurses' responsibilities

The key responsibility for nurses caring for patients participating in clinical trials is safety by minimizing risk and maximizing benefit. The role and responsibilities for nurses working in clinical trials are multi-faceted and include education, advocacy, coordination, care giving, and paperwork/administration.

Education

- **Clinical staff**: educating clinical staff about the trial protocol, specific study requirements, and treatment plan. Where new agents or combinations are being used, education on expected and potential side effects is needed.
- **Patients and families**: all information required for informed consent, which will include randomization and registration process, explanation of the treatment, its mode of action, treatment goals, study requirements, e.g. how frequently hospital/clinic visits occur, potential side effects, and complications.

Patient advocate

- Assess patient understanding of clinical trial and participant rights.
- Assess patient ability to adhere to the demands of the trial protocol.
- Communicate assessments of specific issues and concerns to study personnel and the patient's clinician.
- Support patient withdrawal from the trial—it is important that patients understand their right to withdraw from the study at any point, without affecting their future care.

Coordination of trial

- Ensure necessary regulatory approval is in place.
- Ensure patients are suitable and eligible for trial entry.
- Ensure the trial protocol is adhered to by patients and clinicians.
- Day-to-day organization of participant pathways—patient and researcher in the right place at the right time, treatment available when needed, registration of patient, and, where appropriate, randomization.
- Once a patient is in the trial, ensure trial investigations and activities are carried out in a timely fashion, e.g. coordinating scan dates, blood tests, and patient follow-up visits.
- Liaison with other agencies such as drug companies.

Care giver

- Support with diagnosis and prognosis.
- Administration of trial agent(s).
- Assessment of side effects and toxicity.
- Collecting blood and urine samples, recording observations, further tests, such as electrocardiograms (ECGs), as required by the study protocol.

Paperwork/administration

It is essential to keep complete documented records of all trial information. Source data must be available, and every trial record must be completed in full. Data are transferred from medical notes or a specifically designed data capture record onto case report forms.

Essentials include:
- Case report form completion
- Adverse event reporting
- Management of investigator and study files
- Production of data collection tools, e.g. brief study guide or patient diary card, specific for each clinical trial and suitable for use in their own area.

See the Medical Research Council website[1] for further guidance.

Research nurses may have the greatest working knowledge of the protocol and, as such, may be utilized in a consultancy role for the duration of patient recruitment and treatment.

Ward, clinic, and day unit nurses

The responsibilities of department nurses are very similar to those of the research nurse. The challenge for these nurses is that trial activity is only a limited aspect of their role, yet they need to understand the trial protocol, treatment schedule and intent, possible side effects, and trial risks and benefits. Each clinical area is likely to be caring for patients entering a broad spectrum of trials, and therefore, the nurses need to have enough knowledge of each trial to ensure patient safety.

Vulnerable patients

Vulnerable patients can be defined as those who may suffer harm, abuse, or maltreatment as a result of ↓ capacity, disempowerment, or minority grouping.

Vulnerability may be due to:
- Physical or mental illness, including incurable disease
- Low education level
- Position in health-care hierarchy
- Physical surroundings, e.g. hospital environment
- Age—both elderly and children
- Ethnic minorities
- Homelessness.

Anyone currently in receipt of health care may be considered to be vulnerable, by the nature of their dependence on professional support. In addition to this, no clinical trial is free from risk, and every clinical research patient may therefore be considered to be vulnerable. It is the responsibility of both researchers and ethics committees to reduce the levels of vulnerability by ensuring that the principles of minimizing risk, whilst maximizing benefit, are adhered to.

Reasons for trial participation

Willingness to participate in clinical trials may be due to many factors, which include:

- Financial gain—many healthy volunteers are paid for participating in clinical trials
- Expectation of benefit associated with participation
- To please health-care professionals or the family
- To gain access to medicinal agents which may otherwise not be available
- To participate in the development of future treatments.

Reducing risk

These factors may increase vulnerability, particularly the patient's desire to please clinicians in charge of their care and expected benefits associated with participation. Patients may fear rejection by clinicians if they do not agree to participate in trials or may see participation as a means of thanking clinicians for previous care. Other patients may agree to take part, as they believe they will receive the best treatment and may have unrealistic expectations of the impact the treatment may have on their disease.

Gaining valid informed consent attempts to minimize vulnerability and ensures that clinical trial participants are fully aware of what they are agreeing to. Information regarding study participation should be given to the potential recruit at least 24 hours before they consent to taking part, except in emergency situations, though these are rare in cancer clinical trials. Information should be both written and verbal, giving the patient the opportunity to ask questions, and they should be encouraged to discuss their participation with family or friends or with health-care professionals not associated with the research, e.g. GP, district nurse, CNS.

The researcher must ensure that, prior to participation in the trial, the patient understands what taking part will involve. Participation may include not only exposure to novel agents, but additional investigations and tests, extra hospital and clinic visits, or prolonged hospital admissions. The researcher must also ensure that participants are free from duress. This may be due to a sense of obligation to clinicians or because of limited availability of potential treatments outside of a clinical trial. This is often relevant in randomized controlled trials where a new treatment has been found to be effective but is not yet licensed for general use. Patients need to clearly understand the randomization process, as they may be randomized to an arm of the trial which does not include the new treatment.

Informed consent is an ongoing process and is a means of continuing to protect vulnerable patients. The responsibility for ensuring valid consent rests with each individual engaged in the research process. It is also essential that patients understand that they can withdraw from clinical trials at any time without giving a reason and that this decision will not negatively impact on their future care.

Researchers have a duty of care towards research participants, and in most cancer trials, this relationship is complicated by the fact that the researcher is also the clinician in charge of the patient's treatment. Awareness of issues influencing vulnerability and adherence to clinical trial guidelines and legislation will minimize the risk of harm, abuse, or maltreatment. Minimizing vulnerability in groups such as palliative care patients or those near the end of life can enable participation in clinical research, therefore preventing exclusion and disadvantage of the whole cohort.

Further reading

Medicines and Health Care Products Regulatory Authority. *Good Clinical Practice Guide*. London: Stationary Office; 2012.

NHS National Institute for Health Research. Clinical Research Network. Available at: ℘ https://www.nihr.ac.uk/about-us/how-we-are-managed/managing-centres/crn/

References

1 Medical Research Council. Available at: ℘ https://mrc.ukri.org

Management of Major Cancers

Bone and soft tissue cancers

Bone sarcomas

Bone sarcomas are extremely rare, with around 500 new cases per annum in the UK. They are most common in older children, accounting for only 0.1% of all new cancers, but 4% of childhood cancers and 5% of all cancers in teenagers and young adults. As with all cancers affecting younger people, it is essential to have a good awareness of the nursing needs of this group (➲ see Teenage and young adult cancer, pp. 454–8). Sarcomas of the bone are twice as common in ♂ as in ♀.

The main types of bone sarcoma/tumour are:
- Osteosarcoma
- Chondrosarcoma
- Ewing's sarcoma
- Malignant fibrous histiocytoma of bone.

Osteosarcoma is the most common primary bone tumour, accounting for 20% of all cases.

Risk factors

Most patients have no known risk factors. Bone sarcomas are occasionally associated with genetically inherited disease, e.g. Li-Fraumeni syndrome or hereditary retinoblastoma (osteosarcoma).

Presentation

- Painful bony swelling, with warm and red overlying tissues—can be associated with local trauma.
- Axial lesions may cause pain—with compression of abdominal organs, urinary tract, or nerve.
- 10% of Ewing's sarcomas develop fever and a hot swollen limb, presenting similarly to osteomyelitis.
- The most common site for a bone sarcoma is in the long bones of the lower limb. This site accounts for 30% of all cases.

Diagnosis

- Plain X-ray and isotope bone scan.
- CT chest and abdomen. MRI scan of primary lesions and hotspots.
- Trephine or core biopsy.
- In Ewing's sarcoma, a bone marrow aspirate (×2) and trephine from sites distant from known disease.
- Staging is through TNM (➲ see Diagnosis, classification, and staging of cancer, p. 176) plus whether or not the tumour is confined within or beyond the cortex. The cell type (pathological grade) is also important.
- Poor prognostic factors include tumours in the axial skeleton, poor initial response to chemotherapy, high grade, and local recurrence.

Note: within the UK, patients with any suspected bone malignancy must be referred to a specialist reference centre for biopsy and further management, as inappropriate biopsy siting can result in tumour spillage and unnecessary requirement for limb amputation.

Osteosarcoma

This occurs predominantly in adolescence—its peak incidence coincides with the growth spurt. Vascular invasion is common, and it typically spreads to the lung and bone. Overall, the 5-year survival rate is 55–70%.

Management of patients with osteosarcoma

- 2–3 cycles of chemotherapy usually delivered, followed by limb-sparing surgery, followed by further 3–4 cycles of chemotherapy. The most active agents are doxorubicin, cisplatin, high-dose methotrexate, and ifosfamide.
- ~80% of osteosarcomas are treated successfully with limb-sparing techniques. A wide variety of endoprosthetic devices are available, including extendable prostheses for growing children.
- The use of radiotherapy is limited to non-resectable axial osteosarcomas—for those who refuse surgery or who have poor excision margins—and palliative treatment of bone metastases.
- Around 15% of new cases have metastatic disease at presentation. Combined with treatment as above, a subset of these patients can benefit from resection of the metastatic disease, enabling long-term survival in around 20–30% of cases.

Risk versus benefit of limb-sparing surgery

In large, poorly differentiated tumours, the QoL benefits of limb-sparing surgery need to be carefully weighed against the risk of local recurrence.

Ewing's sarcoma

This is a highly malignant rare primary bone tumour, with peak age of 10–20 years. It may affect any bone with 55% arising in the axial skeleton. Blood-borne spread to the lung and bone is common.

Management of Ewing's tumours

Management consists of six cycles of preoperative chemotherapy, followed by limb-sparing surgery ± adjuvant radiotherapy. Further chemotherapy is continued—up to another eight cycles of conventional chemotherapy or HDT with PBSC support.

Note: the intensification of chemotherapy regimens has led to significant improvement in the outcome of treatment, but at the cost of significant toxicities such as severe myelosuppression, risk of neutropenic sepsis, mucositis, and risk of graft-versus-host reaction. Late effects of treatment include cardiomyopathy, nephrotoxicity, infertility, and second malignancy (e.g. leukaemia, osteosarcoma).

Management of metastatic disease

Metastatic disease is initially managed as above (➲ see Management of Ewing's tumours, p. 279), with induction chemotherapy, followed by local therapy to the primary tumour.

- Patients with lung metastases may then be treated with conventional chemotherapy and whole lung irradiation or high-dose chemotherapy with PBSC support (➲ see High-dose therapy (autologous transplant), pp. 250–2).

- Patients with bone or marrow metastases have a poorer prognosis, and high-dose chemotherapy may be considered for many of them.

Chondrosarcoma

- This is a cartilage-forming malignancy of middle to late age. It is the second most common primary bone tumour, accounting for 15% of the incidence.
- Chondrosarcoma typically presents with a painful enlarging mass in the pelvis, proximal femur, humerus, shoulders, or ribs. It is unusual in the distal bones.

Management of chondrosarcoma

Treatment is surgical resection, with limb conservation, if possible. There is no proven role for adjuvant chemotherapy. Radiotherapy is used after incomplete resection or for palliation of advanced disease. The tumour grade is the best prognostic indicator. Grade 1 has a 90% 5-year survival. Grade 3 has a 40% 5-year survival.

Soft tissue sarcomas

Epidemiology and aetiology
- These are rare tumours, with around 3300 cases per annum being diagnosed in the UK in 2010. They account for about 1% of adult cancers and 6% of childhood cancers.
- There are over 70 different histological subtypes.
- Soft tissue sarcomas are occasionally associated with genetically inherited disease or previous radiation exposure.
- The incidence of soft tissue sarcomas has ↑ since the mid 1990s. This is likely to be due to improved diagnostics and data recording.

Presenting symptoms and signs
Most patients present with a painless soft tissue mass. In the UK, the most common sites are on the limbs (25%) and soft tissue of the trunk (10%). Other more common sites are the H&N and retroperitoneum.

Staging system
A combination of grading, tumour size, and evidence of metastatic spread is used. Histological grading and tumour size are crucial. Low-grade sarcomas rarely metastasize and may be dealt with successfully by surgery alone. High-grade sarcomas are locally invasive and typically metastasize via blood supply to the lung.

Pathological classification of soft tissue sarcomas
- Liposarcoma
- Fibrosarcoma
- Malignant fibrous histiocytoma
- Rhabdomyosarcoma
- Leiomyosarcoma
- Angiosarcoma
- Extraosseous Ewing's tumour
- Synovial sarcoma
- Epithelioid sarcoma
- Clear cell sarcoma
- Alveolar soft part sarcoma
- Malignant peripheral nerve sheath tumour
- GIST

Investigations
(➔ See Bone sarcomas, pp. 278–80.)

Management
Surgery
- Ideally, localized sarcomas are managed by complete excision, with clear excision margins, together with removal of any biopsy tract.
- A radical excision—dissection of the tumour and the muscular compartment as one unit, in a major operation, reduces the risk of local recurrence, but it may lead to unacceptable loss of function.

Post-operative radiotherapy may enhance the opportunity for limb preservation. If the disease cannot be completely excised with the conservation of a functional limb, amputation is infrequently indicated.

- For the majority of soft tissue sarcomas, surgery is the main local treatment. Surgery may also be appropriate for local recurrence and metastatic disease, in particular solitary pulmonary metastasis.
- Locally advanced disease not amenable to primary surgery may be treated with preoperative radiotherapy or chemotherapy, in order to facilitate resection.

Chemotherapy

The majority of adult sarcomas are only moderately chemosensitive. The most active agents are doxorubicin and ifosfamide, with response rates of 10–30% in advanced disease.

In 2010, in England, NICE approved the cytotoxic alkylating agent trabectedin for use in treating soft tissue sarcomas. The drug is available on the NHS for patients who have lapsed following standard chemotherapy.

The role of adjuvant chemotherapy remains controversial. For some disease, e.g. extraosseous Ewing's, chemotherapy has a major impact on survival. The benefits of chemotherapy in other adult sarcomas are less clear—it reduces the risk of disease recurrence but has no impact on overall survival.

Radiotherapy

Most adult soft tissue sarcomas are only moderately radiosensitive. The most important role for radiotherapy is in the post-operative adjuvant setting, particularly for high-grade sarcomas that have been treated by wide excision, as microscopic tumours may still be present within the muscle compartment.

Treatment outcome and prognostic factors

Overall, the 5-year survival rate is around 70%; it is nearer 20% for those with metastatic disease at presentation. Treatment outcomes are worse with high-grade disease, large tumours, deep tumours, and visceral/retroperitoneal and metastatic disease at presentation.

Surgical treatments

The main treatments for bone and soft tissue sarcomas are surgery, radiotherapy, and chemotherapy. Support of individuals receiving radiotherapy and chemotherapy is covered in ➲ Radiotherapy, pp. 200–1 and ➲ Systemic anti-cancer therapy, p. 206. This section will look at the surgical treatment and nursing care of these patients.

Types of surgery

- **Endoprosthesis**: removal of diseased bone, usually close to a joint, and insertion of a prosthesis into the body, e.g. to replace part of the femur. An endoprosthesis tends to be very much like a custom-made joint replacement, with a longer stem inserted into the remaining bone left after excision of the diseased bone.
- **Wide excision**: this surgical procedure is used to completely excise the tumour, including a clear margin of normal tissue. This is the most common procedure used in the removal of soft tissue sarcomas. It allows clear removal of the tumour. Wide excision surgery is not always undertaken, e.g. if the tumour involves nerves or blood vessels that cannot be removed without serious loss of function to the patient. If wide excision is not an option, it usually means the only option for surgery is an amputation.
- **Amputation**: removal of a limb in order to completely excise the tumour and disease. Not commonly used, but it may be necessary if the tumour cannot be fully excised with other surgical procedures.
- **Plastic surgery**: the use of plastic surgery is very important in cases where patients have had major soft tissue surgery to remove a tumour. Some patients have flaps moved from other parts of the body to fill the gap left by tumour removal.

Preoperative care

If an amputation is being performed, it is important for the patient to have been seen by a specialist from the prosthetics service. The prosthetics specialist will deal with the patient's concerns and answer questions relating to prosthetics options following surgery.

Issues that will be covered include:
- The exact nature of the surgery
- Prosthetic options
- Phantom limb pain due to nerve damage
- Altered body image.

Having an amputation does not automatically mean that a prosthesis will be available. It depends on the nature of the surgery and how much bone and tissue are left.

It is important to ensure issues of altered body image have been addressed with the patient. Patients can be concerned about how friends and family will react. Sometimes it can be useful to get them to talk to patients who have gone through similar surgery (➲ see Body image, p. 607).

Preoperative exercises are also very important. It can be useful to build up the muscles that are going to be used significantly after amputation, e.g. building up arm muscles if using crutches to mobilize.

Post-operative care

Immediate post-operative care for patients who have undergone limb surgery is largely the same for any post-operative patient (➔ see Surgery, pp. 186–7). However, with limb surgery, it is very important to:

• Observe the limb and surgical site
• Ensure that blood flow and nerve conduction have not been compromised by the surgery
• For patients who have undergone plastic reconstruction with flap surgery, it is **vital** that flap observations, including temperature, Doppler, and capillary refill, are done regularly, beginning with quarter-hourly observations
• If flaps are going to fail, it can happen very quickly. Plastic surgeons need to be contacted directly about any concerns with the flap.

Upper limb surgery

Patients who have undergone upper limb surgery are encouraged to mobilize as soon as possible, to reduce the risk of DVT. Nursing care of these patients may include assistance with all activities of daily living. It is important to remember that having upper arm surgery may mean the patient is unable to do even simple things like drinking from a cup; it is therefore important to ensure that all aids are in place to help the patient.

Lower limb surgery

Patients who have had lower limb surgery will require a longer period of bed rest. Lower limbs support the body weight (unlike upper limbs), and support will be required to recover full walking function.

Infection

It is very important to prevent wound infection, if at all possible, as the consequences can be severe and disabling. If a patient's endoprosthesis gets infected, it could mean the prosthesis will need to be removed. Revision of an endoprosthesis is difficult since:

• More bone may need removing, reducing its function and stability
• If a patient has undergone radiotherapy, they are less able to heal effectively post-surgery
• Patients receiving chemotherapy may be neutropenic or immunosuppressed.

Psychological care

As with all cancers, psychological care of patients and their families is of utmost importance. For patients who have had an amputation, it is important to remember they may well need counselling to help with problems such as altered body image and loss of the limb.

Patients who have undergone proximal femoral endoprosthetic replacement, for example, may need support in terms of sexual health. They may need advice about other ways of enjoying their sex lives, as intercourse may not be possible for a number of weeks. This is because the implant needs time to become completely stable (➔ see Sexuality and cancer, p. 606).

Rehabilitation

Rehabilitation of patients who have had surgery for bone and soft tissue tumours depends on the extent and type of surgery performed. Some patients who have surgery to remove a soft tissue tumour from a forearm, for example, may be back to normal activities in a number of days. Patients having had femoral endoprosthesis insertion may be unable to walk without aids for a number of weeks, and unable to drive for at least 4–6 weeks. Physiotherapy and occupational therapy are very important, as well as nursing care of these patients.

Post-amputation rehabilitation can last for a matter of months or years. For an amputation of the leg, patients may require fitting of a prosthesis. Limb swelling must have gone, in order for the prosthesis to fit correctly. Once fitted, a number of sessions with both physiotherapists and occupational therapists are undertaken to get full and safe use of the prosthesis.

With an upper limb amputation, physiotherapy and occupational therapy are important, as it may be the patient's dominant arm that is missing. Some patients may spend years learning to do everyday routines in a completely different way to what they were used to preoperatively.

There are many makes and models of prosthetic limbs around on the market, and patients need to have guidance as to which would be best for them. It is also seen in practice that many patients who have prostheses made actually find them hard work and manage very well without them.

It is also important for the patients to have contact details of someone, e.g. the CNS. This allows them to feel that they are still being cared for. It gives them a contact for any questions or enquiries that they may have.

Websites

National Cancer Intelligence Network. *Bone Sarcomas: Incidence and Survival Rates in England—NCIN Data Briefing*. Available at: ⅏ http://www.ncin.org.uk/publications/data_briefings/bone_sarcomas_incidence_and_survival

PathologyOutlines.com (2018). *Bone Chapter*. Available at: ⅏ http://pathologyoutlines.com/bone.html

Further reading

Chauhan A, Joshi GR, Chopra BK, Ganguly M, Reddy G. Limb salvage surgery in bone tumors: a retrospective study of 50 cases in a single center. *Indian J Surg Oncol* 2013;3:248–54.

Clark MA, Fisher C, Judson I, Meirion-Thomas J. Soft tissue sarcomas in adults. *N Engl J Med* 2005;353:701–11.

Hogendoorn PC; ESMO/EUROBONET Working Group, Athanasou N, *et al*. Bone sarcomas: ESMO Clinical Practice Guidelines for diagnosis, treatment and follow-up. *Ann Oncol* 2010;**21**(Suppl 5):v204–13.

National Institute for Health and Care Excellence (2006). *Improving Outcomes for People with Sarcoma*. Cancer service guideline [CSG9]. Available at: ⅏ https://www.nice.org.uk/guidance/csg9.

Gastrointestinal stromal tumours

GISTs are sarcomatous tumours which occur largely in the lining of the digestive tract, most commonly (in around 60% of cases) in the wall of the stomach.

Epidemiological data are relatively scanty but suggest that GISTs are a rare cancer, with <1000 cases diagnosed in the UK each year. It is more common in patients over 50 years old but can affect people of any age. It is unclear if there are any risk factors associated with developing GISTs, but very rarely GISTs can occur as part of genetic syndromes. The most important factor in determining the prognosis of a patient with a GIST is resectability of the tumour, which is determined by its size, location, and whether it has metastasized.

Presenting symptoms and signs

- Early disease: tends to be symptom-free. May be found incidentally.
- Larger tumours: common symptoms include bleeding, anaemia, and abdominal pain and/or swelling.

Treatment

Surgery

The ideal primary treatment for GISTs is **surgery**. This should be carried out by an experienced GI surgeon who is working as part of an MDT. Surgery is not without risk, as GISTs can be very friable tumours and prone to bleeding.

Metastatic disease

For tumours which have metastasized and are not operable, **targeted therapies** can be very effective (➔ see Targeted and biological therapies, p. 227). Occasionally, these therapies may also be used in the neo-adjuvant setting to reduce the size of a tumour prior to surgery.

The TKI imatinib (Glivec®) has proven to be a successful treatment for GISTs, often controlling the disease for a number of years. Side effects can include nausea and vomiting, diarrhoea, skin rashes, and myelosuppression.

Sunitinib, another TKI, can be used either if imatinib is not tolerated or as second-line therapy. It has been shown to further extend survival for patients with GISTs for an average of 3 months.

A third TKI regorafenib (Stivarga®) has been shown to have some benefit in patients with GISTs who have progressed on imatinib and sunitinib.

Treatment outcome and prognostic factors

Currently, no survival data are available from the UK, but in the USA, with similar treatment options, the 5-year survival rates for early GISTs are around 90%, falling to around 45% for metastatic disease.

Metastatic bone disease

Bone is the third most common site of metastases, after the liver and lung. Metastatic bone disease (MBD) is actually far more common than primary bone cancer. The most common sites of MBD are the vertebrae, pelvis, ribs, femur, and skull. MBD is particularly common in the following cancers:
- Breast
- Prostate
- Lung
- Kidney
- Thyroid
- Myeloma.

Aetiology

Bone destruction due to metastatic cancer is a complex process, involving:
- Tumour-produced osteoclast (cells that break down bone) factors
- Direct destruction by the tumour cells
- ↑ osteoblast (bone-forming cells) activity, producing unstable bone matrix.

Presenting symptoms

- Pain (most common presentation).
- Impaired mobility.
- Hypercalcaemia (➲ see Malignant-induced hypercalcaemia, pp. 637–40).
- Pathological fracture.
- Spinal cord compression (➲ see Metastatic spinal cord compression, pp. 641–4).
- Bone marrow suppression (➲ see Chapter 37, Bone marrow suppression).

Diagnosis

- History, physical examination.
- X-rays—can miss small lesions.
- MRI or CT scan.
- Bone scans.

Management of bone metastases

Bone metastases are a sign of progressive and advanced disease. Management is therefore based around the principles of effective symptom management and palliative care. Effective pain and mobility management can lead to an improvement in QoL.

Treatment of the underlying disease

This may improve the symptoms of bone metastases. Approaches include chemotherapy, hormonal manipulation, or radiotherapy.

Bisphosphonate therapy

For people with known metastatic bone cancer, bisphosphonates have been shown to reduce bone pain, reduce the incidence and rate of skeletal events (e.g. lytic lesions, pathological fractures), and improve the QoL in a number of different cancers.

Options include IV pamidronate, zoledronic acid, or ibandronic acid. Oral options include sodium clodronate or ibandronic acid. The specific drug, the route, and the dose will depend on the specific disease, as well as the patient's health status and wishes.

Denosumab

This monoclonal antibody targets RANK ligand (RANK-L), which controls the action of osteoclasts. If RANK-L is blocked, osteoclasts are not able to break down bone, thus maintaining the strength of bone, even when cancer is present. Denosumab has been found to be effective in preventing fractures and other bone problems, such as spinal cord compression (➔ see Metastatic spinal cord compression, pp. 641–4), in people with known bone metastases, other than those resulting from prostate cancer.[1]

The drug is administered as a single SC injection, making it a convenient option for controlling bone metastases. However, in the UK, the main factor which prevents denosumab from being used as widely as bisphosphonates. is the comparative cost of the drug. NICE has judged that the drug could be used as an option in preventing skeletal matastases.

Side effects

- Infusion-related reactions are rare but include high temperature and chills, headache, and a temporary increase in bone pain.
- Other side effects are usually mild. They include renal toxicity (zoledronic acid), stomach upset, and nausea and vomiting.
- Denosumab can cause diarrhoea, breathlessness, and rarely, as with bisphosphonates, osteonecrosis of the jaw.

Bone pain

This usually develops progressively over weeks and months. It is often described as dull and unremitting, and is generally worse at night and on weight-bearing. It can include a nerve pain component and can be difficult to fully resolve.

Analgesic management includes:

- Non-steroidal anti-inflammatory drugs (NSAIDs) and opioids, often used in conjunction
- Localized short doses of radiotherapy—can be completely effective in around one-third of patients and give some relief in up to 80% of patients. Strontium-89, a radionuclide which is given IV, is also used to treat multifocal bone pain in prostate cancer. The main side effect is mild bone marrow suppression
- Bisphosphonate therapy (➔ see Bisphosphonate therapy, pp. 287–8) can reduce bone pain as an adjunct to other pain management
- Pain on weight-bearing may require the support of mobility aids such as walking sticks or walking frames. Adapting the individual's home environment with physiotherapy and occupational therapy involvement may also be required.

The nurse's role in assessing the individual's functional ability, including their mobility, is essential to planning effective care. Maintaining maximum independence and the level of desired mobility is an important goal.

Pathological fractures

Bone integrity can be severely reduced due to MBD, leading to bone fractures. Pathological fractures in long bones can cause severe pain and disability. Untreated pathological fractures rarely heal. Rib fractures and vertebral collapse are the most common. Implications of these are pain, restricted breathing, reduced mobility, and risk of spinal cord compression (➲ see Metastatic spinal cord compression, pp. 641–4).

Management

- Orthopaedic surgical stabilization of long bones and pelvic/shoulder area can be successful in reducing pain and re-establishing mobility/function. The aim should be to stabilize the bone for the lifespan of the patient. Careful patient selection is required due to the potential morbidity of such procedures.
- A single dose of post-operative radiotherapy can be given to the site of the fracture.
- Some patients with MBD may be candidates for prophylactic fixation, if they are at high risk of pathological fractures.

Quality of life issues

Bone metastases can have a huge impact on patient and family QoL. Pain and reduced mobility can impact on personal role function, body image, and self-concept, and are also risk factors for anxiety and depression. Individuals can become housebound and isolated. Psychological assessment and support are key elements of care.

Nurses have an important role in discussing the risks of pathological fractures and the possible treatment options with patients and their families. Nurses also need to liaise with other health professionals, such as occupational therapists and physiotherapists, to assist with fracture prevention, e.g. walking aids, education, and environment adaptations.

Spinal cord compression and hypercalcaemia are potential emergency consequences of bone metastases. Nurses have a key role in educating patients and their families about the signs and symptoms of both, and the need to urgently contact a health professional if any of these signs and symptoms develop.

Further reading

British Association of Urological Surgeons (2013). *Multi-disciplinary Team (MDT) Guidance for Managing Prostate Cancer*. Available at: ⅋ http://www.baus.org.uk/_userfiles/pages/files/Publications/MDT%20Prostate%20Cancer%20Guidance.pdf

McQuay HJ, Collins SL, Carroll D, Moore RA, Derry S. Radiotherapy for the palliation of painful bone metastases. *Cochrane Database Syst Rev* 2013;11:CD001793.

Wong MH, Stockler MR, Pavlakis N. Bisphosphonates and other bone agents for breast cancer. *Cochrane Database Syst Rev* 2012;2:CD003474.

References

1 National Institute for Health and Care Excellence (2013). *Review of TA265; Denosumab for Treating Bone Metastases from Solid Tumours*. Available at: ⅋ http://www.nice.org.uk/guidance/ta265/documents/ta265-bone-metastases-from-solid-tumours-denosumab-appendix-b-proposal-paper-presented-to-the-institutes-guidance-executive2

Chapter 22

Breast cancer

Introduction

Epidemiology

- Breast cancer is the most common cancer in ♀ in the UK and Europe—accounting for almost 1 in 3 of cancers in ♀ in the UK.
- In 2011, 49,500 cases of breast cancer were diagnosed in the UK. Currently, there are 12,000 breast cancer deaths per year.
- The incidence of breast cancer in the UK has ↑ by around 72% since the mid 1970s, but since its peak in the mid 1980s, UK ♀ breast cancer mortality has fallen by around 40%.
- ♂ breast cancer is rare, with about 350 cases per annum in the UK.

Risk factors

- Age—the incidence of breast cancer doubles every 10 years until the menopause. After 50 years of age, the rate of increase slows.
- Early menarche and late menopause.
- Having had no children or late age at first pregnancy.
- Genetic predisposition accounts for around 10% of ♀ and 20% of ♂ breast cancers.
- HRT.
- Associations have been shown with obesity and alcohol consumption. It is thought that around 27% of all UK breast cancers might be linked to lifestyle.
- Breastfeeding and physical activity protect against developing breast cancer.

Hereditary breast cancer

Around 25% of ♀ breast cancers is due to hereditary factors with the inheritance of a mutated copy of either the *BRCA1* or *BRCA2* gene, accounting for between 5% and 10% of the total. These mutations bring with them an ↑ risk of breast cancer at an early age and an elevated lifetime risk of breast cancer—to between 45% and 65% by the age of 70 years. There is also an associated risk of ovarian cancer (greater with *BRCA1*). ♂ carriers of either *BRCA1* or *BRCA2* are at ↑ risk of prostate cancer, and for *BRCA2* carriers breast cancer.

The management of hereditary breast cancer is essentially the same as that of non-hereditary disease, though *BRCA1* cancers may be more aggressive.

Pathology

- 85% of breast carcinomas arise in the ducts of the breast. Over 80% of these are invasive.
- DCIS remains within the confines of the ductal basement membrane.
- Lobular carcinomas account for 15% of breast cancers. About 20% of these develop contralateral breast cancer.
- ER and PR status varies between cancers and impacts on prognosis and treatment options.
- In some individuals, the normal protein HER-2 can be found at very high levels on the surface of breast cells. These high levels of HER-2 can be associated with faster-growing breast cancers and cancers that are ER- and PR-negative.

Routes of spread

- Lymphatic regional nodes—most commonly, the axillary; less often, the internal mammary.
- Systemic spread—breast cancers can most commonly metastasize to bone, the lung or pleura, the liver, the skin, and the CNS.

Prognostic factors

(See Table 22.1.)

The most important independent prognostic factors are:

- Tumour size
- Number of histologically positive axillary lymph nodes
- Tumour grade (a lower-grade tumour has a better prognosis)
- Other prognostic factors include:
  - Hormone receptor status (ERs and PRs)
  - HER-2 over-expression
  - Histological subtype
  - Lymphovascular invasion
  - Proliferative index (rate of cell division in the tumour).

Table 22.1 Nottingham prognostic index (NPI) calculation

NPI = (0.2 × pathological tumour size in cm) + grade (1–3) + axillary node score

This scale combines tumour size, histological grade, and lymph node involvement to give a predictive prognostic score.

Axillary node status	Score
No lymph nodes positive	1
1–3 lymph nodes positive	2
>3 lymph nodes positive	3
NPI	**Prognosis**
<3.41	Good
3.41–5.4	Intermediate
>5.4	Poor

Reprinted from Todd J.H. *et al* (1987) Confirmation of a prognostic index in primary breast cancer *Br. J. Cancer* **56**:489–492, with permission from The Macmillan Press.

Further reading

Dixon JM. *ABC of Breast Diseases*, 4th ed. Oxford: BMJ Publishing Group; 2012.

Early Breast Cancer Trialists' Collaborative Group. Effect of radiotherapy after mastectomy and axillary surgery on 10-year recurrence and 20-year breast cancer mortality: meta-analysis of individual patient data for 8135 women in 22 randomised trials. *Lancet* 2014;383:2127–35.

Foxson S, Lattimer J, Felder B. Breast Cancer. In: Yarbro CH, Wudjcik D, Gobel B (eds). *Cancer Nursing: Principles and Practice*, 7th edn. Sudbury: MA: Jones and Bartlett; 2010. pp. 1092–137.

Diagnosis and staging

Presentation

- Abnormal screening mammogram results in 28% of cases. (This is increasing due to increase in screening up to 70 years of age.)
- Breast lump or thickening.
- Axillary tumour.
- Breast skin changes such as dimpling, puckering, or erythema.
- Nipple changes such as inversion or discharge.
- Persistent breast tenderness or pain.

Note: less commonly, there may be symptoms from metastatic disease such as bone pain, pathological fracture, or spinal cord compression. (See Box 22.1 for criteria to refer urgently to a breast clinic.)

In the UK, 43% of breast cancers are diagnosed following an urgent ('2-week wait') referral for suspected cancer, and a further 16% are diagnosed following a non-urgent GP referral. Only 5% of breast cancers are diagnosed following an emergency presentation, which is low, compared to other tumour types. As with other tumour types, diagnosis as an emergency presentation is associated with higher levels of social deprivation.

Diagnosis

The diagnosis of breast cancer is made by 'triple assessment', including:
- A full clinical examination
- Bilateral mammography, often combined with US
- Fine-needle aspiration (FNA) cytology and/or core biopsy.

Box 22.1 Indications for referral to breast clinic

Screen-detected breast cancer
- Breast lump:
  - Any new discrete lump
  - New lump in pre-existing nodularity
  - Asymmetrical nodularity persisting after menstruation
  - Abscess/inflammation which does not settle after one course of antibiotics
  - Persistent or recurrent cyst
- Pain:
  - Associated with a lump
  - Intractable pain which interferes with the patient's life and fails to respond to simple measures (well-supporting bra, simple analgesics, abstinence from caffeine, trial of evening primrose oil)
  - Unilateral persistent pain in post-menopausal women
- Nipple discharge:
  - In any women aged >50 years
  - In younger women if bloodstained, persistent single duct or bilateral, sufficient to stain clothes
  - Nipple retraction, distortion, or eczema
- Change in breast skin contour
- Axillary lump and strong family history

In a few cases where there is still uncertainty, excision biopsy of the breast lesion may be required. The axilla is staged surgically in patients with invasive disease. A CXR and blood tests are done preoperatively; a bone scan or CT scan may be done if there is advanced local disease or signs/symptoms of metastatic spread.

Breast cancer is staged using the TNM staging system (➔ see Diagnosis and classification, p. 184). (See Table 22.2 for prognostic relevance of different stages.)

Table 22.2 Breast cancer survival rates—based on stage of disease

Stage	5-year survival (%)
1	99
2	88
3	55
4	15
Overall	86

Management of non-invasive breast cancer

Ductal carcinoma *in situ*

Treatment options
Surgery/radiotherapy
- Options are a simple mastectomy or lumpectomy and breast irradiation.
- Mastectomy remains the standard treatment for large *in situ* cancers, multifocal disease, and recurrence of DCIS.
- The risk of recurrence is <10% at 5 years for either treatment.

Adjuvant hormone therapy
Half of local recurrences are invasive. Clinical trials with aromatase inhibitors are under way to assess their role in preventing recurrence.

Lobular carcinoma *in situ* (also referred to as lobular neoplasia)

The management of lobular carcinoma *in situ* (LCIS) is controversial. Strictly speaking, it is not a pre-malignant condition, but it does identify women at ↑ risk of developing invasive breast cancer, in either breast.

Many cases are managed by wide local excision and regular mammogram surveillance.
- Problems include:
  - LCIS commonly missed on mammograms
  - Risk of multifocal disease in the same breast (ipsilateral)
  - Risk of disease in the other breast (contralateral).

Risks of overtreatment of '*in situ*' breast cancer

Screening programmes have led to many more early-stage non-invasive breast cancers being diagnosed and treated surgically. There has been recent criticism of the trend for aggressively treating these '*in situ*' breast cancers. Recent research has questioned whether many of these would not have developed into more invasive cancers in many cases and that a more careful monitoring policy for these cancers might be more appropriate.[1]

For all patients with breast cancer, the key to selecting the optimum treatment is multidisciplinary discussion, including radiology, pathology, surgery, oncology, and CNS input. Appropriate treatment options can then be presented to the patient to help them choose, according to their individual circumstances and preferences.

References

1 Is Observation Without Surgery a Viable Strategy for Managing Ductal Carcinoma in Situ? available at ℘ http://www.ascopost.com/issues/november-10-2016/is-observation-without-surgery-a-viable-strategy-for-managing-ductal-carcinoma-in-situ/?utm_source=TrendMD&utm_medium=cpc&utm_campaign=The_ASCO_Post_TrendMD_0

Management of early breast cancer

Introduction

Early breast cancer is defined as disease that can be completely removed by surgery (T1–3 and N0–1 tumours). The management of early breast cancer involves:

- Surgical treatment of the breast and axilla
- Pathological assessment and staging to help direct adjuvant therapy, including chemotherapy, radiotherapy, and endocrine therapy.

Breast surgery

- The options are:
  - Wide local excision followed by breast irradiation
  - Mastectomy.
- The local recurrence rate for each is <10% after 10 years' follow-up.
- The preferred treatment for the majority of T1–2 breast cancers is wide local excision, followed by breast irradiation.
- Breast conservation may not always be appropriate, e.g.:
  - Multifocal disease
  - Large tumour in a small breast
  - Where breast irradiation would be contraindicated
  - Some patients prefer mastectomy, not least because of the possible avoidance of radiotherapy.

Breast reconstruction can be offered after surgery, either at the time of primary surgery or at a later date (➲ see Breast reconstruction, pp. 305–7).

Axillary surgery

Minimal surgery, rather than lymph node clearance, should be performed to stage the axilla for patients with early invasive breast cancer and no evidence of lymph node involvement on US or a negative US-guided needle biopsy. Pre-treatment US evaluation of the axilla should be performed for all patients being investigated for early invasive breast cancer.

Sentinel node biopsy

This is now the preferred technique for assessing the involvement of the axilla and is standard practice across the UK. The aim is to identify node-negative patients and to spare them axillary clearance by providing more effectively targeted treatment.

Axillary sampling

A minimum of four lymph nodes are sampled from the lower axilla.

If positive, they are treated by axillary clearance or, more commonly, by axillary radiotherapy. There is less morbidity for node-negative patients, with equivalent local control rates and survival to total axillary clearance.

Total axillary clearance

Offers good regional control but has a high risk of lymphoedema and arm pain, both of which can be disabling. It also leads to overtreatment of some women, i.e. after clearance, they will be found to be node-negative and therefore will have had this procedure unnecessarily.

Loco-regional radiotherapy

Breast irradiation

Whole breast radiotherapy reduces the risk of local recurrence after breast-conserving surgery to <10% at 10 years. Care must be taken to minimize the volume of lung and heart irradiated.

Post-mastectomy radiotherapy to the chest wall increases survival in patients at high risk of relapse and is recommended for patients with at least two of the following:

- Size >4cm
- Grade 3
- Lymph node positive
- Vascular invasion.

Axillary radiotherapy

This is indicated after positive lymph node sampling. It is generally avoided after axillary clearance because of the high risk of lymphoedema and brachial plexopathy.

Radiotherapy timing

Normally, radiotherapy should begin as soon as possible after surgery. However, enhanced normal tissue damage can result when radiotherapy and adjuvant chemotherapy are given together, and radiotherapy is often postponed until chemotherapy is completed.

Adjuvant treatment of early breast cancer

Adjuvant systemic therapy

- Many women have occult micrometastases at diagnosis. If untreated, these can cause metastatic disease.
- Effective systemic treatment at the time of the breast cancer diagnosis produces a significant survival benefit in the majority of women.
- HER-2 and ER status should be available for all patients when discussion of adjuvant therapy options takes place.
- The risk of micrometastatic disease correlates well with the prognostic factors summarized by the NPI (➋ see Introduction, p. 293).
- In the UK, NICE recommends the genetic typing of patients (using the Oncotype DX assessment) if they are ER-positive, have no affected lymph nodes, and are assessed as being intermediate risk. This information is used to guide therapy decisions, specifically the risk of breast cancer recurrence and the benefit of adjuvant chemotherapy.

NICE recommends the calculation of the potential benefit from adjuvant chemotherapy for individual patients via approved websites such as ✎ http://www.adjuvantonline.com

Adjuvant chemotherapy

Combination chemotherapy reduces recurrence and mortality in most groups of women and should be considered in:
- All but very good-prognosis pre-menopausal breast cancer (almost always recommended in women under the age of 35)
- Post-menopausal women with intermediate- or poor-prognosis breast cancer

Current practice is to give six cycles of FEC-T chemotherapy (three cycles of 5FU/epirubicin/cyclophosphamide, followed by three cycles of docetaxel), unless contraindicated.

Trastuzumab should be offered to women with HER-2-positive disease, following cardiac assessment. This assessment should be carried out by calculating the left ventricular ejection fraction (LVEF) prior to commencing treatment and at 3-monthly periods. Women with significant levels of cardiovascular impairment are not offered trastuzumab. The drug is normally given every 3 weeks for 1 year in the adjuvant setting and can be given IV or SC.

Adjuvant endocrine therapy

- 60% of breast cancers are ER-positive, and in these women, adjuvant hormone therapy confers survival benefits, in some cases greater than with chemotherapy. Toxicity is less than chemotherapy, although menopausal symptoms can be distressing for some.
- In post-menopausal women with ER-positive early breast cancer, aromatase inhibitors (➋ see Aromatase inhibitors and breast cancer, p. 300) should be offered to women, in preference to tamoxifen, unless they cannot be tolerated, in which case tamoxifen should then be offered.

In pre-menopausal women with ER-positive early breast cancers, tamoxifen should be offered to patients.

- 20mg of tamoxifen daily for 5 years improves survival in pre-menopausal women, reducing the risk of contralateral breast cancer.
- Tamoxifen offers no benefit in ER-negative breast cancer.
- It increases the risk of thromboembolic disease and endometrial cancer (× 2.5).

Note: tamoxifen should only be commenced after completion of chemotherapy, as it reduces the effectiveness of chemotherapy.

Aromatase inhibitors and breast cancer

AIs are more effective than tamoxifen alone in reducing recurrence and have a reduced risk of thromboembolic disease and endometrial cancer. They can cause fatigue, joint pain, and reduction in bone density. At the time of writing, recommendations are:[3]

- The AIs anastrozole, exemestane, and letrozole are the preferred option for the adjuvant treatment of early ER-positive invasive breast cancer in post-menopausal women.
- Primary adjuvant treatment with an AI should be utilized, but where a patient has been receiving tamoxifen, then:
  - Switching from tamoxifen to an AI should be an option after 2–3 years of tamoxifen where a woman has moderate- or high-risk disease
  - Use of an AI is recommended after completion of 5 years of tamoxifen treatment in all women with lymph node-positive disease.

Women with questions about the use of AIs should be referred to their breast care clinician and CNS.

Breast cancer treatment guidelines

Treatment guidelines for breast cancer change frequently, as new research comes through into clinical practice.

You can check for the latest national guidelines on the NICE website (℞ http://www.nice.org.uk and ℞ https://pathways.nice.org.uk). You should also check for local guidelines.

Ovarian ablation

For pre-menopausal women, ovarian ablation can provide a 10.6% improvement in 10-year survival. It can be offered, in addition to tamoxifen, to pre-menopausal women with ER-positive early invasive breast cancer who have been offered chemotherapy but have chosen not to have it.

Neo-adjuvant therapy (preoperative treatment)

Preoperative treatment downstages the primary tumour, and in some women, it facilitates breast-conserving surgery where mastectomy would otherwise be required. No difference in survival has been shown between people given pre- or post-operative chemotherapy.

References

3 National Institute for Health and Care Excellence (2015). *Early and Locally Advanced Breast Cancer: Adjuvant Therapy.* Available at: ℞ https://pathways.nice.org.uk/pathways/early-and-locally-advanced-breast-cancer

Management of locally advanced breast cancer

Locally advanced disease is defined by the presence of infiltration of the skin or chest wall or fixed axillary nodes, e.g. T4 or N2–3.

The risk of metastatic disease is >70%. Long-term survival is possible, and the median survival of these patients exceeds 2 years.

Staging investigations should assess possible metastatic disease and include:
- A CXR
- An isotope bone scan
- A liver US or CT scan.

Local control of the tumour and prevention of tumour fungation are of major importance to the QoL of these women, irrespective of the presence of metastases.

A combination of primary systemic treatment and radiotherapy is commonly used.

Neo-adjuvant systemic therapy

There is an increasing tendency to use primary or neo-adjuvant systemic treatment in patients who would otherwise require major breast surgery, in an attempt to reduce the complexity of the surgery. This would include chemotherapy and, in HER-2-positive disease, the use of trastuzumab and pertuzumab.

Pertuzumab is a monoclonal antibody which targets HER-2-positive breast tumours. In the UK, it has been approved by NICE for neo-adjuvant treatment of HER2-positive breast cancer, in combination with chemotherapy and trastuzumab.[4] The combination with trastuzumab is more effective than trastuzumab alone, as two different parts of the HER-2 protein are targeted by the drugs.

Older patients and those with ER-positive disease

- First-line therapy in this group should be with one of the AIs (anastrozole, letrozole, or exemestane), which may downstage the disease to make it operable.
- Radiotherapy is reserved to control bleeding or other uncontrolled symptoms such as lymphoedema.

Younger patients and those with ER-negative disease

- First-line therapy is primary chemotherapy, usually an anthracycline-based combination.
- Surgery may be feasible in some patients with a good response to systemic treatment, followed by loco-regional radiotherapy.
- Hormonal therapy is started after chemotherapy for ER-positive tumours:
  - Pre-menopausal—tamoxifen and add in ovarian suppression (LHRH agonist) for poor-prognosis patients. May also use bisphosphonates (➔ see Bisphosphonate therapy, pp. 287–8)
  - Post-menopausal—AI.

Patients with HER-2-positive disease

- Patients with locally advanced HER-2-positive breast cancer should be offered trastuzumab, as for patients with early-stage HER-2-positive disease.
- Patients with locally advanced HER-2-positive breast cancer should be offered pertuzumab where neo-adjuvant therapy is indicated, in combination with trastuzumab and chemotherapy (⊃ see Neo-adjuvant systemic therapy, p. 300).

References

4 National Institute for Health and Care Excellence (2016). *Pertuzumab for the Neoadjuvant Treatment of HER2-Positive Breast Cancer*. Technology appraisal guidance [TA424]. Available at: ℛ https://www.nice.org.uk/guidance/ta424

Management of metastatic breast cancer

Twenty per cent of patients with metastatic breast cancer survive for at least 5 years. ER-positive disease and bone metastases have the best prognosis. Visceral metastatic disease generally has a poor prognosis, and the aim of treatment with these patients is palliation.

Endocrine therapy

This is preferred over chemotherapy in older patients and for non-visceral metastatic disease.

First-line treatment should be as follows:
- Pre-menopausal women—ovarian suppression (LHRH agonist) plus tamoxifen
- Post-menopausal women—AI (anastrozole, letrozole, or exemestane)
- Subsequent further therapy with agents to which the patient has not been previously exposed can be of benefit.

Chemotherapy

- Combination chemotherapy is the preferred treatment for patients with visceral disease and ER-negative tumours.
- Despite the toxicity of chemotherapy, the quality of life of women improves, as they respond to treatment. Around 50% of women will respond, with a median time of 8 months to further disease progression.
- Following disease progression, second- or third-line chemotherapy can be offered, although tumour responses will reduce and fewer patients will remain fit to tolerate such regimes.

Targeted therapy

- 25–30% of breast cancers over-express HER-2, a growth factor receptor associated with poor-prognosis disease.
- Trastuzumab is a monoclonal antibody targeted against HER-2, which is administered 3-weekly IV or SC. It has shown improved response rates over chemotherapy alone in HER-2-positive breast cancer. It can be given alone or in combination with chemotherapy (it is contraindicated with anthracyclines due to cardiotoxicity) (➔ see Introduction to targeted and biological therapies, p. 227; ➔ see Adjuvant treatment of early breast cancer, pp. 299–300).
- It seems very likely that pertuzumab, when given in combination with trastuzumab, in metastatic HER-2-positive breast cancer offers significant advantages in overall survival. In the UK, this has been the subject of a long-running NICE appraisal, resulting in NICE guidance TA458 (2017).

Radiotherapy

Low-dose radiotherapy (e.g. 20Gy/5#) provides effective palliation for:
- Painful bone metastases
- Soft tissue disease
- Spread to the brain or choroid.

Bisphosphonates (e.g. pamidronate or zoledronate)

- These drugs have an important role for patients with bone metastases from breast cancer. This includes:
  - Treatment and prevention of malignant hypercalcaemia
  - Healing of osteolytic metastases
  - Reducing bone pain
  - Reducing progression of bone disease.
- Prolonged treatment is recommended, starting from the time of diagnosis of bone metastases and continuing even in the face of progressive disease.
- Denosumab, a monoclonal antibody, has been shown to be effective in preventing the development of further skeletal metastases in patients with breast cancer and known bone metastases. In the UK, NICE has recommended it as an option in patients who would normally receive bisphosphonates (➲ see Bone and soft tissue cancers, pp. 287–9).

Breast reconstruction

- Breast reconstruction should be made available to all suitable patients, as part of their cancer treatment.
- It may be done immediately post-mastectomy/partial mastectomy or as a delayed procedure after adjuvant therapies, such as chemotherapy/ radiotherapy, are completed.
- It is also available for women having prophylactic surgery to reduce the risk of developing either familial breast cancer or contralateral disease.
- There is no evidence to show that reconstruction delays the identification of local recurrence, and it can reduce the psychological and emotional impact of a mastectomy.

Aims

- Replaces breast tissue volume.
- Provides women with a breast mound (does not recreate their breast).
- Provides symmetry in volume and projection and sometimes ptosis (sagging), leading to a more natural appearance.
- Removes the need for an external prosthesis.
- Reduces the impact of a mastectomy on the patient's body image.
- Provides an oncologically safe operation.

Immediate versus delayed reconstruction

Reconstruction can provide immediate psychological benefit. However, without tumour histopathology, it is not known what adjuvant therapies are required. Radiotherapy is contraindicated with certain types of reconstruction.

In delayed reconstruction, patients will have completed all of their adjuvant therapies. There can be a long recovery period post-reconstruction, which can be exacerbated by adjuvant therapies. Some patients prefer to complete the cancer side of their treatment first.

Types of surgery

- Implants—most commonly tissue expanders.
- LD (latissimus dorsi) muscle flap reconstruction.
- TRAM (transverse rectus abdominis muscle) flap reconstruction.
- DIEP (deep inferior epigastric perforator) flap.
- SGAP (superior gluteal artery perforator) flap.

Tissue expanders

A part silicone and part saline implant is placed under the pectoralis major muscle in a deflated state. Once the incision has healed, the implant is gradually inflated over a number of weeks with saline. This can be done as an outpatient procedure. In order to produce a more natural, supple contour, the implant is overinflated for 2–3 months and then deflated to achieve symmetry in volume. The inflation procedure can be uncomfortable. It can sometimes be done as a two-stage procedure where the expander implant is replaced with a fixed-volume implant. It is the simplest type of reconstructive surgery, with no additional scarring. Suitable for smaller-breasted patients and bilateral surgery.

Disadvantages

Formation of scar tissue around the implant can cause it to become mis-shapen and uncomfortable for the patient. Not suitable post-radiotherapy due to lack of elasticity of the skin and muscle. It is less suitable for fuller-breasted women, as difficult to provide symmetry.

Latissimus dorsi flap

This involves movement of the skin, fat, and muscle to replace breast tissue. The flap is rotated onto the mastectomy site. The muscle remains attached to its original blood supply in the axilla. It takes 3–4 hours and produces additional scarring. This can provide a more natural shape and is very suitable post-partial mastectomy. It offers the possibility of avoiding an implant, though an implant may be required to provide additional volume and projection.

Disadvantages

Flap necrosis, though rare, can occur. Seroma formation under the donor site may require repeated aspirations. It may not be suitable for patients who enjoy certain activities such as rock climbing or surfing.

TRAM flap

Movement of the transverse rectus abdominis muscle with overlying fat and skin to re-create breast volume. The blood supply to the muscle is attached to the inframammary vein and artery with microsurgery. This produces the most natural cosmetic result, as no implant is required—can achieve more ptosis and greater symmetry for fuller-breasted women. Suitable procedure for immediate bilateral reconstruction.

Disadvantages

Can take up to 8 hours, with lower abdominal scarring and longer recovery period of 2–3 months. Flap necrosis is more frequent than with LD flap. Can get abdominal hernia. Synthetic mesh can be used to strengthen the abdominal wall. Not suitable for smokers or women with a body mass index of over 30.

DIEP and SGAP flaps

These involve moving fat and skin from the lower abdomen or buttocks. There is no abdominal weakness from the procedure. There is a higher risk of flap necrosis, due to the need to surgically establish new microvascular blood supply. It is not widely available.

Nipple preservation

Some patients wish to preserve the nipple. This is not recommended if the nipple is inverted due to the cancer, if there is evidence of disease in the ducts behind the nipple, or if there is evidence of Paget's disease of the nipple. Patients should be made aware that nipple preservation increases the risk of disease recurrence by 5–10%.

Nipple reconstruction

This is often done as a delayed procedure, once the new breast has settled in volume and shape. Skin may be grafted from the other nipple/areola or from the inner thigh where the skin is naturally darker. The areola may be tattooed to enhance the cosmetic effect.

Prosthetic nipples

A cast can be taken of the remaining nipple to make a silicon replica. This can be colour-matched with the remaining nipple. The nipple is attached to the breast with surgical glue.

Surgery to contralateral breast

Women can be offered surgery on the contralateral breast, e.g. mastopexy—breast lift or mammoplasty—breast reduction. This can be offered during initial surgery, preventing the need for surgery at a later date.

Patient education issues

Patient education and support from a breast care nurse and the rest of the clinical team are essential in preparing women for any possible reconstructive surgery. Key issues to cover include:

- The individual's expectations and beliefs about the outcome
- Potential risks of surgery, including failure of flaps, or possible need for further surgery
- Altered sensation and prolonged post-operative neuropathic pain
- The relationship between surgery and further anti-cancer treatment.

Prophylactic (risk-reducing) mastectomy

In recent years, there has been an increasing number of women who have chosen to have a mastectomy on a healthy breast in order to reduce the chances of developing breast cancer. Normally, these women are particularly at risk of developing the disease, e.g. in high-risk disease in the contralateral breast or those with an extensive family history of breast cancer and/or genetic risk factors. In the UK, women who would meet the criteria to have such an operation on the NHS would have:

- A strong and reliable family history of breast or ovarian cancer—especially if breast cancer was diagnosed among several close blood relatives on the same side of the family before the age of 50
- Any of the main gene mutations linked to an ↑ risk of breast cancer, e.g. *BRCA1* or *BRCA2, TP53*, or *PTEN*
- Had breast cancer and have a high risk of developing it in the other breast.

In any of these cases, women will need to be counselled carefully prior to undergoing any surgery, particularly with respect to:

- Alternatives to mastectomy (e.g. ↑ levels of surveillance via the breast screening service and radiographic monitoring)
- The percentage reductions in the risk of developing breast cancer—risk-reducing mastectomy does not entirely reduce the risk of developing the disease but can significantly reduce it
- Surgical risk and morbidity
- The types of reconstruction available and how these might look and feel
- Potential changes in body image.

Further reading

National Institute for Health and Care Excellence (2013). *Familial Breast Cancer: Classification, Care and Managing Breast Cancer and Related Risks in People With a Family History of Breast Cancer.* Available from: ℘ https://www.nice.org.uk/guidance/cg164/chapter/recommendations#risk-reduction-and-treatment-strategies

Nursing management issues

Nursing people with breast cancer can be challenging in many different ways. Due to the improving prognosis, women, even with locally advanced or metastatic disease, may survive for many years with the disease. Breast cancer has been likened to a chronic disease trajectory for some, with periods of relapse and intensive treatment, followed by long remission or more benign treatment.

Women will need different levels and types of support throughout this process. Supporting women to set and achieve realistic goals at different stages requires skilled and knowledgeable nursing care.

Treatment decision-making

Women face difficult decisions about treatment at diagnosis, after surgery, or at disease recurrence. This may include what type of surgery to have and choices of chemotherapy or endocrine therapy. The potential benefit of treatments may be slight, and they all include some risk. Anxiety and fear may also reduce a woman's ability to make effective decisions.

- Good information and emotional support can aid decision-making. Nurses can help clarify the differences between treatment options, explain why these options exist, and give women access to information.
- Acting as a liaison between patients and medical staff can also be a supportive role for the nurse.
- Many women will appreciate a shared approach to decisions, reducing the burden on them at a difficult time.
- Good emotional support can aid decision-making. A specialist palliative care team referral may be helpful for those with advanced disease.
- Excellent breast cancer charities, such as Breast Cancer Care, offer specific support to younger women with breast cancer and partners of breast cancer patients (Partner Volunteer service).
- Breast cancer has a very high media profile, and nurses can help patients to work through the plethora of information available through the various media.

Surgery

After surgery, the nurse can offer advice on appropriate exercises to prevent shoulder stiffness and lymphoedema, as well as assess for complications such as seroma or infection.

Note: early referral to a lymphoedema specialist is important to establish the most effective management of lymphoedema (see Lymphoedema, pp. 626–8).

Adjuvant treatment

Chemotherapy and radiotherapy treatment often lasts for 6 months or more and can be exhausting. For many women, this is followed by years of endocrine therapy. Preparing women for what to expect is essential.

- Common side effects of chemotherapy are: fatigue, hair loss, risk of infection, nausea and vomiting, and mucositis (see Chemotherapy: side effects and complications, p. 225).

- Radiotherapy side effects include fatigue and sore skin. Axillary radiotherapy can also contribute to lymphoedema and brachial plexopathy (➔ see Radiotherapy, pp. 200–1).
- Hormonal therapy such as tamoxifen can give severe menopausal side effects. AIs can cause fatigue, nausea, headaches, and joint pains (➔ see Hormonal therapy alone, pp. 241–5).
- Both chemotherapy and hormonal therapy can affect fertility. All breast cancer patients should have access to a fertility expert to discuss treatment options).

Psychosocial issues

These can be prominent throughout the disease process. Early and continuous assessment of potential psychological problems is essential. Referral to psychological support services may be appropriate for further advice or support (➔ see Psychological support, p. 130).

- Surgery, hair loss, and weight change all impact on an individual's body image and sexuality (➔ see Body image, p. 607).
- Depression and anxiety are not uncommon and are often underdiagnosed (➔ see Anxiety, pp. 586–7; ➔ Depression, pp. 581–2).
- Recurrence of the disease is a particularly difficult time, with all the implications it holds and the impact of advanced cancer.
- A significant group of patients will be young or have young children.
  - The potentially hereditary nature of breast cancer may add to fears women have for their children.
  - Support from genetic counsellors or specialists can help clarify issues around genetic cancer links (➔ see Genetic testing, p. 65).

Advanced cancer symptom issues

Common problems experienced with advanced breast cancer include:

- Fungating breast tumours: radiotherapy can be helpful in reducing bleeding. Topical antibiotics, e.g. metronidazole, and regular dressings can help maintain dignity. Use of deodorizers may also reduce the smell
- Lung metastases can cause breathlessness and cough (➔ see Breathlessness, pp. 514–15)
- Liver metastases can cause capsular pain, which responds to NSAIDs and steroids. Also nausea and vomiting, reduced appetite, and ascites
- Brain metastases: can cause a range of problems, including confusion and change of personality (➔ see Acute confusional state or delirium, pp. 594–5).
- Bone metastases: these cause a range of problems, including:
  - Bone pain: radiotherapy, bisphosphonates, NSAIDs, and opioids can all be effective (➔ see Metastatic bone disease, pp. 287–9)
  - Pathological fractures: these may need treatment with radiotherapy or orthopaedic surgical intervention (➔ see Metastatic bone disease, pp. 287–9)
  - Hypercalcaemia: treatment with hydration and bisphosphonates can be helpful (➔ see Malignant-induced hypercalcaemia, pp. 637–40)
- Spinal cord compression: it is essential to diagnose this early to try and prevent major morbidity (➔ see Spinal cord compression, pp. 641–4).

Central nervous system cancer

Introduction

Primary malignancies of the CNS are uncommon but are difficult to treat when they occur. They are often characterized by a marked deterioration in the patient's functional ability and mental state. This can be devastating and life-changing for the patient and their family, friends, and carers.

There are many types of CNS malignancy, and unfortunately the most common tumours have a poor prognosis. Recent advances in cancer treatment, imaging, and surgical modalities have largely failed to improve overall survival for this group of patients.

The management of brain tumours presents a considerable challenge for the MDT, both in the hospital and in the community, and an integrated approach is essential.

Note: the management of metastatic brain tumours and leptomeningeal carcinomatosis are also covered briefly within the chapter.

Epidemiology

- CNS cancers account for 3% of all cancers diagnosed.
- CNS cancers account for 20% of cancers diagnosed in children under the age of 15.
- The incidence of CNS cancers peaks in childhood, falls, and then rises exponentially until the age of 75.
- The incidence and age profile of CNS cancers are consistent across the world.
- The 5-year survival rate for all brain tumours is 15–20% across Europe.

Risk factors

- The majority of primary CNS tumours are sporadic.
- The main risk factors are increasing age and higher socio-economic status.
- There are a number of rare familial syndromes associated with primary CNS tumours.
- Speculation that exposure to non-ionizing radiation, e.g. from mobile telephones, increases the risk of developing brain tumours remains unproven.
- Increasing incidence is likely to be due to better detection and imaging and an ageing population.

Common presenting symptoms

Intracranial tumours: neurological dysfunction or symptoms of raised ICP. Pituitary tumours can present with visual field defects or symptoms of hormone secretion. Common symptoms include:

- Seizures
- Headache
- Change in personality, cognitive and speech disturbance
- Motor disturbance and/or loss of sensation in limbs
- Collapse
- Tiredness and fatigue.

Investigations

- Neurological assessment and medical interpretation of signs and symptoms.
- Preferably MRI scan of the head or spine, otherwise cranial or spinal CT scan.
- Tissue diagnosis may be required in order to determine the exact nature of the tumour, e.g. whether it is a primary or a metastatic tumour, and to assess histology.
- Most brain tumours do not metastasize, apart from, very rarely, to the spinal cord.

Biopsy

The following should be considered before making a decision to obtain a tissue sample:

- Should the tumour be excised, a biopsy taken, or neither?
- Is the patient fit for either or one of these procedures?
- Is the tumour safely accessible by surgery?

These decisions are complex and are ideally made within a multidisciplinary setting, with the involvement of the patient and carers. They should include specialist neurological and neurosurgical input.

Stereotactic biopsy is the approach of choice. It is a minimally invasive technique that utilizes imaging in order to obtain a tissue sample. It may be used where a tumour is likely to be malignant and is in a functionally important or inaccessible area. It is normally followed by radiotherapy.

Classification of primary CNS tumours

The pathophysiological classification of CNS tumours is complex. It is based on the type of cell from which the tumour originates. Only the most common CNS malignancies are covered here (see Table 23.1). By far, the most common primary CNS malignancy is the brain tumour, with spinal cord tumours accounting for only 10–15% of primary tumours.

Gliomas

Gliomas—including astrocytomas, oligodendrogliomas, and ependymomas—are the most common brain tumours. They arise from neuroepithelial (or glial) cells within the brain. These are one of the few groups of neural cells that divide. Gliomas are further classified by the malignancy of the cells within the tumour and their ability to cause necrosis. Grade 1 is the least malignant, and grade 4 the most.

Astrocytomas

In England, astrocytomas account for around 34% of all brain tumours. They generally arise within the cerebral hemispheres but can occur in the spinal cord. Grade 1 and 2 tumours are typically well differentiated, whilst grade 3 and 4 tumours show far higher levels of necrosis and vascular changes.

The most malignant form of astrocytomas (grade 4) is also called glioblastoma multiforme. It is the most common subtype, accounting for eight out of ten of all astrocytomas. These tumours are resistant to surgical and non-surgical treatment and are associated with a particularly poor prognosis.

Oligodendrogliomas

These gliomas are typically slow-growing tumours that occur within the frontal lobes. They account for around 5% of primary brain tumours and tend to be more chemosensitive than other gliomas.

Ependymomas

These gliomas arise from ependymal glial cells and account for around 6% of all brain tumours. They can occur in adults but are more common in children. They are unusual in that they can spread [via the cerebrospinal fluid (CSF)] to the spinal cord. Patients may present with a cerebral ependymoma and lesions in the spinal cord. Spinal ependymomas account for >50% of all primary spinal tumours.

Non–glioma tumours

Meningiomas

These tumours are the most common type of non-glioma brain tumours, and they arise from the cells of the meninges—the inner lining of the brain. They tend to be slow-growing, low-grade tumours. They can often be successfully excised surgically, because of their more superficial nature.

Table 23.1 Survival chart for different tumour types

Tumour group	Treatment	5-year survival (%)
Low-grade astrocytoma (grades 1 and 2)	Surgery radiotherapy	50–60
High-grade astrocytoma (grades 3 and 4)	All treatments	<5
Oligodendroglioma	Surgery + radiotherapy	35
Ependymoma	Surgery + radiotherapy	56–80
Meningioma	Surgery	45–80
CNS lymphoma	Chemotherapy + radiotherapy	3

Primary CNS lymphomas

These account for <1% of primary brain tumours. They are much more common in immunosuppressed patients, e.g. after an organ transplant or people with long-term HIV disease (➔ see HIV-related malignancies, pp. 428–30). Primary treatment is generally chemotherapy, with radiotherapy held in reserve as a second-line treatment. Primary CNS lymphomas are associated with a poor long-term prognosis.

Spinal tumours

Eighty per cent of spinal tumours are metastatic in origin, with the sites of origin being myeloma, breast, lung, or lymphoma. The remainder are typically as a result of ependymomas, meningiomas, or more rarely astrocytomas. Diagnosis of spinal tumours is determined by clinical examination, followed by MRI scan. Recognition and swift treatment of metastatic spinal tumours are important, as they can result in spinal cord compression, an oncological emergency (➔ see Spinal cord compression, pp. 641–4).

Management of primary CNS malignancy

Treatment modalities

Surgery

Surgery can be used as a primary treatment (full or partial resection) or used to facilitate non-surgical treatments (debulking or stereotactic biopsy). Surgery is often the primary treatment of choice for patients with a CNS malignancy, and it offers the best chance of long-term survival.

The aim is to excise the tumour with as wide a margin as possible, to avoid an incomplete excision. The extent to which this is possible depends on:

• The type of tumour and the degree to which it is encapsulated
• The location of the tumour and its proximity to key functional areas within the brain and/or CNS
• The general fitness of the patient.

The extent to which the margins of a tumour can be excised in neuro-surgery is limited by possible damage to healthy brain tissue and the re-sulting possible long-term neurological damage inflicted on the patient. Where a complete resection is not possible, a tumour may be excised as much as possible, or debulked and then followed up with post-operative radiotherapy.

With any neurosurgery, the main post-operative risks are cerebral oedema, intracranial bleeding, and infection. All of these can be life-threatening or may leave the patient with neurological deficits and dis-ability. Patients should therefore be cared for in a specialist neurosurgical unit in the immediate post-operative period, as their condition can deteri-orate rapidly.

The degree to which surgery is successful in improving survival de-pends largely on the tumour type; 80% of meningiomas are successfully treated with surgery alone, whereas grade 4 astrocytomas (glioblastoma multiforme) will almost certainly recur.

Chemotherapy

The success of chemotherapeutic agents has been very limited in the treat-ment of CNS malignancy. Therapy is limited by many tumours being intrin-sically chemoresistant and the presence of the blood–brain barrier, though this can be disrupted in many primary CNS tumours.

Most cytotoxic agents do not pass through the blood–brain barrier and are therefore rendered ineffective. Procarbazine and lomustine are exceptions to this general rule—they can bypass the blood–brain bar-rier and are frequently employed in treating brain tumours, together with vincristine.

Temozolamide is an oral cytotoxic, which has been found to be effective, particularly when combined with radiotherapy.

There is currently interest in developing biological, or genetic, therapies which might be more effective against brain tumours. There have been some trials using the TKI erlotinib, but at the time of writing, results have been inconclusive.

The blood–brain barrier

The blood–brain barrier consists of tightly joined linings of cells surrounding cerebral capillaries. These prevent the exchange of water-soluble ions, proteins, and drugs between the vessel and the surrounding neural tissues. Smaller molecules and fat-soluble ions diffuse more readily. The blood–brain barrier protects the sensitive neural tissue from potentially damaging fluctuations in the biochemical environment.

The blood–brain barrier can be bypassed by administering chemotherapy directly into or around a brain tumour—using a reservoir system, usually an Ommaya reservoir. This is placed under the scalp and has a fine tube that passes into the CSF or into a cystic tumour. It can also be used as a drainage device to prevent build-up of fluid within a cystic tumour. These devices should only be used by specially trained staff.

Other techniques which have been used include intraoperative wafers containing slow-release carmustine, which can be placed in the tumour bed, following excision of the tumour, to try and reduce the incidence of local recurrence.

Radiotherapy

For the most common types of CNS malignancy, the main role of radiotherapy is as an adjunct to surgical resection, rather than as a primary treatment. However, advanced and improved modes of delivering radiotherapy to brain tumours might offer the best hope for improving survival. Examples of these include:

- Proton therapy: a slower-moving beam of radiotherapy is used, which reduces damage to surrounding tissue. In the USA, this method is already used for treating brain tumours, and in the UK paediatric brain tumours can be treated with proton therapy.
- Boron neutron capture therapy (BNCT): boron is injected into the patient and then congregates in the cells of the brain tumour. The boron molecules can then be made to produce targeted radiation by stimulating them with low-energy external radiotherapy.
- Stereotactic radiotherapy and radiosurgery: these are two different methods of delivering high-dose radiotherapy to a tumour without destroying adjacent healthy tissue. They require specialist equipment and skills and are not available in all hospitals.

Giving radiotherapy to a brain tumour is a highly skilled element of clinical oncology. This is because exceeding the maximum tolerance of nerve tissue can cause tissue necrosis, with accompanying loss of brain tissue and neurological damage.

Steroids

Steroids have a vital role in the management of CNS tumours, particularly brain tumours, as they can stabilize a patient's condition at many stages throughout their illness. Dexamethasone is generally used.

Steroids are powerful anti-inflammatory agents and can dramatically improve a patient's overall condition by reducing cerebral oedema.

TABLE 23.2 Common steroid side effects and their management

Side effect	Management strategies
Gastric ulceration	Administer regular proton pump inhibitor (PPI)
Sleep disturbance	Administer steroids in the morning, rather than the afternoon
Diabetes	Monitor urine daily for sugar, and treat diabetes if necessary
Weight gain	Monitor dietary intake and provide guidance
Confusional state ('steroid psychosis')	Reduce steroid dose if acute and distressing, and treat with benzodiazepines or haloperidol if severe
Addisonian crisis	Reduce steroids gradually, rather than stopping them

Steroids have a wide range of side effects—the guiding principle is to keep steroid dosage down to a minimal level and to reduce the dose of steroids once the patient's condition has stabilized (see Table 23.2).

Note: it should also be remembered that steroids can mask pyrexia, making a potential infection more difficult to assess.

Metastatic brain disease

The presence of brain metastases is a poor prognostic factor in most types of tumour, with patients rarely surviving >3–6 months, even with treatment. Many patients also have an accompanying low quality of life, with significant neurological or cognitive deficits. The viability of any treatment is often based upon the performance status of the patient and the number and/or size of metastases within the brain.

Aetiology

- Brain metastases are ten times more common than primary malignant CNS tumours. However, many patients are asymptomatic (found only on autopsy).
- Most occur in cerebral hemispheres, with a minority in the cerebellum or brainstem. Over half have multiple lesions.
- Caused by haematological spread from the primary cancer. Most commonly lung and breast primaries. Also melanoma and kidney and colon cancers.

Presenting symptoms

- Focal neurological disturbances: hemiparesis, dysphasia, cranial nerve palsies.
- Raised ICP, headache, nausea and vomiting, lethargy.
- Epileptic seizures.
- Cognitive behaviour change.

Management

Surgery

In a small group of patients with single lesions, surgery may be appropriate, particularly if it is a radiotherapy-resistant tumour. A specialist neurosurgeon can assess the risks and potential benefit of surgery, normally as part of a specialist MDT. It is therefore vital that patients who are likely to benefit from surgery are identified and referred to the neurosurgical team for discussion.

Radiotherapy

For most patients, surgery is not an option due to multifocal brain lesions, tumour inaccessibility, widespread systemic disease, performance status, and comorbidity.

Options include:

- Whole brain radiotherapy and steroid therapy are the standard treatment. These provide symptomatic improvement in about 70% of patients.
- Stereotactic radiotherapy: fractionated treatment which accurately targets the tumours, reducing the impact on healthy tissue.
- Radiosurgery (single high-dose stereotactic radiotherapy) can be used to treat small lesions.

Note: radiosurgical treatment is not available in all treatment centres.

Symptoms of radiotherapy include somnolence and long-term memory/cognitive impairment (not always relevant due to short life expectancy) of many of these patients.

Chemotherapy

Adjuvant chemotherapy can be considered in chemotherapy-sensitive disease, e.g. germ cell, haematological, or small cell lung cancers.

Leptomeningeal carcinomatosis

This is diffuse seeding of cancer cells throughout the CSF and the meninges. It is generally caused by progressive systemic cancers, most commonly haematological disease such as leukaemia and lymphoma. It can also occur in breast, lung, and GI cancers.

Common presenting symptoms

• Cranial nerve problems, headache, back pain, leg weakness.

Diagnosis

• Lumbar puncture, with cytology of CSF.
• MRI scan.

Management

• Leptomeningeal carcinomatosis can be treated with intrathecal chemotherapy, as well as localized radiotherapy, to deal with specific symptoms.
• Median survival is very poor, other than in a few curative haematological cancer patients.

Nursing management issues

Nursing patients with tumours of the CNS can be extremely challenging due to invasive treatments, complex symptom management, and often poor prognosis. The long-term changes in an individual's behaviour and personality can be very distressing for family members.

Common nursing challenges include:
• Hemiparesis or other neurological deficit
• Aphasia or dysphasia
• Depression (➔ see Depression, pp. 581–2)
• Confusional state (➔ see Acute confusional state or delirium, pp. 594–5)
• Fluctuating level of awareness
• Swallowing difficulties and aspiration
• Cerebral oedema (caused by disease, surgery, or radiotherapy).

Management of cerebral oedema

Cerebral oedema is swelling of the brain caused by build-up of fluid within the brain tissue. It occurs as a result of irritation to the brain, either by the effects of the tumour itself, by invasive surgery and other procedures, or by radiotherapy.

If allowed to proceed unchecked, cerebral oedema can damage brain tissue, causing deterioration in the patient's condition, and ultimately proving fatal.

The key aspects in managing this problem are:
• Patient assessment—noting that the patient's condition has changed either by formal assessment (neurological observations) or, more informally, by knowing your patient and the significance of any change
• High-dose steroid treatment (up to 16mg of dexamethasone per day) and reducing once the patient's condition has stabilized
• Management of steroid side effects (see Table 23.2)
• Occasionally high-dose diuretics, e.g. mannitol.

MDT working and team approach

It is vital that care for a person with a CNS tumour is planned and coordinated in a holistic and consistent way, and that carers are supported. This is best managed via a responsive and regularly reviewed multidisciplinary plan of care.

The role of the key worker is vital in coordinating the plan and referring to other specialists as the patient's condition changes.

Key referrals for individuals with CNS tumours

• Speech therapy (swallowing and dysphasia)
• Dieticians (poor oral intake, steroid-induced diabetes)
• Occupational therapists (functional assessment and forward planning)
• Social services (care management)
• District nurses (community support and care)
• Palliative care teams (acute, Trust, and community)
• Psychological services (advice on management of acute confusional states)

Ethical issues

(→ See Chapter 13, Ethics in cancer care.)

The treatment of patients with CNS tumours is an area where ethical issues are often brought into sharp focus. This is because:

• It is often not clear whether a patient can consent to treatment or not
• Patients are often treated with long, and potentially taxing, regimens of chemotherapy or radiotherapy, with an overall poor prognosis
• The perception of the patient may differ widely from that of the carers or health-care professionals
• Because swallowing can often be impaired and there may be issues around supported feeding and hydration (via NG or PEG) for patients with severe disabilities.

Many of these issues do not have an overall right or wrong answer. What is in the best interest of a patient may vary with time and circumstance, and may not be applicable to another patient. What is crucial is involving the patient and, where possible, the carers in decision-making and raising the issues in an open and inclusive manner (→ see Patient and family involvement in decision-making, pp. 120–1).

Further reading

Kaye A, Laws E. *Brain Tumors: An Encyclopedic Approach*, 3rd ed. New York, NY: Saunders Elsevier; 2012.

National Institute for Health and Care Excellence (2006). *Improving Outcomes for People With Brain and Other Central Nervous System Tumours*. Cancer Service Guideline [CSG10]. Available at: ℛ https://www.nice.org.uk/guidance/csg10

Colorectal cancer

Introduction

Incidence
- Colorectal cancer is the fourth most common cancer in the UK, with over 41,000 cases diagnosed annually.
- It affects men and women almost equally, with 53% of cases being in ♂.
- It is rare under 40 years of age, with 95% of colorectal cancer diagnoses occurring in the over 50s and 57% of deaths in the over 75s.
- More people are diagnosed with advanced disease (55% at stage 3 or 4) than earlier-stage disease.
- Most cases are diagnosed in the lower colon and rectum, with 47% of all tumours occurring in the rectum or sigmoid colon.

Risk factors
- Around half of bowel cancers are linked to lifestyle factors, including eating high levels of red or processed meat, obesity, alcohol, and smoking.
- Exercise seems to confer some protection against developing bowel cancer, with colon cancer risk being 27% higher in the most sedentary population, compared with the least sedentary.
- 7% of cases are associated with genetic predisposition syndromes such as FAP and HNPCC.

Presenting symptoms
These are partly dependent on where the tumour occurs in the bowel.
- **Early**: rectal bleeding, persisting change in bowel habit, and anaemia.
- **Late**: weight loss, nausea, anorexia, and abdominal pain.

Common sites of spread
- Liver, lungs, and peritoneum.
- Local recurrence at anastomosis site or pre-sacral.
- Liver metastases are the most common because the colon's venous drainage is mainly via the portal system.

Staging and diagnosis
Commonly staged using TNM classification (traditionally, Dukes is used as well) (➲ see Diagnosis, classification, and staging of cancer, p. 176).
   Useful investigations include:
- Full colonoscopy or procto-sigmoidoscopy (barium enema now rarely used, as other imaging more useful)
- CT colonography (low-dose radiation CT scanning used to produce a clear picture of the colon). This is also known as a 'virtual colonoscopy' and is increasingly becoming a mainstay of colorectal cancer diagnosis. This does require some bowel preparation
- Liver US
- CT scan of the chest, abdomen, and pelvis
- MRI and US of the pelvis for rectal cancers.

Treatment approaches to colorectal cancer

Surgery

- Surgery is the main curative therapy for colorectal cancer. Curative resection requires the excision of the primary tumour and its lymphatic drainage, with an enveloping margin of normal tissue.
- Minimally invasive (laparoscopic) colon surgery is becoming a commonly used technique, except where there is concern over adequacy of clearance in patients with more advanced cancers.
- The 'Enhanced Recovery Programme' has been shown to reduce both the length of stay after surgery and complication rates.

Rectal cancer

- TME is considered essential. This has been shown to effectively reduce local relapse rates.
- About 5% of rectal cancers may be removed by non-radical transanal surgery.

Hepatic metastases

- Patients with solitary, multiple, and even bilobar liver metastases may be eligible for liver resection.
- The aim is to remove all macroscopic disease with a clear resection margin and leave sufficient functioning liver.

Complications of surgery

- Infection and intra-abdominal abscesses.
- Anastomotic leak and GU tract injury—both require immediate surgical intervention.
- Large bowel obstruction—may respond to conservative management (→ see Bowel obstruction, p. 510).
- Sexual dysfunction—abdominoperineal resection can cause impotence due to surgical nerve damage (→ see Chapter 50, Sexuality and cancer).

Stoma formation

About 15% of patients diagnosed with colorectal cancer end up with a permanent colostomy. Many others will require a temporary colostomy or ileostomy, whilst they recover from their surgery (→ see Care of the patient with a stoma, p. 328).

Non-surgical

Adjuvant therapy of colorectal cancer

Fifty per cent of patients who undergo apparently curative resection of bowel cancer will have residual micrometastases that are invisible at the time of surgery and not evident on any imaging investigation. These eventually lead to locally recurrent or distant metastatic disease. Adjuvant chemotherapy aims to eradicate these micrometastases and thereby prevent future relapse.

It is normally offered to those with stage 3 disease cancers. Adjuvant therapy for rectal cancer may include both radiotherapy and chemotherapy, aimed at local and systemic micrometastases, respectively.

Chemotherapy used in adjuvant setting

5FU ± oxaliplatin (FOLFOX) or its oral equivalent capecitabine ± oxaliplatin (CAPOX) is standard therapy in many countries.

Targeted therapies, such as cetuximab, bevacizumab, and panitumumab, have been investigated in the adjuvant setting, but these are not thought to be useful.

Chemo-irradiation

For patients with rectal cancer, preoperative pelvic radiotherapy can be given concurrently with chemotherapy in order to reduce the size of the tumour, thereby making surgery more successful. This may be followed by a more prolonged course of standard adjuvant chemotherapy aimed at distant micrometastases.

Side effects of treatment

Side effects vary considerably from patient to patient and depend on the dose and schedules used. Side effects should be tolerable for most patients, and chemotherapy can normally be given to the elderly.

Common side effects

- Nausea and vomiting.
- Oral mucositis.
- Diarrhoea.
- Red, painful palms and soles (palmar–plantar syndrome).
- Peripheral neuropathy (when oxaliplatin is included).

Chemotherapy in advanced colorectal cancer

- The median survival time for such patients without further therapy is 6–9 months.
- In most cases, the aim of therapy is palliation.
- Survival has been prolonged by using modern chemotherapy agents and targeted therapies.
- A few patients have advanced disease, which could be made resectable by volume reduction (downstaging) using chemotherapy.

First-line chemotherapy

- Infusional 5FU or capecitabine with either oxalipatin (FOLFOX/ CAPOX) or irinotecan (FOLFIRI/Cape-IRI).
- Survival improvements of about 6 months over best supportive care alone.
- If a patient responds to all available chemotherapy agents, then median survival can be ↑ by 2.5 years.
- Capecitabine is frequently utilized, as the convenience of oral treatment can be an important factor in advanced disease (➔ see Oral chemotherapy, p. 219) but can cause ↑ levels of diarrhoea in combination therapies, when compared to 5FU.

- Debate still continues in colorectal cancer chemotherapy in terms of:
  - Which combination is best
  - The optimum duration of therapy
  - If continuous or intermittent exposure to treatment is best.

Second-line chemotherapy
- Irinotecan is standard second-line therapy in patients who relapse following 5FU or progress whilst on this therapy.

Novel biological agents
- These have been shown to be useful in colorectal cancer in combination with cytotoxic agents, particularly in advanced disease. Cetuximab and panitumumab are monoclonal antibodies which target EGFRs. Cetuximab has now been suggested as an option as first-line treatment in patients with wild-type *K-RAS* gene.
- Bevacizumab is an anti-angiogenic compound, which has been widely used in various combinations and schedules in both first-line and second-line treatments. Aflibercept is an anti-VEGF angiogenesis inhibitor, which has shown some survival advantage in second-line chemotherapy.

Note: neither of these is funded in the UK at the time of writing.

Radiotherapy in colorectal cancer
- Preoperative radiotherapy is becoming standard practice in rectal cancer to reduce the risk of recurrence. It can increase the chance of complete surgical resection in some patients with large tumours that have not yet metastasized.
- Pelvic chemo-radiotherapy reduces the risk of relapse for patients with stage II and III rectal cancer.
- Radiotherapy is also used in palliative situations, e.g. recurrent rectal cancer.

Care of the patient with a stoma

A stoma is the result of a surgical intervention in which the stream of faeces or urine is diverted away from its normal route.

There are three main types of stoma:

- Ileostomy: loop or end-ileostomy, sited on the right side of the abdomen. Can be temporary or permanent. Output from an ileostomy is primarily liquid
- Colostomy: loop or end-colostomy, sited on the left side of the abdomen. Can be permanent or temporary. Output is generally solid
- Urostomy: always permanent and sited on right side of abdomen. Output is urine.

Uses of different stomas

Temporary ileostomy

- To protect an anastomosis (join in the bowel) following removal of low rectal cancer.
- As a palliative procedure to relieve obstruction in inoperable tumours.
- To relieve obstructive symptoms during long-course downstaging chemotherapy or radiotherapy.

Permanent ileostomy

- When the patient has multiple tumours or hereditary polyposis and the entire large bowel has to be removed.

Temporary colostomy

- When the patient has presented as an emergency and the tumour has been removed, but the bowel not rejoined (Hartmann's procedure).
- To relieve obstructive symptoms during long-course downstaging chemotherapy/radiotherapy.

Permanent colostomy

- When a low rectal tumour cannot be removed, leaving disease-free margins. To enable the bowel to be joined (anastomosis). This operation would be an abdominal-perineal excision of the rectum.
- As a palliative procedure to alleviate symptoms of obstruction.

Urostomy

- Used when the bladder cannot be preserved either because of trauma or disease, e.g. bladder cancer.

Nursing management

Preoperatively

It is essential that all patients are referred to a stoma therapy CNS for pre- and post-operative information and for a clear discussion about the potential impact of the stoma on a patient's lifestyle. This prepares the patient and their family and allows the nurse to assess the patient prior to surgery for any potential difficulties they may have, both physically and psychologically, adjusting to life with a stoma.

Post-operatively
- **Surgical complications**: a range of surgical problems can occur with stoma formation. If the stoma does not have adequate blood supply, it can become necrotic and appears a maroon or black colour. This may require further surgery. It is important to observe the stoma for colour, which should be a dark pink and have a wet appearance, similar to the inside of the mouth.
- Other complications include:
  - Stenosing (narrowing) due to extensive scar tissue, which may require further surgery or use of dilatation
  - Prolapsing due to herniation of the stoma. This can be caused by over-exertion and may need surgical repair
  - Para-stomal hernia due to herniation around the stoma—may need surgery to correct
  - Retraction of the stoma where it recedes back into the abdomen. It becomes difficult to seal appliances, and it may need surgical repair.

Stoma care
Sore skin is a common problem if the appliance is incorrectly applied and has been leaking; this, in turn, creates further problems with appliance adherence. Teaching patients the management and application of pouches and the importance of maintaining skin care and a high level of personal hygiene is essential. The aim is for independence in stoma care upon discharge.

Note: patients should be assessed by a stoma therapy CNS prior to discharge, to ensure that they are independent in stoma management.

It is important to observe stoma output for amount, colour, and consistency. For colostomies, this should be faecal brown colour and formed stool. Ileostomies should produce loose stool, faecal-coloured, and the appliance should be emptied 5/6 times in 24 hours. Urostomies should drain straw-coloured urine, ~3L volume a day. Whenever stomas drain blood, it needs to be reported and investigated.

Patients with an ileostomy can become dehydrated, caused by stoma overactivity, leading to readmission for IV fluids. Patients are encouraged to have a higher intake of salt in their diet or to take 1L of isotonic drink daily.

Note: constipation and diarrhoea can still be a problem for patients with stomas and should be treated in the usual way.

Dietary advice
- Colostomy patients should be encouraged to have a normal diet, including high-fibre foods.
- Ileostomy patients should take a low-fibre diet and caution with some fruit and vegetables, to reduce bowel action.
- Urostomy patients are encouraged to drink 3L of fluid a day (to include a mixture of drinks, not just water). Some patients are encouraged to drink one glass of cranberry juice a day (to alter the pH of the urine and reduce the incidence of stone formation and infection), although evidence for the effectiveness of this is limited.

Exercise

Exercise (including driving) should not be undertaken for at least 1 month if the patient has a large abdominal wound, and heavy lifting should not begin until after 3 months. This is to avoid rupture of internal repairs and for the patient's long-term recovery and comfort. If key-hole surgery has been performed, driving may commence after 2 weeks, and lifting after 6 weeks.

Psychological issues

Having to cope with a stoma can be very difficult for some patients. A stoma can impact on body image and social and sexual functioning, and feelings of disgust, anger, embarrassment, or shame can occur. Allow patients time to express and talk about their feelings, and include partners/relatives. Remember that the patient will be watching you for your response, whilst you are undertaking stoma care. Patients can be reassured that these feelings, although new to them, are normal following stoma surgery. The cancer site-specific CNS or stoma specialist are excellent sources of support both for the patients and their families.

Sexual function

Ensure that the patient is informed preoperatively that sexual function may be affected following surgery.

- Explain that following surgery, chemotherapy, or radiotherapy, sexual function can take weeks or months to regain.
- Encourage patients to discuss any fears and anxieties that they may have by giving them time and privacy to discuss sexuality issues.
- Advise them when referral to a psychosexual counsellor is an option.
- Men who have urostomies will be impotent and will therefore need advice on the use of medication and penile implants.
- Practical advice can include:
  - Empty appliance before sex
  - Use of underwear/lingerie to cover appliance.
- Reassure that a stoma will not be damaged during sex (➔ see Chapter 50, Sexuality and cancer).

Further reading

Beets-Tan R et al. Rectal cancer and the systemic therapy of colorectal cancer. In: Kerr DJ, Haller DG, van de Velde CJH, Baumann M (eds). *Oxford Textbook of Oncology*, 3rd ed. Oxford: Oxford University Press; 2012. pp. 408–43.

Cancer Research UK. *Bowel Cancer Statistics*. Available at: http://www.cancerresearchuk.org/health-professional/cancer-statistics/statistics-by-cancer-type/bowel-cancer

Nursing management issues

A number of specific challenges face nurses supporting individuals with colorectal cancer. Body image and psychosexual issues often emerge, both from the nature of the disease and from treatment side effects. Those patients with advanced cancer may also have complex and difficult symptoms such as bowel obstruction, pain, and bowel fistulae. Effective multidisciplinary management is crucial to support these patients effectively.

Treatment issues

Post-surgical

Many men will suffer a level of impotence and/or ejaculatory problems after colorectal surgery, whilst colorectal surgery, particularly low anterior or abdominoperineal resection, is among the most important causes of sexual dysfunction in women. Women may also suffer from urinary problems such as dysuria and incontinence. Patients requiring stoma formation also report many problems with body image and sexuality. Faecal incontinence or ↑ bowel movements are also a problem (⊃ see Care of the patient with a stoma, p. 328).

- Patients can become socially isolated and face periods of depression. Many of these difficulties can occur months after surgery.
- It is essential to assess patients' social and psychosexual well-being regularly, to pick up issues early and to offer support both in hospital and in the community.
- Nurses can play an important part in offering advice on lifestyle changes, coordinating care, and referring to appropriate specialist services.

Radiotherapy

Radiotherapy can be debilitating. Common problems include:
- Diarrhoea
- Fatigue
- Sore skin
- Perineal wound infection if used pre-surgery.

Chemotherapy

Chemotherapy regimens are generally well tolerated. Particular issues are:
- Severe diarrhoea (irinotecan-/capecitabine-based regimes)
- Nausea, infection, and fatigue.

Pain

- **Liver metastases** can cause capsular pain, which responds to NSAIDs and steroids.

Local rectal recurrence

- Can cause severe neuropathic perineal and pelvic pain, as well as tenesmus (painful sensation of rectal fullness).
- Each can be difficult to manage successfully and only partially responds to opioids.

- Management options include analgesics, anti-convulsants, radiotherapy, and local nerve blocks.
- Skilled nursing pain management is required to support these patients effectively (➲ see Chapter 46, Pain management). Specialist palliative care teams can be invaluable for these symptoms.

Altered bowel habit

Diarrhoea and constipation

- Patients can suffer from diarrhoea and/or constipation on a regular basis.
- For patients with diarrhoea, it is important to rule out faecal impaction.
- Alternating diarrhoea and constipation could be a warning of developing bowel obstruction.

Bowel obstruction

- Can be a major problem after surgery (where it normally responds to conservative approaches) and in advanced cancer.
- Nurses have a key role in early diagnosis by assessing patients for signs of obstruction.

Nutritional issues

- Many colorectal patients will suffer from weight loss, anorexia, and malnutrition, with associated fatigue and weakness.
- It is important that the MDT, and especially the dietician and the patient's family, are fully involved in managing nutritional disorders.

Further reading

Colorectal cancer. *BMJ Best Practice* (updated Feb 2015). Available at: ℜ http://bestpractice.bmj. com/best-practice/monograph/258/treatment/step-by-step.html

Health and Social Care Information Centre (2014). *National Bowel Cancer Audit Report – 2014*. Available at: ℜ https://digital.nhs.uk/data-and-information/publications/statistical/national-bowel-cancer-audit/national-bowel-cancer-audit-report-2014

Sheldon LK. *A Nurse's Guide to Caring for Cancer Survivors: Colorectal Cancer*. Sudbury, MA: Jones and Bartlett; 2010.

Chapter 25

Cancer of unknown primary

Introduction and prognosis

Introduction

There are two main groups of patients who are often termed as having 'cancers of unknown primary' (CUP).

The larger group of these patients comprise those who have a metastatic malignancy with an unknown primary at the point of initial imaging or clinical examination. In real terms, they could be more accurately described as having **malignancy of unknown origin** (MUO). If initial, but not exhaustive, investigations, do not find a primary site, then these are classified as **provisional CUP**.

Many subsequently obtain a working diagnosis, but a significant proportion of these patients are not fit enough for treatment, or even to complete investigations.

The second, smaller group is made up of those patients whose primary cannot be identified, despite full investigation, and they are treated without this being known.

Confirmed CUP

- Confirmed CUP is now a relatively rare phenomenon, with only around 3% of all cancers diagnosed in the UK, as a result of advances in diagnostic methods and registration methodology.
- CUP disproportionally affects older people. More than 50% of patients with a CUP are older than 75 when diagnosed, and >75% of all patients diagnosed are older than 65 years. More men than women are diagnosed with CUP.[1]
- CUP are twice as likely to present as emergencies (57%, compared to an average of 23% for other cancers).

Prognosis

In general, the prognosis for patients with both CUP and MUO is very poor.
- Patients with CUP make up 3% of the cancer population but account for around 8% of cancer mortality.
- By definition, all CUP/MUO disease is metastasized at diagnosis.
- Average survival is 4–6 months. However, there are subgroups of patients with CUP who perform significantly better:
  - Patients with a single metastasis—radical surgical treatment can be successful
  - Cervical neck node, with unknown primary—radical treatment, presuming a cancer of the H&N region, can lead to 5-year survival of over 30%
  - Women with peritoneal adenocarcinoma—can be treated as a gynaecological cancer. Median survival is around 16 months, with 15% surviving longer term
  - Younger patients (<50 years) with poorly differentiated mediastinal metastases—50% respond to platinum chemotherapy, and some respond longer term. Median survival is around 13 months.
- The characteristic most likely to lead to a poor prognosis is the presence of liver metastases without a known primary.

References

1 Cancer Research UK. *Cancer of Unknown Primary Statistics*. Available at: ℛ http://www.cancerresearchuk.org/health-professional/cancer-statistics/statistics-by-cancer-type/cancer-of-unknown-primary

New approaches to managing CUP

The CUP multidisciplinary team

In 2014, in order to address poor prognosis of CUP and MUO in the UK, the NHS set up specialist CUP MDTs. These measures were based on NICE guidelines first produced in 2010[2] and incorporating aspects of ESMO's guidelines produced in 2011 (updated in 2015).[3]

These measures established parity with other site specialist MDTs, e.g. a named oncologist, imaging and pathology experts, and a CNS with responsibility for giving advice and support to patients with CUP/MUO.

Other key measures include a core member of the CUP MDT providing a face-to-face assessment of patients with a CUP/MUO within 1 working day (for inpatients) or 2 weeks (for outpatients).

Links with other services

• Acute Oncology Services: as CUP patients are frequently diagnosed and/or investigated as a result of an emergency admission, strong formalized links for referral and discussion with the acute oncology service are essential (➔ see Acute Oncology Services, pp. 651–3). In some locations, the acute oncology team is also part of the CUP MDT. In others, the services are entirely separate.

Palliative care services

Palliative care plays a crucial role in caring for this patient group. A palliative care consultant should be a core member of the CUP MDT. Patients often face a short prognosis, have multiple symptoms, and can benefit from the skills and resources of palliative care teams.

Further reading

NHS England (2014). *Manual for Cancer Services: Cancer of Unknown Primary Measures*, Version 1.1. Available at: ⅊ https://cupfoundjo.org/wp-content/uploads/2016/05/CUP-Measures-V1.1.pdf

References

2 National Institute for Health and Care Excellence (2010). *Metastatic Malignant Disease of Unknown Primary Origin in Adults: Diagnosis and Management*. Clinical guideline [CG104]. Available at: ⅊ https://www.nice.org.uk/guidance/cg104

3 Fizazi K, Greco FA, Pavlidis N, Daugaard G, Oien K, Pentheroudakis G; ESMO Guidelines Committee. Cancers of unknown primary site: ESMO Clinical Practice Guidelines for diagnosis, treatment and follow-up. *Ann Oncol* 2015;**26**(Suppl 5):v133–8.

Diagnosis and treatment

Investigations

It is important to identify potentially curable malignancies, such as germ cell tumours and lymphomas, and also those who fit better performance groups such as women with axillary lymph nodes, men with retroperitoneal lymph nodes, or patients with cervical or inguinal lymph nodes.

It is important to only carry out investigations that may change clinical outcome. There is a danger of exhausting the patient with extensive, but futile, investigations.

We should ensure:
- The patient is fit enough and is prepared to accept treatment and that there exists a clear treatment option
- The results of any investigation are likely to affect treatment decisions
- The patient understands the purpose of the investigation and any risks/ benefits of investigations and treatment.

Note: it is unethical to carry out multiple tests on a patient with irreversible symptoms who is never likely to be fit enough to be treated.

Initial investigations
These should include:
- Full history, including family history
- Full physical examination
- Blood profiling—FBC, LFTs, serum biochemistry. Include tumour markers, based on the clinical scenario, e.g. PSA in men with bone metastases, CA-125 in women with ascites.

Further investigations
Imaging
As CUP can present in a large variety of different forms and affect a wide range of organs, a similarly wide range of imaging tests are often used to accurately stage patients with CUP. These can include X-rays, CT, PET, MRI, US, and various forms of endoscopy.

It is vital that there is an element of coordination of this pathway in order to obtain the best picture of the patient.

Biopsy
This will determine whether the primary tumour can be identified or at least the tissue type categorized. It can guide the MDT on which treatment strategy to employ.

Gene profiling
This is not currently in routine clinical practice. However, there is much interest in utilizing profiling in order to more accurately identify a primary tumour and to target chemotherapy.

In principle, gene profiling is able to identify primary tumours in around 80% of CUPs.[4] For these reasons, it is likely that genetic profiling will become more important in correctly diagnosing and treating patients with CUP.

Treatments

Chemotherapy (SACT)

SACT can be used to treat patients where they are well enough to receive it. In real terms, this tends to be patients who fit into WHO performance status categories 1 or 2 (➔ see Clinical performance status, p. 194). The choice of agents employed is governed by:

- Available histology
- Whether patients fit into previously identified high performance categories (e.g. women with peritoneal adenocarcinoma who could be treated with gynaecological regimes)
- Comorbidities (e.g. renal or cardiac impairment)
- As with all palliative treatments, it is important that patients are reviewed and monitored regularly to ensure that the benefits of chemotherapy outweigh possible side effects.

Radiotherapy

Radiotherapy in the palliative setting is generally well tolerated and is commonly used in patients with CUP/MUO to palliate symptoms (➔ see Use of radiotherapy, p. 194).

Surgical interventions

Surgery can be considered if only solitary metastasis can be identified after full staging.

Otherwise surgery is palliative, e.g. a defunctioning stoma in bowel obstruction or to stent an obstructed ureter in hydronephrosis.

Trials in the treatment of CUP

In recent years, poor survival of patients with CUP has led to ↑ interest in providing trials for this group of patients, in order to improve longer-term survival and promote more active treatments, though currently the number of trials remain low.

Further reading

Hainsworth J, Greco E. Gene expression profiling in patients with carcinoma of unknown primary site: from translational research to standard of care. *Virchows Arch* 2014;464:393–402.

References

4 Horlings HM, van Laar RK, Kerst JM, *et al*. Gene expression profiling to identify the histogenetic origin of metastatic adenocarcinomas of unknown primary. *J Clin Oncol* 2008;26:4435–41.

Nursing management

The lack of certainty around diagnosis means that it is difficult to give the patient and their family adequate information about potential outcomes of the disease or treatment.

It is essential to remain honest about the uncertainties and the general poor prognosis. This uncertainty may cause high levels of anxiety, distress, and anger, for both the patient and their family (➔ see Living with cancer, pp. 83–4).

It is therefore important to focus also on what is known, e.g. results of biopsies, where metastases are, and plans of treatment.

Information-giving issues will include:
- Clarifying reasons for a particular treatment approach
- Potential further approaches if initial treatment is unsuccessful
- The balance between full investigations and the potentially futile nature of such investigations.

For many patients, a crucial step will be involvement of the palliative care team, either within an acute environment or in the community. Most patients will benefit from an early referral to these teams, as this will help in patients' decision-making around treatment and symptom control.

The Cancer of the Unknown Primary Foundation (Jo's Friends) has now established a supportive patient-focused website for people with a diagnosis of CUP and their families. This contains information and a patient forum. This can be accessed at ℅ https://cupfoundjo.org/support

Endocrine cancers

Introduction

Endocrine tumours arise from glands that secrete endocrine hormones. This includes the pituitary, thyroid, parathyroid, and adrenal glands, as well as the gonads and the islets of Langerhans in the pancreas.

Endocrine tumours are rare and benign in most cases. Benign tumours can still cause significant morbidity, but they are not covered in this book.

The causes of most cases of endocrine cancer are unknown. There is an autosomal dominant inheritance disorder called multiple endocrine neoplasia (MEN), in which individuals can develop multiple endocrine tumours, generally earlier in life, with multicentric and bilateral presentation due to a dominant mutation in the *MEN1* gene.

Nursing people with these cancers requires knowledge of the hormones secreted and their effects on body systems. Nursing management needs to focus both on the symptoms caused by these hormones and the symptoms caused by the mass effect of the tumours.

Thyroid cancer

Thyroid cancer accounts for 90% of endocrine tumours. The most common are differentiated thyroid cancers (DTCs) such as papillary thyroid carcinoma (PTC) and follicular thyroid cancer (FTC), which have a 10-year survival rate of over 90%. However, about 5–20% will have regional/local recurrence and around 10% will have distant metastases, commonly to the lung or bone.

High risk for poorer survival includes older patients, ♂ gender, poorly differentiated cells, larger tumour, and extra-thyroidal invasion.

Differentiated thyroid cancers

Presentation

The most common clinical presentation is with a painless lump in the neck—a solitary thyroid nodule.

Urgent signs include associated hoarseness, cervical lymph nodes, or a rapidly enlarging mass (possible signs of anaplastic thyroid carcinoma).

Anaplastic cancer generally presents with a rapidly enlarging neck mass and enlarged lymph nodes.

Risk factors

- Nuclear fallout—e.g. massive increase in childhood thyroid cancer post-Chernobyl.
- Childhood exposure to radiation examination.

Treatment

Surgery is the most common treatment, involving partial or total thyroidectomy. Potential complications of this include hypoparathyroidism and laryngeal nerve injury.

If the lesion is <1cm, then a partial thyroidectomy is normally the treatment of choice. PTC of >1cm or high-risk FTC require near-total or total thyroidectomy. This may include node dissection if high risk or if node involvement. The majority of these cases will also require adjuvant [131]iodine ablation therapy.

Lifelong thyroid-stimulating hormone (TSH) suppression will be required post-thyroidectomy. EBRT may be used to downstage some tumours and for palliation of symptoms from advanced local or metastatic disease.

The TKI sorafenib can be used in advanced DTC when it no longer responds to[131] iodine ablation therapy. Other biological therapies are also being trialled in a number of studies.

Follow-up

This should be life-long—the disease has a long natural history, late recurrences can be successfully treated, and ongoing monitoring of treatment and for potential hypocalcaemia. Surveillance includes clinical examination, thyroid function tests, and diagnostic imaging or FNA, if indicated.

Anaplastic thyroid carcinoma

Anaplastic thyroid cancer is far rarer. It is generally too advanced at diagnosis for surgery and is not responsive to iodine therapy. Median survival is between 4 and 7 months. Chemotherapy or combined chemo-/radiation may slightly prolong survival. The mainstay of treatment is EBRT for palliation of symptoms.

Medullary thyroid cancer

Medullary thyroid cancer (MTC) accounts for 5–10% of thyroid cancers; 25% of MTCs are familial. Common genetic syndromes include MEN 2 and 3, previously known as MEN 2a and 2b. All patients with MTC should be offered genetic counselling and *RET* mutation analysis (which identifies mutations in the *RET* oncogene), whether or not there is an evident family history.

Presentation
- Neck lump.
- Metastatic disease symptoms.
- Dysphagia.
- Vasomotor flushing and diarrhoea (↑ calcitonin).

It is important to exclude phaeochromocytoma and primary hyperparathyroidism by measuring 24-hour urine catecholamines and metanephrines and serum calcium.

Treatment
Surgery
Patients may survive for many years, even with significant tumour burden.

Minimum treatment is normally total thyroidectomy and node dissection. The aim is for loco-regional control and, if possible, biochemical/clinical cure. There may be value in thyroid surgery, even if there are distant metastases, to prevent future compromise of the trachea or oesophagus.

External beam radiotherapy
This may reduce relapse rates of gross macroscopic disease and is also used to palliate local symptoms.

Other treatments
Chemotherapy is generally ineffective. If used, the most common agents are doxorubicin and cisplatin. Vandetanib is also available for inoperable MTC that is causing symptoms. Peptide receptor radionuclide therapy, using either somatostatin or metaiodobenzylguanidine (MIBG), is an option, though there is limited research evidence of long-term benefit. Gastric symptoms, such as chronic diarrhoea, can be treated with long-acting somatostatin analogues.

Prophylactic surgery in familial conditions
Prophylactic surgery should be considered in carriers of germline *RET* mutations. In MEN 2a, surgery is recommended in patients before the age of 5 years, and in MEN 2b, ideally by the age of 12 months. Life-long follow-up is essential.

Palliative care in thyroid cancer

Though most thyroid cancers have a good prognosis, those who have progressive disease may have a number of extremely distressing symptoms, e.g. stridor, superior vena cava obstruction (SVCO) (see Superior vena cava obstruction, pp. 645–6), fear of choking, and bleeding (see Bleeding in advanced cancer, p. 486), and will require input from specialist palliative care services.

Adrenal cancer

Adrenal tumours are rare, with an incidence of about 1–1.5 per million in the adult population. Peak incidence occurs in childhood and then again in the fourth and fifth decades. Most are sporadic, though a number of cases link to inherited syndromes, e.g. MEN 1, Li-Fraumeni.

Presentation

About two-thirds of patients will present with symptoms from one of a number of hormonal syndromes, e.g. Cushing's syndrome or virilization.

Prognosis

Overall prognosis is poor, with 5-year survival of around 20–30%. Key factors are stage of the disease at diagnosis and resection-free margin post-surgery.

Even after surgery, >50% of patients will subsequently relapse.

Diagnosis

- Endocrine assessment.
- Imaging: CT/MRI. Functional PET imaging in selected cases.
- Avoid biopsy in potentially resectable cases, due to risk of disease spread.

Treatment

Surgery

Mainstay of treatment: adrenalectomy for local disease. If locally advanced, resection of other nearby organs may be required to try and obtain resection-free margins. Surgery can also be repeated for local recurrence, particularly if >12 months from original diagnosis and resection-free margins are possible.

Mitotane

The mechanism of action not fully understood, but it is known to directly suppress the adrenal cortex. It should be offered as adjuvant treatment in those with no clear resection margins or a faster mitotic rate (Ki67 >10%). Low-risk patients should be considered for a trial of adjuvant mitotane.

The most effective length of adjuvant treatment is uncertain; suggested for 1–2 years, as this is the most common time for relapse. It can be difficult to tolerate, due to CNS and GI side effects. Patients must remain on glucocorticoids throughout to cover for adrenal insufficiency; 50% will need to remain on these life-long, even after stopping mitotane.

Metastatic disease

Poor prognosis, with 5-year survival of <15%. If the patient is fit enough, then offer chemotherapy with etoposide, doxorubicin, and cisplatin (EDP) ± mitotane. Patients with poorer performance status can have single-agent mitotane.

Further reading

Berruti A, Baudin E, Gelderblom H, et al. Adrenal cancer: ESMO Clinical Practice Guidelines for diagnosis, treatment and follow-up. Ann Oncol 2012;23(Suppl 7):vii131–8.

Mihai R. Diagnosis, treatment and outcome of adrenocortical cancer. Br J Surg 2015;102:291–306.

Perros P, Colley S, Boelaert K, et al.; British Thyroid Association, Royal College of Physicians (2014). Guidelines for the Management of Thyroid Cancer, 3rd ed. Available at: ℅ http://onlinelibrary.wiley.com/doi/10.1111/cen.12515/pdf

Neuroendocrine tumours

Epidemiology/aetiology

Neuroendocrine tumours (NETs) originate from a wide range of cells, including pancreatic islet cells and diffuse neuroendocrine cells distributed throughout the gut and respiratory epithelium. Historically, often known as carcinoid tumours.

- Relatively rare tumour, possibly between 4.5/100,000 and 9/100,000.
- Prevalence of NETs is relatively high, due to many NETs being slow-growing and having relatively prolonged survival.
- Common sites for NETs include the lung, small intestine, colorectal, and pancreatic.
- Most are sporadic, but some occur as part of MEN 1, MEN 2, and NF1 familial syndromes.

They are a heterogenous group of tumours, ranging from indolent to aggressive. Though often slow-growing, many NETs will have metastasized at diagnosis. Over half of small bowel and colonic NETs will have metastasized, most commonly to local lymph nodes and secondly to the liver.

Survival

Those with low-grade NETs (well and moderately differentiated) may live for a number of years, even with metastatic disease. High-grade tumours have a far worse prognosis. The 5-year survival, based on the grade of the tumour is grade 1: 96%, grade 2: 73%, and grade 3: 28%. Staging of tumours shows survival rates for stages I, II, III, and IV are 100%, 90%, 79%, and 55%, respectively.

Presenting features

- Often through incidental radiology/surgery.
- Pain, often intermittent and present for many years.
- Nausea and vomiting.
- Anaemia due to intestinal blood loss.
- Hormone-related clinical features such as flushing, diarrhoea, palpitations, wheeze (carcinoid syndrome), or specific pancreatic peptide syndromes (e.g. insulinoma, gastrinomas).
- Carcinoid syndrome occurs in 20% of cases of midgut NET.
- Chest symptoms for lung NETs.

Functioning versus non-functioning tumours

The term **functioning tumour** is used to describe patients with tumours that cause hormonal syndromes, such as carcinoid syndrome (small intestinal NETs) or Zollinger Ellison syndrome (gastrinomas). Patients without any hormone-related features will be described as having a 'non-functioning tumour'.

Diagnosis

There is often a delay between the appearance of first symptoms and a diagnosis of NET. This could be typically as long as 7 years. A number of specialist tests may be required, including:

- Biopsy
- Endoscopy

- Radiological imaging: CT, MRI, endoscopic US (EUS)
- Scintigraphy, including PET/CT, octreotide/single-photon emission CT (SPECT CT), gallium-68 dotatate/PET scan.
- Biochemistry: urinary 5-hydroxyindoleacetic acid (5-HIAA), chromogranin A and B markers, fasting gut hormones.

Treatment

The aim of treatment should be curative, where possible, but it is palliative in the majority of cases. Patients may often survive for many years with metastases, so the aim should always be to maintain a good QoL for as long as possible.

General approach

Surgery

Surgery is the only curative treatment for NETs. Surgery with intent to cure depends on the stage of disease and the general health state of the patient. Assessment for risk of carcinoid crisis is also essential (see Box 26.1).

Palliative surgery may also be used, e.g. to prevent possible bowel obstruction or to reduce symptoms from liver metastases which may be producing high levels of hormones. Valve replacement may be carried out for patients with carcinoid heart disease.

Somatostatin analogues

The majority of NETs express somatostatin receptors. Long-acting somatostatin analogue injections (octreotide or lanreotide) can be administered to reduce the release of various peptide hormones. They produce symptomatic benefit in the majority of patients with 'functioning tumours' (➔ see Functioning versus non-functioning tumours, p. 346), particularly reducing flushing and diarrhoea. Recent studies have also shown an anti-tumour effect, with ↑ progression-free survival. Their use is therefore increasing in non-functional tumours as well.

Peptide receptor radionuclide therapy

Radiolabelled peptides (generally labelled with a somatostatin analogue) can be used to deliver radiotherapy directly to tumour cells. The most commonly used radionuclides are yttrium-90 or lutetium-177 therapy.

Box 26.1 Carcinoid crisis

Carcinoid crisis is characterized by profound flushing, bronchospasm, tachycardia, and widely fluctuating blood pressure. It is caused by the release of high levels of serotonin and other vasoactive peptides. It is often precipitated by anaesthetics, intraoperative handling of the tumour, or other invasive procedures such as embolization.

Prophylactic administration of short-acting octreotide should be used to prevent this, even in patients who are receiving long-acting somatostatin analogues. Typical protocols give an IV infusion at a dose of 50–100 micrograms per hour, started 12 hours before, and given for 24–48 hours after, surgical intervention. Antihistamines and corticosteroids may also be helpful.

Liver-directed therapies

Liver metastases in NETs often cause pain and hormonal symptoms. A number of treatment approaches are available:

- **Partial hepatectomy**: isolated metastases, within one area of the liver can be resected
- **Hepatic artery embolization**—using microspheres: useful when there are numerous metastases in the liver or if the tumours are producing a lot of hormones
- **Selective internal radiotherapy treatment (SIRT)**—embolization with radioactive microspheres
- **Radiofrequency or microwave ablation**: this may be used when a patient has relatively few liver metastases and if they are fairly small.

Chemotherapy

Mainly used with higher-grade NETs and certain pancreatic or bronchial NETs.

Commonly used regimens include:

- Streptozotocin (STZ)—with 5FU or capecitabine
- Cisplatin and etoposide (mainly higher-grade NETs)
- Temozolamide.

Biological therapy

Everolimus and sunitinib have shown efficacy in pancreatic NETs.

Nursing issues with NETs

NET patients have often spent years with distressing symptoms, going through a multitude of investigations before being diagnosed. If not managed in a specialist centre, there may be a continuing lack of knowledge and support in managing their illness.

Patients should be able to access a specialist NET MDT to guide treatment. This can lead to long distances travelling to appointments or for treatment. Other models include specialist MDTs guiding local hospitals to support patients with NETs. In both models, patients will benefit from support from nurses who have a clear understanding of the illness, treatment options, and management of ongoing symptoms.

European centres of excellence

It is recommended that all patients with a NET are reviewed by, or referred to, a European Neuroendocrine Tumour Centre of Excellence. These 'centres of excellence' can be contacted for advice or direct input. There are now ten such centres in the UK, with numbers likely to increase in the near future (see ℘ http://www.enets.org/coe.html)

Abdominal symptoms

NETs affect digestion and the body's ability to extract nourishment from food. Patients may have distressing symptoms, including frequent diarrhoea, bloating, flatulence, and abdominal pain. This often leads to malnourishment, weight loss, and fatigue. It can also cause low mood and isolation. These symptoms are often chronic; they have had them for a number of years, and they are often resistant to a number of treatments. There are often multiple reasons for these symptoms, including the mass effect of the tumours themselves, hormonal release, treatments including surgery, and medication such as somatostatin analogues and chemotherapy. Diet may also contribute to symptoms, with some patients having 'trigger' foods that set off flushing and/or diarrhoea.

Specialist assessment, preferably with dietician support, is essential. Common issues that need managing are weight loss, steatorrhoea, diarrhoea, bloating, flatulence, and vitamin and mineral deficiencies.

Patients may typically need some or all of the following: anti-diarrhoea treatments, pancreatic supplements, specialist diet advice, and calorie supplementation

Quality of life

Patients with NETs often describe having a fairly good QoL. However, the physical symptoms they often have, plus living with the uncertainty of a chronic illness that may progress in the future, can lead to a number of problems such as anxiety and depression. Diarrhoea and other abdominal symptoms can often lead to social isolation. Chronic fatigue is common and can be debilitating. Social issues, such as having to reduce or give up work, financial concerns, including issues with insurance, all impact on patients living with what is often a chronic illness.

Specialist nurses can support patients with information, understanding, and providing access to a range of specialist services. This may include referring on to specialist NET centres to offer appropriate expertise and support.

Further reading

European Neuroendocrine Tumor Society (ENETS). *ENETS Guidelines*. Available at: ℰ http://www.enets.org/enets_guidelines.html (website for up-to-date European guidelines).

NET Patient Foundation. Available at: ℰ http://www.netpatientfoundation.org/

Ramage JK, Ahmed A, Ardill J, *et al*. (2012). Guidelines for the management of gastroenteropancreatic neuroendocrine (including carcinoid) tumours (NETs). *Gut* 2012;61:6–32.

The Carcinoid Cancer Foundation (2012). *Neuroendocrine Tumors: A Guide for Nurses*. Available at: ℰ http://www.carcinoid.org/content/neuroendocrine-tumors-guide-nurses

Upper gastrointestinal cancers

Introduction

Cancers of the upper GI tract are a diverse group of cancers, accounting for around one-fifth of all cancers diagnosed in the UK. Improved surgical treatment and, for some, endoscopic treatments of early-stage disease can offer excellent survival rates. However, the majority of patients present with locally advanced or metastatic disease. The symptoms of many of the upper GI cancers are vague and non-specific and often occur late in the course of the disease. Combined with poor overall responses to chemotherapy and radiotherapy, this makes them difficult to treat; as a result, long-term survival rates tend to be low.

For some diseases, such as pancreatic cancer, the outcome may be bleak, with a short life expectancy and rapid physical deterioration not unusual.

Accurate oncological staging and evaluation of fitness for treatment, including potentially radical treatment with surgery or chemoradiotherapy, are essential. Over the past few years, improvement in preoperative staging, centralization of upper GI services to high-volume centres, improvement in perioperative care, a specialist multidisciplinary approach to care, and a multimodal approach to treatments have resulted in a better selection of patients for radical treatment, prolonged post-operative survival, and reduced post-operative mortality.

Oesophageal cancer

Incidence

The incidence of oesophageal cancer is increasing, especially lower-third and oesophagogastric junction adenocarcinomas, with ~9200 people diagnosed in the UK each year. It is at least twice as common in ♂ than in ♀. Early lymphatic spread is common before symptoms occur. Most people therefore present with advanced disease, and the overall prognosis is poor, with around 15% surviving for 5 years or more. Distant spread to the liver, adrenal glands, lung, bone, and brain is common in advanced disease.

Risk factors

- Gastro-oesophageal reflux disease (GORD).
- Barrett's oesophagus (dysplastic changes in the lower oesophagus).
- Obesity: may increase oesophageal reflux and incidence of Barrett's oesophagus.
- Alcohol and smoking: heavy smokers and drinkers have a 100-fold ↑ risk.

Presenting symptoms

- Typically presents with progressive dysphagia; initially solids, later liquids.
- Often combination of weight loss, anorexia, and cachexia.
- Other symptoms include odynophagia, hoarseness, chest pain, regurgitation, and dyspepsia.

Diagnosis and staging

- Endoscopy with tissue biopsy is the investigation of choice.
- CT scan to detect distant metastases and local spread and metastatic disease. Fluorodeoxyglucose positron emission tomography (FDG PET) can improve detection of distant metastases, therefore reducing futile surgical resection.
- EUS—shows the extent of local invasion and lymph node involvement.
- Staging laparoscopy may be indicated to assess peritoneal disease if surgery or radical treatment is being considered.

Treatment

A specialist multidisciplinary approach is recommended for optimum patient management. This should involve surgeons, oncologists, site-specific CNS, radiologists, histopathologists, palliative care specialists, dieticians, and the MDT coordinator.

Endoscopic treatments

Endoscopic treatments, including endoscopic mucosal resection (EMR), are suitable in a highly selected patient group with high-grade dysplasia or early gastro-oesophageal intramucosal cancer.

Radical treatments for cancer of the oesophagus

Radical treatments commonly include: surgery alone, a combination of chemotherapy and surgery, a combination of chemoradiotherapy and surgery, or a radical course of chemoradiotherapy.

Around 10–20% of all cases in the UK are treated by surgery, with transthoracic oesophagectomy plus local and regional lymph node removal. An oesophagogastrectomy may be required for cancers of the GOJ and the proximal stomach.

There is a considerable risk of post-operative morbidity, including pulmonary complications and anastomotic leak. Post-operative mortality rate is <4% in specialist centres. Long-term effects of treatment include the need for major dietary adjustment, dumping syndrome, and malabsorption.

Radical chemoradiotherapy

A radical course of chemoradiotherapy is a gruelling treatment. It may be a possible treatment option for those patients who have SCC or are unfit for surgery or those who choose not to undergo surgery. However, radical chemoradiotherapy has a cure rate in its own right.

Neo-adjuvant treatments

Neo-adjuvant chemotherapy prior to surgical resection has become a common treatment strategy, with trials showing an increase in overall survival.

Neo-adjuvant chemoradiotherapy in oesophageal cancer is currently used in selected patients.

Adjuvant treatments

Adjuvant chemotherapy is not routinely given following surgery and has not been shown to improve survival. It may be offered in a clinical trial setting. Adjuvant radiotherapy is sometimes offered to patients, who have positive surgical resection margins.

Palliative treatments

Palliative treatments, such as chemotherapy, radiotherapy, or oesophageal stent insertion, may be given singly or in combination, though median survival for stage IV disease remains poor at around 8 months. Palliative chemotherapy can offer improvement in symptoms such as dysphagia and pain, with a 3-month improvement in median survival. Palliative radiotherapy can assist in the relief of dysphagia and bleeding. Oesophageal stenting is the treatment of choice in patients with severe dysphagia or aphagia.

Gastric cancer

Epidemiology

This is the fifth most common cancer worldwide and the 17th most common in the UK, accounting for 10% deaths per annum from cancer worldwide. In most countries, the incidence of stomach cancer is declining due to improved refrigeration The incidence rises steeply after 55 years.

Adenocarcinoma of the stomach accounts for >90% of all gastric cancers.

Aetiology

- *Helicobacter pylori* infection has a 3- to 6-fold increase in risk and causes chronic gastritis.
- Other environmental factors include smoking, diet (high in salt, low fruit and vegetable consumption), heavy alcohol intake, and lower socio-economic class.
- Barrett's oesophagus: associated with an increase in gastro-oesophageal cancer.
- Pernicious anaemia: 3-fold increase.

Presenting signs and symptoms

- In early disease, symptoms are non-specific. Dyspepsia is the most common symptom reported.
- In more advanced disease, weight loss, anorexia, early satiety, and vomiting may occur. Gastric outflow obstruction will cause persistent vomiting.
- Dysphagia in proximal stomach or oesophagogastric cancers.
- Other symptoms may include upper and lower GI bleeding, upper abdominal pain, ascites, and jaundice.

Diagnosis and staging

- History and examination.
- Endoscopy and biopsy.
- CT scan to assess local involvement, including lymphadenopathy and distant metastases.
- PET/CT scan—to assess local and nodal involvement and distant metastatic disease.
- Staging laparoscopy may be indicated to assess peritoneal disease if surgery is being considered. Biopsies can also be obtained from suspicious lesions in the abdomen.
- Stomach cancer is usually advanced at diagnosis. Commonly see local extension to the pancreas, liver, or oesophagus, and local and distant nodes. Distant spread most common to the liver, peritoneal cavity, adrenal glands, lung, and bone.

Treatment

Resectable disease

Surgery remains a potentially curative option for early disease. The extent of a surgical resection is dependent on the position and extent of the tumour. A partial or total gastrectomy and regional lymphadenectomy are most commonly undertaken.

A minimally invasive gastrectomy can offer improved post-operative pain control, enhanced mobility, and a reduced hospital stay.

Surgery can have long-term effects on QoL, including adjustment to a reduced capacity and diet, with associated dumping syndrome and malabsorption. Those who have a total gastrectomy will require life-long replacement of vitamin B12.

Neo-adjuvant and adjuvant treatment

A standard treatment strategy is neo-adjuvant chemotherapy prior to a surgical resection, followed by adjuvant chemotherapy.

The standard chemotherapy regime for resectable gastric cancer in the UK is three cycles of preoperative epirubicin, cisplatin, and capecitabine, followed by surgery and post-operative chemotherapy.

The 5-year survival benefit over surgery alone is 36% versus 23%.

Adjuvant radiotherapy may be offered to patients where the surgical resection margin has been breached or within 1mm of the margin.

Palliative treatments

Advanced disease

- **Endoscopic stenting** is used to palliate an obstructing gastric cancer.
- **Surgical** gastrojejunostomy or enterostomy may be offered to bypass a locally advanced and obstructing tumour. A palliative surgical resection may be used to resect an obstructing or bleeding tumour.
- **Palliative radiotherapy** can be used for managing bleeding tumours or persistent anaemia and pain.
- **Palliative chemotherapy** can offer an improvement in symptoms and a modest benefit in life expectancy in patients who respond to chemotherapy.
- One-fifth of patients have gastric cancers with a high HER-2 expression. Targeted treatment with trastuzumab may show a median overall survival of 16 months, compared to 9.3–11.2 months with standard chemotherapy.

Cancer of the liver (hepatocellular cancer)

Epidemiology

There is a low incidence of liver cancer in the UK and Europe. It is most common where hepatitis B is endemic, e.g. in sub-Saharan Africa, South East Asia, and China. There is a correlation within areas of increasing deprivation. The majority of cases of liver cancer are under the age of 50, with ♂ affected more frequently than ♀.

Risk factors

- >90% of cases arise in patients with chronic liver disease or cirrhosis. Hepatitis B or C infection accounts for the majority of worldwide cases.
- Cirrhosis secondary to alcoholic liver disease often associated with a poor socio-economic status.
- Non-alcoholic fatty liver disease may be a risk factor, but further research is needed on diet and activity risk factors.

Symptoms

- Can be vague, particularly when the patient has chronic liver disease.
- Right upper quadrant abdominal pain, abdominal distension, fatigue, anorexia, and weight loss.
- Jaundice is uncommon.
- Paraneoplastic effects include: hypoglycaemia, erythrocytosis, hypercalcaemia, and hypercholesterolaemia.

Diagnosis and staging

- History.
- CT scan.
- Laparoscopy and US.
- Biopsy.
- Angiography.
- CXR and CT chest to exclude metastases.
- AFP—useful for diagnosis and monitoring recurrence.
- LFTs—to assess functional reserve.

Treatment options

Surgical resection

Surgery offers the only hope of cure for HCC. However, resection is not possible in many patients due to multifocal disease and liver failure associated with cirrhosis.

Liver transplantation

This is appropriate for some cirrhotic patients with HCC of <3cm. It is preferred in the treatment of HCC arising from hepatitis C because of the high likelihood of further tumour development in these patients.

Systemic chemotherapy

Systemic chemotherapy has been used for unresectable tumours, but response rates have been poor. Sorafenib (a TKI) is commonly offered in advanced HCC. Trials of combined treatments with SIRT and sorafenib are also ongoing.

Ablative techniques

- Radiofrequency ablation (RFA) and microwave ablation can be used to destroy tumour cells using heat. Causes minimal damage to surrounding tissue. Can be performed percutaneously in a radiology suite.
- More recently, irreversible electroporation, a non-thermal technique, has been used. May cause less damage to surrounding tissues.

Transarterial embolization

- Small embolic particles are injected selectively through a radiologically placed catheter in the hepatic artery.
- This can include chemoembolization (TACE) or radio-embolization (SIRT).
- Repeat embolization is performed at 2- to 3-monthly intervals. This may render some tumours resectable.
- Can be complicated by acute abdominal pain and fever (self-limiting) and liver failure (uncommon).

Prognosis

Overall survival is poor, with <10% of patients alive at 3 years. Survival for unresectable disease is about 2–6 months.

Pancreatic cancer

Epidemiology

Pancreatic cancers arise from the exocrine pancreas, of which adenocarcinomas are the most common (80%). In the UK, over 9900 cases are reported every year, and it is the sixth most common cause of cancer death in the UK. Around 44% of cases of pancreatic cancer present as an emergency, and 80% of patients have unresectable disease at the time of diagnosis. Disease spread is mainly to local lymph nodes, retroperitoneal tissue, the liver, and the peritoneum. Distant metastases are commonly to the liver, lung, and bone.

Risk factors

- Smoking increases the risk of pancreatic cancer by 30%.
- Diets high in red meat and saturated fats may be important, with obesity also linked.
- Family history of pancreatic cancer. Also hereditary pancreatitis.
- History of pancreatitis (can link to high alcohol intake).
- Diabetes mellitus.

Clinical signs and symptoms

- Early symptoms are non-specific and easily missed.
- Common signs are painless jaundice (dark urine, pale stools, and pruritus secondary to hyperbilirubinaemia), anorexia, weight loss, and back pain.
- Persistent abdominal pain radiating to the back.
- Late-onset diabetes mellitus or glucose intolerance.
- Malabsorption due to an obstructed pancreatic duct.
- Gastric outlet obstruction.

Note: persistent non-specific GI symptoms associated with back pain or recent onset of diabetes should be considered for a diagnosis of pancreatic cancer.

Investigations

- FBC and biochemical LFTs.
- Serum tumour markers: CA19–9, elevated in most, but poor sensitivity. Useful as a surveillance tool following treatment.
- Upper abdominal US scan may suggest a diagnosis.
- Endoscopic retrograde cholangiopancreatography (ERCP)—brush cytology or forceps biopsy.
- EUS scan and FNA of lesions (85–90% accuracy).
- CT, MRI scan—chest, abdomen, and pelvis.
- Laparoscopy—to assess for peritoneal involvement.
- Role of PET/CT scan is yet to be fully ascertained.

Treatment options
Surgery
Surgery is the only option of potentially curative treatment, though <20% of patients present with surgically resectable disease. Even then, the 5-year survival is 10–15%, with a median survival of 11–18 months.

Pancreaticoduodenectomy (Whipple's procedure) is the operation of choice commonly indicated for cancer of the head, neck, or uncinated process of the pancreas. Pylorus-preserving surgery allows some preservation of function.

Distal pancreatectomy is indicated for tumours of the body and tail of the pancreas.

The surgical mortality rate is approaching 10%, though <3% in specialist high-volume centres. Post-operative complications include bronchopneumonia, delayed gastric emptying, pancreatic fistulae formation, anastomotic leak, sepsis, abscess formation, and haemorrhage. Oral pancreatic enzyme supplements may be required for pancreatic exocrine insufficiency causing fat malabsorption.

Adjuvant therapies
Chemotherapy
Gemcitabine is the most commonly used regime. The ESPAC 4 trial has shown that gemcitabine and capecitabine can give a 5-year survival of around 30%.

Radiotherapy
Patients with good performance status and localized resectable tumour may be considered for radiotherapy, with or without chemotherapy.

Palliative treatments
Chemotherapy
Palliative chemotherapy commonly involves a gemcitabine-based regime, with only a modest benefit in life expectancy. Monoclonal antibodies are currently under investigation in patients with unresectable or metastatic disease. The Telovac trial showed that the telomorase vaccine GV1001 was no better than chemotherapy alone in treating pancreatic cancer.

Palliative surgical bypass procedures
These procedures may be possible for some patients. Generally, non-surgical relief of jaundice is indicated. Endoscopic or percutaneously inserted stents to relieve biliary tract or duodenal obstruction have relatively low morbidity rates.

Prognosis
The median survival rate in advanced disease is poor—between 3 and 6 months; the overall 5-year survival rate is 0.5%.

Cancer of the biliary tract

Epidemiology and aetiology

Cholangiocarcinoma is the second most common primary liver tumour worldwide. In the UK, 1500 people die annually from cholangiocarcinoma, with approximately equal numbers of men and women. However, >80% of people with early-stage tumours survive for 5 years.

There has been a rise in the incidence of cholangiocarcinoma, the cause of which is unexplained.

Risk factors

- Primary sclerosing cholangitis.
- Chronic intraductal gallstones.
- Cirrhosis of any cause.
- Other factors may include obesity, diabetes, fatty liver disease, smoking, high alcohol intake, and inflammatory bowel disease.

Presenting signs and symptoms

- Typically symptoms of biliary obstruction, i.e. jaundice, pale stools, dark urine, and pruritus.
- Malaise and fatigue.
- Anorexia and weight loss.

Routes of spread

Commonly infiltrates the muscular wall of the gall bladder and the neighbouring liver tissue, and spreads to regional lymph nodes and the liver. Distant metastases occur late.

Diagnosis

- US scan is the standard first-line investigation.
- CT scan may reveal intrahepatic mass lesions, dilated ducts, localized lymphadenopathy, and metastases.
- LFTs.
- MRI scan, combined with magnetic resonance cholangiopancreatography (MRCP), to assess bile duct involvement and resectability.
- CEA, CA19-9, and CA-125 are often elevated.
- EUS scan—accurate assessment of the bile duct. Can enable biopsy of distal lesions and nodes.
- Invasive ERCP is reserved for histological diagnosis, therapeutic decompression of cholangitis, and stent insertion.

Treatment

Surgical treatment

- Ten to 20% of patients are resectable at presentation.
- Intrahepatic cholangiocarcinomas are usually treated by resection of an involved lobe or segments of the liver, with associated removal of lymph nodes.
- A pancreaticoduodenectomy is recommended for distal cholangiocarcinomas or ampullary cancer.

- An open cholecystectomy is recommended for gall bladder cancers. If gall bladder cancer is detected following a simple cholecystectomy, then an additional resection should be considered.
- Risks: there is a risk of liver failure if there is a remaining small liver remnant.

Adjuvant treatment
- Adjuvant chemotherapy and radiotherapy are not routinely used.

Palliative treatments

- **Stenting**: palliation of biliary obstruction by biliary stenting using plastic or metal stents.
- **Chemotherapy**: cisplatin and gemcitabine are commonly recommended for locally advanced or metastatic cholangiocarcinoma.
- **Palliative radiotherapy** is used in the palliation of bleeding or localized metastatic disease.
- **RFA**: percutaneous US-guided thermal ablation is used for unresectable intrahepatic cholangiocarcinoma.
- **Loco-regional treatments**, such as radio-embolization and TACE, need further evaluation.

Nursing management issues

Specialist nursing care is required to support patients with upper GI tumours and their families. Treatment morbidity and common symptoms of dysphagia, severe weight loss, and malnutrition, amongst others, can create high levels of physical and psychological distress.

Accurate assessment and coordination of care are required for effective support of patients and their families. A multidisciplinary approach is essential throughout, with early involvement of specialist palliative care services recommended for many patients.

Nutritional issues

This is probably the biggest single management issue for individuals with upper GI cancer. Dysphagia, severe weight loss, anorexia, and malnutrition are all common. Malnutrition can arise from the behaviour of tumour metabolism, the obstructive effects of the tumour, and the side effects of treatments. It can result in reduced survival and impact on the clinical decision to consider potentially curable radical treatment and the response to cancer treatments.

The impact on the patient, their family, and their QoL can be enormous. Social activities may be curtailed; body image is affected, and fatigue and weakness may be severe. It is important that the MDT, especially the dietician and the patient's family, are fully involved in managing nutritional disorders (see Nutritional support, pp. 542–5).

Many patients require modification of their diet, in terms of texture and consistency of foods; others will require the prescription of oral supplements. Pre- and post-surgery patients may require a jejunostomy tube or nasojejunal feeding. Post-surgery, there is considerable adjustment to reduced capacity, possible dumping syndrome, and malabsorption problems.

Pain

Patients with upper GI cancers face a range of different pain due to their disease. Liver pain caused by stretching of the liver capsule, due to primary liver disease or liver metastases, is common. This pain is only partially responsive to opioids but responds well to NSAIDs and oral steroids.

Coeliac plexus involvement occurs in some upper GI cancers, including pancreatic cancer. This can create abdominal and mid-back pain, which is often difficult to control. Anaesthetic nerve blocks can be useful.

Bleeding

Liver involvement may cause clotting abnormalities. Locally advanced tumours can also occasionally cause bleeding, which can be severe or even life-threatening. This can often be reduced by local treatment such as endoscopic laser treatment or localized radiotherapy (see Bleeding in advanced cancer, p. 486).

Liver failure

Patients may have ascites (➔ see Malignant ascites, pp. 526–7), periph-eral oedema, and, in advanced stages, encephalopathy (➔ see Acute confusional state or delirium, pp. 594–5).

Further reading

Allum WH, Blazeby JM, Griffin SM, *et al.* Guidelines for the management of oesophageal and gastric cancer. *Gut* 2011;60:1449–72.

Bond-Smith G, Banga N, Hammond TM, Imber CJ. Pancreatic adenocarcinoma. *BMJ* 2012;344:45–50.

Cancer Research UK. Oesophageal Cancer Statistics. Available at: ℜ https://www.cancerresearchuk.org/health-professional/cancer-statistics/statistics-by-cancer-type/oesophageal-cancer

Cancer Research UK. *Oesophageal Cancer Statistics*. Available at: ℜ http://www.cancerresearchuk.org/cancer-info/cancerstats/keyfacts/oesophageal-cancer

Khan SA, Davidson BR, Goldin RD, *et al.* 2012 guidelines for the diagnosis and treatment of cholangiocarcinoma: an update. *Gut* 2012;61:1657–69.

Thrumurthy SG, Chaudry MA, Hochhauser D, Mughal M. The diagnosis and management of gastric cancer. *BMJ* 2013;347:27–33.

Chapter 28

Genitourinary cancers

Renal cancer

Epidemiology and aetiology
- There are 10,000 cases annually in the UK; 10-year survival of 50%.
- It is 1.5 times more common in men than women.
- Frequency increases with age—75% are 60 years or older.
- Smoking doubles the relative risk.
- Inherited predisposition causes 2% of renal cancers—often multifocal/bilateral.

Pathology
- 85% of renal cancers are adenocarcinomas and arise from the renal tubular epithelium.
- Approximately one-third of patients have metastatic spread at diagnosis. Common sites are the lungs, soft tissues, bones, and the liver.
- Transitional cell carcinomas (TCCs) can arise within the urothelium of the renal pelvis and represent the majority of the remaining tumours.

Presenting symptoms and signs
- Haematuria.
- General malaise.
- Night sweats.
- Loin pain.
- Anaemia.
- Weight loss.
- Pyrexia.
- Syndromes of hypertension, hypercalcaemia, and polycythaemia.

About 50% of renal cancers are diagnosed via their GP. About 25% present as an emergency, whilst around 25% are asymptomatic and are discovered during imaging for other reasons.

Investigations
- US scan or IV urography (IVU).
- Contrast CT scan of the abdomen and chest.
- FBC, biochemical profile.

Staging/prognosis
- Generally staged using the TNM system.[1]

Poor prognostic factors include:
- High blood lactate dehydrogenase (LDH) or high calcium levels
- Anaemia
- Spread to two or more distant sites
- Poor performance status.

Early-stage disease
- For patients who are fit for surgery, complete surgical resection is the only potentially curative treatment. Partial nephrectomy can be considered if the tumour is <7cm. Total nephrectomy if large tumour and/or lymph node involvement.

- Laparoscopic surgery is increasingly common. In specialist cancer centres, assisted robotic laparoscopic surgery may be an option.
- For patients with tumours of <4cm, cryotherapy or RFA can be considered.
- In some elderly asymptomatic patients, conservative management is appropriate as tumour growth may be slow.

Adjuvant therapy

Note: adjuvant immunotherapy in resectable disease has not yet shown clear evidence of improved disease survival.

Patients with a high risk of relapse may be considered for adjuvant biological therapy with sunitinib or possibly local radiotherapy.

Advanced disease

Management of patients with advanced and/or metastatic renal cancer is palliative.

Surgery

- Patients with metastatic disease, but good performance status (0–1), and a resectable primary tumour may benefit from nephrectomy as a palliative procedure to provide:
  - Control of local symptoms
  - Modest survival benefit, combined with immunotherapy.
- Regression of metastases following nephrectomy is reported but is extremely rare (<1%).

Radiofrequency ablation

- Patients with advanced disease may sometimes benefit from this procedure. RFA destroys tumour cells using the heat generated by high-frequency radio waves.
- NICE in the UK has found that there is enough evidence to support its use in renal cancers and that it is safe.

Biological therapy

- First-line treatment of advanced disease includes the use of either sunitinib or pazopanib (TKIs).
- Immunotherapy using interferon alfa or interleukin can also be considered for patients with small tumour burden.
- The TKIs sorafenib or axitinib can be employed second or third line.
- Other second-line treatments include mTOR inhibitors, such as everolimus, or combined treatments such as interferon and bevacizumab.

Prognostic factors that predict higher response rates include:
- Long disease-free interval
- Previous nephrectomy
- Good performance status (0–1).

Chemotherapy/radiotherapy

Renal cancer rarely responds to chemotherapy or radiotherapy. Palliative radiotherapy is appropriate for:
- Painful or bleeding primary tumour
- Non-resectable metastatic disease, e.g. bone, brain, or soft tissue.

Management of transitional cell carcinoma

Their biology, management, and prognosis are similar to those of TCC of the ureter, which is treated as if bladder TCC (see Cancer of the bladder and ureter, p. 369).

References

1 Amin MB, Edge S, Greene F, *et al.* (eds). *AJCC Cancer Staging Manual*, 8th ed. New York, NY: Springer; 2017.

Cancer of the bladder and ureter

Epidemiology
- Incidence of around 10,000 per year in the UK.
- Fourth most common ♂ cancer, with a ♂:♀ ratio of 2:1.
- Two-thirds occur in people aged >70.
- >90% are TCCs.

Risk factors
- Cigarette smoking increases the risk by about three times.
- Industrial chemicals, e.g. aromatic amines and aniline dye, though now better controlled, still account for a small percentage of bladder cancer.
- Previous pelvic radiotherapy, e.g. for gynaecological cancer.

Presentation
- 80–90% present with frank haematuria, usually painless.
- Frequency and dysuria.
- Recurrent UTI.
- Unexplained microscopic haematuria.
- Back, rectal, or suprapubic pain may suggest metastatic disease.

Pathology
- At least 70% of patients present with 'superficial' tumour involving only the bladder epithelium.
- In 25%, there is tumour invasion into the muscle of the bladder.
- 5% present with metastatic disease to the regional lymph nodes, lung, liver, or bone.
- 50% of carcinoma *in situ* can develop quickly into muscle-invasive cancer.

Staging
Both the stage of the disease and pathological grading are important. There is a strong association between well-differentiated tumours and early stage (➔ see Diagnosis, classification, and staging of cancer, p. 176).
- Low-grade tumours rarely progress to advanced disease.
- There is a significant risk of metastatic disease with high-grade disease and with increasing stage of muscle-invasive disease.

Investigations
- FBC, biochemistry profile.
- Cystoscopy and transurethral resection of bladder tumour (TURBT). This should be carried out with either photodynamic diagnosis or narrow band imaging to assist visualization.
- Staging with abdominal and pelvic CT/MRI if high risk of metastases, e.g. muscle-invasive cancer or a suspicion of this.
- FDG PET should be considered if MRI/CT are indeterminate or if there is T3b disease.

Treatment options

Non-muscle-invasive tumours (70% newly diagnosed cases)

- Low-risk tumours: are resected cystoscopically. The specimen should include the detrusor muscle. A single post-resection dose of intravesical mitomycin is given to reduce the risk of recurrence. Follow-up with cystoscopy at 3 months and 1 year.
- Intermediate-risk tumours: post-resection, offer six cycles of intravesical mitomycin. Follow-up with cystoscopy for 5 years.
- High-risk tumours: offer immunotherapy with BCG or radical cystectomy. BCG is a dilute preparation of the tuberculosis vaccine. Directly instilled into the bladder, the vaccine stimulates the immune system within the bladder wall to destroy the tumour.
- Recurrent disease is managed by further surgical resection, intravesical chemotherapy, or immunotherapy with BCG.
- Refractory disease is best managed by cystectomy.

Muscle-invasive bladder cancer

- **Neo-adjuvant chemotherapy**: fit patients should be considered for cisplatin-based combination chemotherapy, e.g. MVAC, Gem/Cis, prior to local treatment.

Local treatment is either:

- **Radical cystectomy**: offer a choice of continent urinary diversion if no contraindications or a urinary stoma. Patients may or may not have a choice, depending on suitability for a diversion. If they do, they should be counselled by both a stoma nurse and a cancer CNS (➔ see Care of the patient with a stoma, p. 328). Offer adjuvant chemotherapy if neo-adjuvant therapy was not already used.
- **Radical radiotherapy** with a radio-sensitizer such as mitomycin and 5FU. This is useful if the patient cannot tolerate surgery.
  - • The side effects of radical radiotherapy include cystitis and diarrhoea (➔ see Diarrhoea, p. 502), plus a late effect of reduction in bladder capacity.
  - • Frail patients who are unfit for radical surgery or radiotherapy may benefit from palliative radiotherapy to the bladder.

Advanced disease

- Gemcitabine and cisplatin or CMV—about 50% of patients respond.
- Second line—MVAC or high-dose MVAC with G-CSF cover can be considered.
- Carboplatin-based regimes if renal function poor—can be used in combination with paclitaxel.
- Regimens can still be toxic, especially for patients with poor performance status and impaired renal function.

Managing symptoms of locally advanced or metastatic bladder cancer

Bladder symptoms

Radiotherapy can be used to palliate symptoms of haematuria, dysuria, urinary frequency, or nocturia when the disease is unsuitable for potentially curative treatment.

Ureteric obstruction
Percutaneous nephrostomy or retrograde stenting can relieve pain or improve renal function.

Pelvic pain
Hypofractionated radiotherapy, nerve block, and palliative chemotherapy can all be considered alongside best supportive care.

Treatment outcomes

The prognosis for superficial disease is good, with 5-year survival rates in excess of 80%. Survival from muscle-invasive disease is 40–60%. For metastatic disease, median survival time is 1 year, with around 10% living 2 years.

Prostate cancer

For many men with this diagnosis, the optimum management is uncertain, with a spectrum of treatment options ranging from no treatment at all to complex surgery or radiation therapy.

Epidemiology

- It is now the most common ♂ cancer in the UK, with >40,000 new cases per annum, accounting for >25% of ♂ cancers.
- 85% of men are diagnosed at age 65 or older. It is rare in men under the age of 50 years, though numbers are increasing due to screening.
- 70% of men >80 years have histological evidence of cancer in the prostate.
- 60% of presentation is early-stage disease, with 10-year survival of >80%.

Risk factors

- Age is the most important risk factor.
- Prostate cancer is androgen-dependent. There is evidence that men with low levels of ♂ hormones are less likely to develop prostate cancer.
- 5–10% of cases appear to be linked to inheritance, i.e. those with a strong family history of prostate or breast cancer.
- African-Caribbean ancestry increases the risk, and these patients are more likely to have micrometastatic disease at presentation.

Pathology

- 95% are adenocarcinomas. Many are multifocal.
- Histological grade, assessed by Gleason score:
  - Low-grade cancers (Gleason 6 or less) are typically small and slow-growing, confined to the prostate gland.
  - High-grade cancers (Gleason >7) grow faster and frequently reflect occult metastatic disease.

Investigations

- Digital rectal examination.
- PSA assessment (◆ see Cancer screening, p. 57).
- High PSA (based on age-related PSA table) or palpable abnormality requires transrectal US scan and prostatic biopsy.
- Consider multiparametric MRI for men with a negative biopsy to determine whether another biopsy is needed. If MRI negative, do not offer another biopsy, unless any of the following risk factors are present:
  - High-grade prostatic intra-epithelial neoplasia (HGPIN)
  - Atypical small acinar proliferation (ASAP)
  - Abnormal digital rectal examination.
- Locally advanced disease, high-grade cancer, and high PSA level at presentation are all indications for more complete staging.
- Isotope bone scans.

Presentation
- Around 50% are asymptomatic, via PSA screening.
- Urinary symptoms, e.g. frequency, nocturia, poor stream, retention, haematuria.
- Advanced disease may cause bone or back pain, lymphoedema in the legs and genitals, or weight loss.
- Haemospermia, erectile dysfunction.

Staging and prognosis
- Staging is carried out using the TNM staging system.[2]
- Risk categories are shown in Box 28.1.

Metastatic spread
- Direct through the prostate capsule into adjacent organs (seminal vesicles, bladder, rectum).
- Regional lymph nodes.
- Distant typically to bone, and rarely to the lung and liver.

Treatment

Organ-confined prostate cancer

There may be several treatment options, based on the following:
- Patient's age and comorbidities
- Disease stage, PSA, and Gleason score
- The patient's concerns about likely toxicities.

Local radical therapy can be considered for intermediate-risk and also high-risk patients if a realistic prospect of long-term disease control.

Radical prostatectomy

Gives excellent disease-free survival rates. Post-operative problems include impotence in ~50%, strictures, penile shortening, and urinary incontinence. For most, the incontinence is minimal and improves over the first 2 years. However, a few will have severe, long-term incontinence.

Radical radiotherapy
- EBRT, combined with 6 months of androgen deprivation therapy before, during, or after EBRT. Can continue androgen deprivation therapy for up to 3 years for high-risk patients.
- Rates of disease-free survival compare favourably with surgery, and EBRT can also be offered if unfit for surgery.

Box 28.1 Prostate cancer, prognostic risk categories (using TNM, PSA, and Gleason score)

Low risk: T1–2a and PSA <10 micrograms/L and Gleason score 6 or less

Intermediate risk: T2b–c, or PSA 10–20 micrograms/L, or Gleason score 7

High risk: T3–4, or PSA >20 micrograms/L, or Gleason score > 7

Toxicities of radiotherapy include acute radiation cystitis/urethritis, proctitis with tenesmus, pain, and passage of mucus and blood. About 50% of those treated will become impotent.

- Brachytherapy to the prostate, using either implanted seeds or high-dose rate (HDR) tubes, has shown itself to be a successful treatment for organ-confined disease, delivering the same results, but with fewer hospital visits and lower rates of side effects in some men.

Hormonal therapy alone

- For patients with high-risk disease, for whom radical treatment is not appropriate or feasible, immediate treatment with androgen deprivation is preferred to 'active surveillance'.
- For metastatic disease, the median benefit is 18 months. However, some patients still have benefits at 10 years.

Active surveillance

- Particularly used for patients with low-risk cancers or patients with higher risk who are concerned with QoL issues arising from treatment.
- Involves initial multiparametric MRI, regular monitoring of PSA levels, and digital rectal examination.
- Changes can be reassessed with MRI and/or biopsy.

Locally advanced disease

Optimum management is controversial. Options include:
- Radiotherapy, with or without androgen deprivation
- Hormonal therapy alone
- Active surveillance.

Relapsed disease

Can consider local salvage therapy, including radiotherapy to the prostatic bed, for local relapse after radical prostatectomy. Hormonal therapy should be based on symptoms, proven metastases, or fast PSA doubling time (<3 months).

Metastatic disease

Advanced prostate cancer is incurable, but most are sensitive to androgen hormones. Excellent palliation can be achieved, with a survival time of 3–4 years with appropriate therapy.

Common hormone treatments include surgical castration (rarely used now), medical castration using gonadorelin analogues, anti-androgen therapy, e.g. bicalutamide, flutamide, or enzalutamide and, more recently, abiraterone.

There is no clear evidence that **maximal androgen blockade** (combining therapies) produces superior outcomes, compared with castration alone. The impact of medical/surgical castration or androgen blockade includes:
- Impotence and loss of libido (➔ see Chapter 50, Sexuality and cancer)
- Fatigue (➔ see Chapter 42, Cancer-related fatigue)
- Mood disturbance
- Muscle weakness
- Flushing and sweats (➔ see Hormonal therapy: background, p. 241)
- Weight gain
- Gynaecomastia (enlargement or tenderness of ♂ breasts)
- Osteoporosis in long-term survivors.

Hormone-refractory metastatic disease

A rising PSA level may suggest local recurrence or advancing disease. This occurs after a median of 2 years. Options are active surveillance, second-line anti-androgen therapy or androgen deprivation, or chemotherapy.

There is controversy surrounding the benefits and timing of these interventions. The most common problem of advancing disease is painful bone metastases (➲ see Metastatic bone disease, p. 287).

Radiotherapy and chemotherapy for metastatic disease

Radiotherapy

- Local radiotherapy can effectively treat painful bone metastases, spinal cord or nerve root compression, or symptomatic soft tissue disease.
- Bisphosphonate therapy is only offered for bone pain relief if analgesia and local radiotherapy have failed. Can be used for patients with osteoporosis on androgen deprivation therapy.
- Radioactive strontium as a single IV injection can be effective in treating multiple bone metastases, but it does cause significant myelosuppression.

Chemotherapy

- Docetaxel, up to ten cycles, is offered to patients with a good performance status.

Treatment outcomes

- Median survival times of >10 years for patients treated with either radical prostatectomy or radiotherapy.
- The natural history of recurrent disease may be very slow.
- For metastatic disease, the median duration of response to hormone therapy is 18–24 months.
- The median survival time after development of hormone-refractory disease is 12 months.

References

2 Amin MB, Edge S, Greene F, *et al.* (eds). *AJCC Cancer Staging Manual*, 8th ed. New York, NY: Springer; 2017.

Testicular cancer

This is one of the few solid tumours for which the majority of patients with metastatic disease can expect to be cured. Overall 10-year survival is around 98%.

Epidemiology

- 95% of testicular tumours are of germ cell origin.
- It is the most common cancer in men aged 25–49 years.
- Incidence has doubled over the last 30 years.
- 40–45% are seminomas—peak incidence age is 30–40 years.
- 40–45% are non-seminomatous germ cell tumours (NSGCTs)—peak incidence age is 20–30 years.
- Some germ cell tumours (10–15%) are a mixture of seminoma and non-seminoma—they are usually classified and treated as non-seminomas.

Risk factors

- History of undescended testis (relative risk 8 times).
- Previous testicular cancer (relative risk 25 times).
- Testicular carcinoma *in situ*.
- Family history of testicular cancer.

Pathology

Testicular cancer is staged using the TNM system, with the addition of an S category, taking account of the levels of LDH, AFP, and HCG proteins in the blood. It calls this the S stage.

Seminomas

Tumour growth can be very slow, and 75% present with disease confined to the testis. The spread tends to be predictable, vertically via the lymph nodes, and then to other metastatic sites. Tumour markers are not very reliable. Only 30% of seminomas present with raised HCG levels. LDH levels may be raised in advanced cancer. Tumours that appear to be seminomas histologically should be treated as NSGCTs if they have elevated AFP levels.

Seminomas are divided into:

- Good prognosis: the seminoma has not spread further than the lymph nodes or lungs; 5-year overall survival of 90%.
- Intermediate prognosis: has spread beyond the lung or lymph nodes; 5-year overall survival of 70%.

Non-seminomatous germ cell tumours

Lymphatic spread occurs earlier. NSGCTs produce markers—HCG and/or AFP in 75% of cases.

NSGCTs are divided into:

- Good prognosis: spread not beyond the lungs or lymph nodes, with marker levels only mildly raised; 5-year overall survival of >90%
- Intermediate prognosis: as above, with moderately raised marker levels; 5-year overall survival of 80%
- Poor prognosis: includes primary mediastinal disease or spread beyond the lungs or lymph nodes, e.g. liver or brain, or highly raised marker levels; 5-year overall survival of around 50%.

Presentation

- Testicular lump, either painless or painful (slightly less common).
  - May be mistaken for infection.
  - If symptoms persist, despite one course of antibiotics, patients should be referred to a urology clinic for assessment.
- Gynaecomastia (swollen breasts in men)—due to HCG.
- Metastatic disease may present with:
  - Lumbar back pain with bulky para-aortic lymphadenopathy
  - Cough and dyspnoea with multiple lung metastases
  - SVCO with mediastinal lymphadenopathy (➔ see Superior vena cava obstruction, p. 645)
  - CNS symptoms/signs with brain metastasis.
- Asymptomatic relapsed spread, often picked up on routine monitoring of serum markers, CXR, or CT scan.

Investigation of testicular germ cell tumours

- US of both testicles.
- CXR.
- Tumour markers (AFP, HCG, LDH).
- Inguinal orchidectomy ± biopsy of other testis.
- Further staging investigations post-operatively:
  - CT scan of the thorax, abdomen, and pelvis
  - Brain or bone scan if clinically indicated
  - Post-operative tumour markers (falling AFP and HCG).

Sperm storage

- Sperm count and storage should be considered at an early stage where patients are likely to require further therapy, though up to 50% of patients with testicular germ cell tumour may be subfertile at presentation.

Treatment of testicular cancer

Stage I seminoma

Primary treatment is inguinal orchidectomy. ~25% of patients develop re-current seminoma, mainly in para-aortic nodes.

- Standard practice in the UK post-orchidectomy is adjuvant radiotherapy to the para-aortic nodes.

Note: almost all patients with relapsed disease are cured by salvage therapy.

Stage I NSGCT

Primary treatment for NSGCT is as above. The relapse rate is around 30%, higher if there is vascular invasion in the tumour.

There are two options post-orchidectomy:

- Surveillance—CXR, tumour marker monitoring, and regular CT scans. Patients need to be motivated to continue regular follow-up
- Adjuvant chemotherapy—particularly if vascular invasion. Two cycles of BEP (bleomycin, etoposide, cisplatin) chemotherapy offers 97% disease-free survival
- Outcome, even for relapsed stage I disease, is excellent, with cure rates of >95%.

All other stages of seminoma and NSGCT

BEP chemotherapy is the current gold standard treatment—three courses for good prognosis, and four for intermediate and poor prognosis. Poor prognostic factors are:
- Mediastinal primary
- Non-pulmonary visceral metastases
- High tumours markers, e.g. AFP, HCG.

BEP chemotherapy is potentially very toxic. Nausea and vomiting, neutropenic sepsis, neuropathy, nephropathy, and pulmonary fibrosis are all common.
- G-CSF is used to avoid dose delays and reductions, if possible.
- Lung toxicity due to bleomycin can be fatal—four cycles of EP chemotherapy can be used in older patients with poor lung function.

Residual tumour masses post-chemotherapy
- Seminomas generally regress on serial scans.
- Surgical resection should be performed for NSGCTs.
- Most are in the retroperitoneum, and extensive and difficult surgery is often necessary. There is an anaesthetic risk due to patient exposure to bleomycin. If the residual mass contains a viable tumour, further chemotherapy is recommended.

Relapse

Patients who relapse or who do not have a complete response can have salvage therapy with further combination chemotherapy regimes. Regular follow-up is necessary as, in those patients who relapse, salvage therapy can be effective in ~25% of cases.

Penile cancer

Epidemiology

This is an uncommon cancer, with around 350 new cases per annum in the UK. The majority occur in people over 70, but up to 20% occur under the age of 40. The disease is relatively more common in Africa, India, and South America.

Risk factors

- HPV 16 and 18 infection.
- Associated with poor hygiene and unretractable foreskin.
- ↑ risk with cigarette smoking and immunosuppression, including HIV infection.
- Neonatal circumcision gives life-long protection.

Pathology

The vast majority are squamous carcinomas. Spread is initially via lymphatics to inguinal, and then pelvic, lymph nodes. Distant spread may include the liver, lungs, bone, and skin.

Staging

The TNM system is commonly used (➲ see Diagnosis, classification, and staging of cancer, p. 176).

Investigations

- Inspection of the penis and biopsy of any lesion.
- Inguinal lymph node palpation—FNA of suspicious lymph nodes.
- Further staging if clinical suspicion of metastatic disease.

Presentation

- Erythema, warty tumour, or ulceration on the glans or foreskin.
- Advanced disease can cause considerable destruction of the penis.
- Metastatic disease, e.g. inguinal and pelvic lymphadenopathy.

Treatment

As penile cancer is a rare cancer, treatment should be coordinated from a specialist regional centre.

Primary tumour

- Early-stage disease may be successfully managed with organ conservation. For tumour *in situ*, topical 5FU, laser therapy, cryotherapy, or local excision are all options. Excision or radiotherapy is used for stage I disease.
- More advanced disease or local recurrence often requires at least partial amputation of the penis. Reconstruction surgical techniques are now excellent. Patients with inoperable disease may be treated with chemotherapy and radiotherapy.

Regional lymph nodes

- With high-grade and stage II tumours, regional lymphadenectomy may be considered. Patients who are unfit for surgery or have

inoperable disease may benefit from chemotherapy and radiotherapy. Lymphoedema is a major side effect of radiotherapy and lymphadenectomy.
• The disease is moderately chemosensitive, and active regimens include methotrexate, bleomycin, and cisplatin (MBP). Chemotherapy is recommended both for advanced disease and as adjuvant therapy for node-positive disease.

Outcomes

Overall, 50% of men with penile cancer survive disease-free beyond 5 years, with better results in node-negative (60%), compared with node-positive (30%), disease. The majority of relapses occur in the first 2 years, and close follow-up is recommended at least during this time.

Nursing management issues

The nursing issues in these cancers will vary considerably, depending on the disease site and on the extent of cancer spread. Common nursing management issues are briefly described below.

Sexuality

There are many potential assaults on an individual's sexuality due to GU cancer and its treatment. Surgery can cause impotence, reduced ejaculate, and incontinence. It may involve the formation of stomas for urinary diversion, removal of the testis or penis, or shortening of the vagina. Hormonal therapy can cause impotence and reduced libido. Chemotherapy and radiotherapy may impact on fertility, and multiple side effects may impact on an individual's body image and sexuality. Nurses need to involve patients and their partners in open discussions about potential problems, as a crucial part of care. In some hospitals, patients can be referred to specialist sexual health clinics or referred to see a specialist sexual therapist.

Pre-surgery

Patients may be extremely anxious about the impact of surgery. Their fears should be openly explored, along with straightforward explanations of likely impacts.

Post-surgery

It is important that nurses feel able to initiate discussions and proactively support patients with what might feel like embarrassing difficulties. Sexual issues may not be uppermost in a person's mind early on after diagnosis and during treatment. Post-treatment follow-up is needed to assess the psychosexual impact of treatment and the disease (➔ see Chapter 50, Sexuality and cancer).

Fertility

Many patients with testicular cancer are young and will not have children at the time of their diagnosis. Sperm banking should be offered as a matter of course, though many patients will be subfertile at diagnosis. BEP chemotherapy causes infertility. Around half of patients will regain normal sperm counts 2 years post-chemotherapy, though others will have long-term damage to their sperm.

Younger prostate cancer and penile cancer patients may also require sperm banking.

Urinary incontinence

After bladder surgery, patients will require support in adjusting to, and managing, their stoma and possible incontinence. This includes skin care, using pouches, signs and symptoms of a healthy stoma, and possible signs of infection. For those with continent pouches, teaching of self-catheterization or rigorous bladder training may also be included. For those with a stoma, support and advice from a stoma therapist will be invaluable at this time (➔ see Care of the patient with a stoma, p. 328).

Radical prostate surgery and radiotherapy for prostate or bladder cancer can all cause long-term continence problems. Nursing management includes accurate assessment of the degree of the problem, teaching the use of pelvic floor and biofeedback exercises, and providing equipment such as pads and condom-like continence devices. Occasionally, urinary catheterization is required. Long-term problems may require medical or surgical input. An incontinence expert is recommended to aid patients and nurses in providing effective support.

Lymphoedema

Advanced pelvic disease in both prostate and bladder cancer can lead to lower limb lymphoedema. This needs to be managed actively, with advice from lymphoedema specialists, to help prevent major complications (→ see Lymphoedema, p. 626).

Pain issues

Patients with advanced bladder and prostate cancer can get pelvic pain, with a neuropathic element, making it complex to manage. Bone pain is also common in advanced prostate cancer, due to bone metastases, and pathological fractures can occur. Pain can often be managed with bisphosphonates and radiotherapy. Physiotherapy and occupational therapy input may assist with mobility and adaptation to bone metastases. Occasionally, orthopaedic surgery can be used to stabilize affected areas (→ see Pain management, p. 550).

Financial issues

Many patients undergoing treatments struggle financially, especially those who are young and supporting a family, e.g. many testicular cancer patients. Advice and contact details should be offered of where to get help and advice (→ see Chapter 6, The social experience of cancer).

Further reading

National Institute for Health and Care Excellence (2014). *Prostate Cancer: Diagnosis and Management*. Clinical guideline [CG175]. Available at: ℜ: https://www.nice.org.uk/guidance/cg175?unlid=

National Institute for Health and Care Excellence (2015). *Bladder Cancer: Diagnosis and Management*. NICE guideline [NG2]. Available at: ℜ https://www.nice.org.uk/Guidance/ng2

National Institute for Health and Care Excellence (2015). *Renal Cancer Overview*. Available at: ℜ: http://pathways.nice.org.uk/pathways/renal-cancer

Prostate Cancer UK. *Sex and Relationships*. Available at: ℜ: http://prostatecanceruk.org/prostate-information/living-with-prostate-cancer/sex-and-relationships

Gynaecological cancers

Introduction

Gynaecological cancers are associated with the ♀ reproductive organs. This includes the ovaries, Fallopian tubes, uterus, cervix, vagina, and vulva. They account for about 15% of cancers in women and about 10% of cancer deaths.

Enhanced cervical screening in the UK has led to a dramatic decrease in the incidence of, and deaths from, cervical cancer. Abnormal development changes (dysplasia) in cervical cells are diagnosed when the disease is still curable. Unfortunately, ovarian cancer is usually diagnosed at an advanced stage, due to its asymptomatic nature in the early stages. Around one-third of women with ovarian cancer are diagnosed following an emergency admission.

There are additional rare tumours called gestational trophoblastic tumours, which arise from pregnancy and include:
- Pre-malignant complete hydatidiform mole (CHM)
- Partial hydatidiform mole (PHM)
- Malignant invasive mole, gestational choriocarcinoma
- Highly malignant placental-site trophoblastic tumour (PSTT).

This section will not look at gestational tumours. Further information on these can be found at: Froeling FEM, Seckl MJ. Gestational trophoblastic tumours: an update for 2014. *Curr Oncol Rep* 2014;**16**:408.

Ovarian cancer

- It is the sixth most common cancer in women in the UK, with 75% of cases in those aged over 55 and around 7,400 new cases annually.
- <5% of cases are clearly hereditary.
- Risk of ovarian cancer is related to an increasing number of ovulatory cycles, thus some protection from the oral contraceptive pill and pregnancy.
- 5-year survival of around 46% for women diagnosed in England and Wales.

Presentation

Eighty per cent of women present with disease that has spread beyond the ovary to involve the peritoneum and other abdominopelvic organs.
Common symptoms include:

- Bloating and early satiety
- Urinary urgency
- Persistently swollen abdomen
- Indigestion
- Ongoing fatigue
- Back/abdominal pain
- Weight change—loss or gain
- Altered bowel function, constipation, diarrhoea, or obstruction.

Note: primary Fallopian tube and peritoneal cancers are rare and behave similarly to ovarian cancer. They can be found on histology when suspicious of ovarian cancer and are treated in the same way.

It is essential that early investigation of these symptoms occurs in primary care, especially in women aged over 50 years. Also investigate any first-time symptoms of irritable bowel syndrome (IBS), as IBS rarely presents first time in women of this age.

Ovarian cancer diagnosis and staging

Investigations

- CA-125 (see Box 29.1).
- US scan of the abdomen and pelvis
- AFP and β-hCG if under 40 years old, to identify possible non-epithelial ovarian cancer.
- Risk of Malignancy Index (RMI) score (see Box 29.2). If >250, refer to specialist MDT.
- Staging CT chest, abdomen, and pelvis.
- If primary debulking surgery is performed initially, then full histological staging is carried out via total abdominal hysterectomy, bilateral salpingo-oophorectomy, omentectomy, lymph node biopsies, and multiple peritoneal biopsies.

Box 29.1 CA-125

Cancer antigen 125 (CA-125) is a protein manufactured by mucus-producing cells and then released into the blood. In 90% of women with ovarian cancer, it is abnormally raised. However, other benign conditions (and even other cancers) can cause the CA-125 level to rise.

Box 29.2 Risk of Malignancy Index (RMI)

A product of US scan score (U), menopausal status (M), and serum CA-125 level:

US scan score (U) × menopausal status (M) × CA-125

The US result is scored 1 point for each of the following characteristics: multilocular cysts, solid areas, metastases, ascites, bilateral lesions.

U = 0 for an ultrasound score of 0 points
U = 1 for an ultrasound score of 1 point
U = 3 for an ultrasound score of 2–5 points

Menopausal status is scored as 1 = pre-menopausal and 3 = post-menopausal. The classification of 'post-menopausal' is a woman who has had no period for >1 year or a woman over 50 who has had a hysterectomy.

Serum CA-125 is measured in IU/mL.

If RMI ≥250, then the patient must be referred to a specialist MDT.

From NICE Clinical Guideline CG122 (2011) Available from ℅ https://www.nice.org.uk/guidance/cg122 all rights reserved. Subject to Notice of Rights. NICE guidance is prepared for the National Health Service in England. All NICE guidance is subject to regular review and may be updated or withdrawn. NICE accepts no responsibility for the use of its content in this product/publication.'

Prognosis

Stage is the most important prognostic factor (see Table 29.1). Also patients with >2cm area of disease after surgery have a poorer prognosis, with only 20% surviving 3 years.

Treatment

Management of suspected early (stage I) ovarian cancer
- Optimal surgical staging (➲ see Ovarian cancer diagnosis and staging, p. 385).

Adjuvant treatment
- **Low-risk disease** (grade 1, stage Ia): no adjuvant treatment required.
- **High-risk disease** (all other grades/stages): adjuvant chemotherapy with carboplatin and a taxane is the usual therapy. Some centres reserve a taxane for relapse.

Table 29.1 Diagnosis and staging (FIGO Ovarian Cancer Staging)

Stage	Level of spread	5-year survival (%)
Stage I	Confined to ovaries	75
Stage II	Tumour spread within the pelvis only	45
Stage III	Peritoneal spread outside the pelvis, e.g. omentum	20
Stage IV	Distant metastases	<5

Staging is a summary from FIGO's staging classification for cancer of the ovary, fallopian tube, and peritoneum: abridged republication (2015) *J. Gynecol. Oncol.* 26(2):87–89.

Advanced (and relapsed) ovarian cancer
- Radical tumour debulking (no tumour of >1cm left) plus adjuvant/neo-adjuvant chemotherapy.

First-line chemotherapy

Platinum/taxane combinations, normally six cycles, are generally regarded as the optimum treatment. Median survival rates are 2–3 years.

In advanced disease, interval debulking can be carried out after three cycles, if appropriate, followed by further chemotherapy. Further tumour debulking is not generally offered in relapsed disease.

Patients with stage IV disease which is deemed highly unlikely to be optimally debulked in the future can be commenced on bevacizumab, with the combination chemotherapy regime continuing with a maintenance dose for up to 18 cycles.

Treatment at relapse

Patients with disease response and remission of at least 12 months should be re-challenged with a platinum-containing regimen. The longer the treatment-free interval, the greater the likelihood of a worthwhile second response. For those relapsing sooner, options including paclitaxel, liposomal doxorubicin, topotecan, and gemcitabine can be used.

Patients with bone metastases

Denosumab can be offered to patients to reduce the risk of skeletal-related events such as fractures, pain, and spinal cord compression.

New approaches

Possible new approaches to improve management include:
- Intraperitoneal chemotherapy
- High-dose systemic chemotherapy
- Biological response modifiers
- Anti-angiogenic agents
- Angiogenesis inhibition (bevacizumab) can be offered to patients with either stage IIIb or stage IV ovarian cancer, in combination with carboplatin/paclitaxel, in the primary setting for patients who are deemed to be inoperable or are suboptimally debulked after initial chemotherapy. Maintenance bevacizumab can be continued for up to 12 months.

Cancer of the cervix

Introduction

Rates of cervical cancer vary enormously between countries. It is the most common ♀ cancer in South East Asia and Africa. Incidence drops rapidly where national screening programmes have been introduced. In the UK, it accounts for around 2% of women diagnosed with a cancer, making it relatively rare, though it is the most common cancer affecting women under 35 years.

Risk factors

- Early onset of sexual intercourse (before 17 years old).
- Non-barrier forms of contraception.
- HPV—particularly HPV types 16 and 18—is present in approaching 100% of cervical cancers seen in the UK. A vaccination programme is under way in the UK for girls aged 12–13 years (➔ see Human papillomavirus vaccine, p. 56).
- Cigarette smoking.

Presentation

- 80–90% are SCC. Adenocarcinoma is less common but increasing in incidence.
- Normally asymptomatic until late presentation.
- ↑ vaginal discharge.
- Post-coital bleeding.
- Inter-menstrual bleeding.
- For management of screening-detected abnormalities, ➔ see Abnormal testing follow-up, p. 55.

Investigations

Colposcopic examination provides an accurate clinical assessment and the opportunity to obtain a biopsy. If the patient is symptomatic, a pelvic and abdomen MRI scan can define tumour size and any lymph node involvement. If this identifies disease outside of the pelvis, then a CT scan is required to assess for more disseminated disease. If imaging cannot exclude bladder or bowel involvement, then cystoscopy and sigmoidoscopy should be used. In inoperable cases, a PET/CT scan is most useful in detecting nodal metastases and determining the appropriate level of therapy.

Staging

Staging is based predominantly on the extent of the primary tumour. The spread is usually from the cervix into the vagina and then into the pelvic wall. Metastatic spread is normally by the lymphatic system and can involve the bladder and rectum, and local or distant lymph nodes (see Table 29.2).

Treatment

Surgery

For very early-stage disease, a simple large loop excision of the transformation zone (LLETZ) can be performed. A radical hysterectomy is the main treatment option for early-stage invasive disease. This generally is carried out laparoscopically by appropriately trained surgeons.

Table 29.2 FIGO staging system for cervical cancer

Stage	Definition
Ia	Microinvasive disease (maximum depth 5mm, maximum width 7mm)
Ib	Clinical disease confined to the cervix
IIa	Disease involves upper one-third of vagina, but not parametrium
IIb	Disease involves parametrium but does not extend to pelvic wall
III	Disease involves lower two-thirds of vagina and/or pelvic wall
IV	Involvement of bladder, rectum, or distant organs

Trachelectomy, where the cervix only is removed, plus pelvic lymph node dissection may be offered to women who wish to conserve their fertility, providing the tumour diameter is <2cm and no lymphatic-vascular space invasion is present. A cerclage suture is placed at the isthmus of the uterus to support future pregnancies. Any future pregnancies should be monitored by a consultant obstetrician, and a Caesarean section is required.

Surgery in disease recurrence

Pelvic exenteration is only used as salvage surgery for a selected group of women with recurrent cervical cancer in the central pelvis whose chemoradiotherapy has failed. It has a high level of morbidity.

Combined chemotherapy and radiotherapy

Combined adjuvant chemotherapy (cisplatin) and radical pelvic radiotherapy should be used in node-positive disease, and node-negative disease with other risk factors, i.e. large tumour and lymphovascular invasion. A combination of EBRT and brachytherapy is used routinely. This can still be a curative treatment.

Pelvic radiotherapy can also be used in very advanced disease to palliate pelvic symptoms.

Radiation side effects

Radiation side effects can be extremely distressing. Late bladder symptoms can include frequency, urgency, dysuria, haematuria, ulceration, reduced bladder capacity, and the potential for perforation and fistula formation. Management requires specialist urological input.

Bowel symptoms can include tenesmus, urgency, diarrhoea, occasional rectal bleeding, adhesions forming around the bowel, and intermittent bowel obstruction.

Sexual problems include loss of libido, altered body image, change in sexual activity, and ↓ orgasm often due to vaginal dryness, vaginal bleeding, stenosis, dyspareunia, atrophic vaginitis, and pain (➔ see Sexual expression, p. 608).

Chemotherapy

Advanced cervical cancer tends to have poor response rates. For advanced disease, platinum-based chemotherapy gives the best results. Patients who have previously undergone cisplatin chemotherapy can be offered carboplatin/paclitaxel in the relapsed treatment setting.

Prognosis

Survival at 5 years is typically: stage Ia, 100%; stage Ib, 70–90%; stage II, 60–80%; stage III, 35–45%; and stage IV, 10–20%. These wide ranges reflect the large variation in disease volume seen within the present staging system; it is based on tissue involvement, rather than volume of disease. Relapse after 5 years of remission is unusual.

Endometrial cancer

Introduction

Endometrial cancer occurs principally in post-menopausal women, and the incidence rises with age. Most cases present in early stage. Its aetiology has not been fully determined, but risks include unopposed oestrogen HRT, endometrial hyperplasia, women with breast cancer taking tamoxifen, diabetes, nulliparity, and obesity.

Presenting features

- 90% present with vaginal bleeding, mainly post-menopausal.
- 10% present with purulent vaginal discharge.
- 5% present asymptomatic after a hysterectomy or follow-up of abnormal Pap smear.
- Pain and pelvic pressure are usually manifestations of advanced disease.

Diagnosis

- Pelvic examination.
- Endometrial biopsy and US scan.
- Further examinations depend on signs and symptoms and grade of disease.
- The preoperative evaluation includes: CXR, clinical and gynaecological examination, transvaginal US, FBC, and biochemistry.

Staging

The main prognostic risk factors are histological subtype, grade 3 histology, myometrial invasion of ≥50%, lymphovascular space invasion, lymph node metastases, and tumour diameter of >2cm.

For grade 3 disease, a CT chest, abdomen, and pelvis is required to complete the staging preoperatively, though it must be noted that final staging is conducted by the pathologist on examination of the specimen.

Treatment

Surgery

Stage I and II disease

The mainstay of treatment in stage I disease is total abdominal hysterectomy and bilateral salpingo-oophorectomy. This can be offered via a laparoscopic approach.

The role of lymphadenectomy is controversial. Further randomized controlled trials will focus on its role in reducing the risk of recurrence. The role of sentinel node biopsy is currently unproven.

If stage II disease is identified preoperatively, then standard practice is to include systematic pelvic lymphadenectomy with or without para-aortic lymphadenectomy. This can guide surgical staging and adjuvant therapy.

Stage III and IV disease

Surgical debulking of the uterus can be considered in good performance patients to palliate pelvic pain.

In high-grade disease, it may be beneficial to perform a palliative hysterectomy to reduce any significant vaginal bleeding.

For stage IV disease, palliative chemotherapy with carboplatin and or palliative pelvic EBRT can be delivered to palliate the patient's symptoms.

Radiotherapy

Radiotherapy can be used as a primary treatment for women unfit to undergo surgery or as adjuvant therapy following hysterectomy if intermediate- or high-risk disease. It is also used to treat local recurrence and advanced disease.

Many centres use a combination of chemotherapy and radiation in advanced-stage disease. Clinical trial involvement should be encouraged for this group of patients.

Chemotherapy

Combination chemotherapy and progesterones can be used in advanced disease to shrink tumours and provide palliation.

Prognosis

Endometrial cancer generally presents early, and 5-year survival rates are around 79%.

Vulval and vaginal cancer

Vulval cancer

- Vulval cancer is rare—the twentieth most common ♀ cancer.
- Predominantly affects older women. One in four tumours occurs in women under the age of 65 years.
- The majority (85%) are squamous carcinoma.
- Other types include basal carcinoma (10%) and malignant melanoma (4%).
- Associations with HPV infection.

Symptoms

- Chronic vulval skin symptoms such as pruritus and irritation.
- Vulval lesions.
- Abnormal vaginal discharge.
- Painful lump.
- Abnormal genital tract bleeding or haematuria may occur.

Note: any change in the vulval epithelium that is not a confirmed infection should be biopsied.

Treatment

Surgery

Surgical excision with clear margins and removal of groin nodes (groin node dissection not required in stage Ia disease) are the mainstay of treatment. Sentinel node biopsy can be considered in squamous vulval cancers where there is no initial evidence of lymph node metastases with tumours of <4cm in size.

Extensive disease may require radical vulvectomy in combination with complex reconstruction. The psychosexual impact of such surgery is high, combined with the morbidity associated with groin node dissection.

Radiotherapy

For those patients not fit enough for surgery, then primary radiotherapy can be used to treat primary vulval and groin nodes. Radiotherapy can also be considered as adjuvant therapy for those at high risk of relapse.

Chemotherapy

Responses are variable, and toxicity may be an issue in this population of patients.

Prognosis

- 5-year survival of >80% if node-negative.
- Survival following regional recurrence is poor.
- <50% survival if inguinal nodes involved, and 10–15% if iliac or other pelvic nodes involved.

Vaginal cancer

Most vaginal cancers are metastatic spread from the cervix, endometrium, or vulva.

Presentation and diagnosis
- Presenting symptoms include abnormal vaginal bleeding, vaginal discharge, and bladder or rectal symptoms.
- It is diagnosed via a vaginal examination and biopsy, with an MRI scan used to evaluate local spread. If distant spread is suspected, then a CT scan is useful for identifying further metastatic disease.

Treatment
For early-stage disease, radiation therapy or surgery, or a combination, is the standard approach. Radical pelvic radiotherapy is the standard of care for all other stages of disease—a combination of external beam and vaginal intra-cavity brachytherapy. There is real uncertainty as to the value of chemotherapy

Prognosis
Overall 5-year survival is 40%, and salvage after a first relapse is uncommon.

Nursing management issues

Treatment support

Many of the treatments available for managing gynaecological cancers are aggressive and can have a profound physical, psychosocial, and sexual impact on women and their families.

Psychosexual concerns

Loss of fertility, onset of menopause, rectal and bladder dysfunction, and vaginal dryness and tightness are all common difficulties that these women face. Changes in body image, sexuality, and fertility may require referral for specialist psychological/psychosexual support.

It is important not to underestimate the significance of loss of fertility. Even if patients had not planned to have children, or to have more children, the knowledge that this is no longer possible can be devastating.

Concerns regarding sexuality may not emerge until well after major treatment is completed and may occur many months to years later. Pre-treatment assessment, education, and counselling, often by the CNS, are therefore essential in preparing individuals and their families.

Post-surgery, patients need to be well informed of what has been removed and the effect this treatment will have on them. It is helpful in planning their care to establish if they are sexually active, planning to have children, or are menopausal.

Appropriate nurse follow-up and PLISSIT assessment are required to ensure any problems are not missed. Primary care involvement may be useful in this area. Early close liaison with the GP and district nursing services is useful (➔ see Chapter 50, Sexuality and cancer).

Other common concerns problems include the following.

Ascites

This is particularly common in ovarian cancer and can be difficult to manage (➔ see Malignant ascites, pp. 526–7).

Pain

Perineal and pelvic pain becomes more common in advanced disease. It often has a nerve-based element, making it difficult to completely resolve (➔ see Classifications of pain, p. 558).

Hormonal symptoms

In most cases where menopause has been induced early because of treatment (surgery to remove both ovaries or radical pelvic radiotherapy), HRT may be given until the average age of the menopause, i.e. 51 years old. Exceptions to this are hormone-dependent tumours such as some endometrial or some cervical tumours (➔ see Management of menopausal symptoms, pp. 246–7). Venlafaxine, an antidepressant, has been shown to control hot flushes for patients unable to have HRT.

Lower limb oedema

When patients have extensive pelvic disease, this is increasingly common. It needs active management, including specialist referral for compression bandaging, specialist massage therapy, and skin care and podiatry advice (➔ see Lymphoedema, pp. 626–8).

Vaginal discharge

This can be offensive and extremely embarrassing. Topical antibiotics and deodorizing dressings can help.

Further reading

Cancer Research UK. *Statistics by Cancer Type*. Available at: ℬ http://www.cancerresearchuk.org/health-professional/cancer-statistics/statistics-by-cancer-type/

Colombo N, Carinelli S, *et al*. Cervical cancer: Clinical Practice Guidelines Cervical Cancer ESMO Clinical practice guidelines for diagnosis, treatment and follow up. *Ann Oncol* 2012;**23**(Suppl 7):vii27–viii32.

Colombo N, Preti E, Landoni F, *et al*. ESMO Clinical Practice Guidelines: endometrial cancer. *Ann Oncol* 2013;**24**(Suppl 6):vi33–8.

Kehoe S, Hook J, Nankivell M, *et al*. Chemotherapy or upfront surgery for newly diagnosed advanced ovarian cancer. Results from MRC CHORUS trial. *J Clin Oncol* 2013;**31**(Suppl):abstr 5500.

National Institute for Health and Care Excellence (2015). *Ovarian Cancer Overview*. Available at: ℬ http://pathways.nice.org.uk/pathways/ovarian-cancer#

Royal College of Obstetricians and Gynaecologists. *Guidelines for the Diagnosis and Management of Vulval Carcinoma*. London: Royal College of Obstetricians and Gynaecologists; 2014.

Chapter 30

Haematological cancers

Introduction

Haematological cancers are cancers of blood cells. All blood cells are made in the bone marrow from a haematopoietic (blood-forming) stem cell. The stem cell divides and gradually turns into one of the mature blood cells, passing first through several immature stages (see Fig. 30.1).

Haematological cancers include acute and chronic leukaemias, high- and low-grade NHL, Hodgkin lymphoma, and myeloma. These conditions can be divided according to the principal site of involvement, the cancerous cell type, and the speed of progression (see Table 30.1).

Investigations

The following tests are useful in diagnosing a haematological cancer:
- FBC
- Blood film
- Bone marrow aspirate from the posterior iliac crest (back of the pelvis)—particularly useful for diagnosing acute leukaemia
- Bone marrow trephine—a piece of intact bone with the marrow is removed from the posterior iliac crest. This is particularly useful in diagnosing lymphoma and myeloma
- Immunophenotyping—can refine diagnosis. It detects surface molecules on a cell and can help define what type of cancer it is. It is useful for distinguishing between AML and acute lymphoblastic leukaemia (ALL)
- Cytogenetics—are vital in diagnosing CML, which is nearly always associated with the presence of the Philadelphia chromosome (➔ see Chronic myeloid leukaemia, p. 404)
- It can also determine how responsive to treatment an acute leukaemia is likely to be
- Lymph node biopsy—a full core or excision biopsy is required
- CT scan—for staging lymphoma
- PET CT scan—particularly useful in Hodgkin lymphoma and diffuse large B-cell lymphoma.

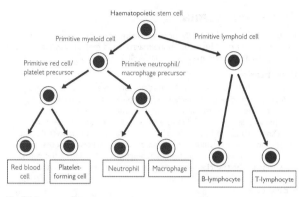

Fig. 30.1 Formation of the cellular components of blood from a single haematopoietic stem cell.

Table 30.1 Outline of the main haematological cancers

Disease	Usual site of involvement	Cell type affected	Speed of progression
Acute myeloid leukaemia (AML)	Bone marrow	Immature myeloid forming blood cell	Rapid
Acute lymphoblastic leukaemia (ALL)	Bone marrow	Immature lymphocyte forming blood cell	Rapid
Chronic myeloid leukaemia (CML)	Bone marrow	Immature neutrophil forming blood cell	Initially slow
Chronic lymphocytic leukaemia (CLL)	Blood, lymph nodes, and bone marrow	Mature lymphocyte	Slow
High-grade lymphoma	Lymph nodes and spleen (but can occur anywhere)	Mature lymphocyte	Rapid
Low-grade lymphoma	Lymph nodes and spleen	Mature lymphocyte	Slow
Myeloma	Bone marrow	Plasma cell (antibody-secreting cell)	Moderate

Acute leukaemia

Acute leukaemia is a rapidly progressive malignancy of an early blood-forming cell. It originates in the bone marrow and may or may not be seen in blood itself. The two main types are AML and ALL.

Presentation

- Bone marrow failure—anaemia (fatigue, breathlessness, headache, dizziness), thrombocytopenia (bruising, bleeding, petechial rash, disseminated intravascular coagulation), leucopenia (infections, sepsis).
- Hyperviscosity of blood due to a very high white cell count—can cause shortness of breath, headaches, alteration in neurological status, confusion, bleeding, kidney dysfunction, and visual disturbances.
- Infiltration of tissues—skin lesions (chloromas), swelling of the gums, swelling of the testicles, enlarged liver and/or spleen, lymph node enlargement, CNS involvement.
- Bone pain.

Acute myeloid leukaemia

This is the most common type of acute leukaemia in adults. Its incidence is 3 per 100,000. The risk increases with age.

Predisposing factors

- In most patients, no cause is found, but smokers are three times more likely to develop AML and exposure to ionizing radiation may also be a risk factor.
- Myelodysplasia, myeloproliferative conditions, previous chemotherapy and radiotherapy, Down's syndrome, and other rare congenital abnormalities can all increase the risk.

Risk/prognosis

AML is divided into good-, intermediate-, and poor-risk disease, based on cytogenetic analysis and other clinical features.

Poor prognostic factors are:

- Older age at diagnosis
- Unfit for intensive chemotherapy
- Gender (men have poorer prognosis)
- Failure to enter a remission after the first course of chemotherapy
- A very high white cell count at presentation
- Leukaemia secondary to previous chemotherapy, radiotherapy, or myelodysplasia.

Treatment

There are three broad approaches to the treatment of AML.

1. *Intensive, potentially curative treatment involving high doses of combination chemotherapy*

- Induction: two courses (but especially course 1) which aim to get the patient into remission.
- Consolidation: two further courses to prevent relapse.
- An allogeneic bone marrow transplant may be used, instead of consolidation for poor-risk disease, particularly if the patient has an HLA-matched sibling (➔ see Chapter 19, Allogeneic haematopoietic stem cell transplant).

- Acute promyelocytic leukaemia (a subset of AML with a specific cytogenetic abnormality) is also treated with all-trans-retinoic-acid (ATRA). These patients are also at risk of disseminated intravascular coagulation (➔ see Oncological emergencies, pp. 635–6) and have a high early mortality risk if the treatment is not started quickly. These patients have a very good prognosis if they get into remission.
- In the event of relapsed disease, a cure is very unlikely with more chemotherapy. An allogeneic stem cell transplant is an option, depending on the age and physical status of the patient and if a suitable donor can be found. Otherwise the outlook is very poor.
- Side effects: these are often severe due to high doses of chemotherapy:
  - General side effects include lethargy, nausea, vomiting, diarrhoea, hair loss, reduced fertility, mucositis, infection, bruising, or bleeding due to profound bone marrow suppression
  - Specific side effects of the chemotherapy agents include conjunctivitis and neurological impairment (high-dose cytarabine) and cardiac impairment (daunorubicin).

2. Palliative chemotherapy

In a patient not fit enough to receive combination chemotherapy, lower-dose chemotherapy, such as azacytidine, may be offered to treat the symptoms. This can induce a remission but will not cure the disease, which will relapse in time.

3. Best supportive care

No specific treatment is offered for AML if patients have very poor performance status, because they are unable to tolerate treatment. In such cases, best supportive care is important. This may include:
- Red cell or platelet transfusions
- Antibiotics to treat infections
- Analgesia and anti-emetics
- Psychological support.

Acute lymphoblastic leukaemia

ALL accounts for only 20% of leukaemias in adults but is the most common type of cancer to affect children. It rarely can arise from CML. The outcome is poor, especially if the Philadelphia chromosome is positive (➔ see Chronic myeloid leukaemia, pp. 404–5).

Risk stratification

The following factors suggest a poor prognosis:
- Increasing age
- Initial white blood cell count of >50 × 10^9/L.
- Adverse findings on cytogenetics, specifically:
  - The Philadelphia chromosome—which is more typically seen in CML (and in adult ALL)
  - Genetic abnormalities—involving chromosome 11
  - <45 chromosomes—termed hypodiploidy
- Slow early response to treatment
- Failure to achieve complete remission by day 28 of treatment.

Treatment

Treatment of ALL is long and complex and often occurs as part of a clinical trial. The various phases of treatment are as follows.

Induction

Combination chemotherapy is used to achieve a remission. Steroids and asparaginase are an important part of treatment but frequently produce severe side effects.

Consolidation—intensification

The aim is to rapidly reduce the burden of leukaemia, which is known to be present, in spite of not being seen by routine testing. Further combination chemotherapy is used.

Central nervous system prophylaxis

ALL can relapse in the CNS, so CNS prophylaxis is essential. Intrathecal chemotherapy (into the spinal fluid) is used, and in some cases, additional cranial radiotherapy in those with CNS disease.

Maintenance

This is used to reduce the risk of relapse. Typically, it involves a combination of oral chemotherapy tablets and intermittent injections, lasting for up to 2 years.

Treatment of relapsed disease

Early bone marrow relapse is particularly hard to treat. Options for treatment include further chemotherapy or an allogeneic stem cell transplant. Stem cell transplantation is also used as first-line treatment in poor-prognosis disease, e.g. Philadelphia chromosome-positive disease.

Nursing issues

Nursing of acute leukaemia patients can present a number of challenges, both in the diagnostic and treatment phases.

Diagnosis

Within 1–2 days of attending the GP for a possible viral infection or other seemingly minor symptom, patients may have been diagnosed and started treatment. This frequently involves the insertion of a CVC, being enrolled into a clinical trial, and commencing chemotherapy, with the prospect of many painful and life-threatening side effects.

It can be a bewildering time, with patients facing a sudden loss of control over their lives, whilst trying to come to terms with a life-threatening illness. Patients and their families will require intensive psychological and informational support to help them through diagnosis and prepare them for the treatment phase.

Treatment

Patients often face a combination of side effects due to the high doses of chemotherapy and their already altered physical state. These include profound neutropenia, mucositis, hair loss, infertility, and nausea and vomiting. Patients are often already acutely unwell due to their disease and can deteriorate very rapidly. Specific risks can include life-threatening infections, leading to septic shock (➲ see Treatment of febrile neutropenia and sepsis/

septic shock, p. 481), bleeding (➔ see Bleeding, p. 483), renal failure, and, in acute leukaemia with a high white count, tumour lysis syndrome (➔ see Tumour lysis syndrome, p. 649). Patients require close regular observations, a strict fluid balance, daily weight, close electrolyte monitoring, multiple IV medications, and blood product support.

Patients who are profoundly neutropenic may be nursed in strict isolation, and the visiting rights of family may be restricted, depending on local policies. Some patients can find isolation reassuring, but other patients will feel lonely and can become anxious and depressed. They may require additional psychological and emotional support.

Chronic leukaemia

There are two main types of chronic leukaemia: chronic myeloid leukaemia (CML) and chronic lymphocytic leukaemia (CLL). These are very different conditions; the only thing they have in common is the fact that they initially progress slowly.

Chronic myeloid leukaemia

CML is rare, affecting 1–2/100,000 per year. The median age at diagnosis is 50–60 years. Individuals exposed to radiation have an ↑ risk of developing CML. In the vast majority of patients, the cause is unknown.

Philadelphia (Ph) chromosome

Ninety-five per cent of people with CML have an abnormal chromosome 22, formed by an unequal exchange of genetic material between chromosomes 9 and 22 [Philadelphia (Ph) chromosome]. This exchange creates a protein which drives the abnormal cell growth.

Presentation

- Abdominal discomfort with nausea and feeling of fullness due to a massively enlarged spleen.
- Hyperviscosity due to a very high white cell count—headaches, breathlessness, visual disturbances.
- Tiredness, weight loss, drenching night sweats.

There are several distinct phases of the disease:

- Chronic phase: most patients first present during this relatively stable, slowly progressive period. It is easily controlled by medications and can now generally last many years (typically 3–4 years). Modern medication (TKIs) allows the vast majority of patients to remain at this state of good disease control.
- Accelerated phase: the disease rarely now becomes more rapidly progressive and difficult to control. It nearly always precedes a blast crisis.
- Blast crisis: this phase represents transformation to an acute leukaemia, either AML or ALL. It is rapidly fatal if untreated, and is often resistant to treatment. If they can be brought back into the chronic phase with chemotherapy, a stem cell transplant should be considered.

Diagnosis

Blood film, and a bone marrow biopsy is taken. The diagnosis is confirmed by demonstration of the Philadelphia chromosome or molecular demonstration of the BCR–ABL fusion protein.

Treatment

There are two main modes of treatment in chronic phase CML.

Imatinib

(➔ See Small molecule inhibitors, p. 228.)

This targets the abnormal protein produced by the Philadelphia chromosome. It is a tablet taken daily and is generally well tolerated.

- The vast majority of patients respond to imatinib. There is, however, currently a debate about whether imatinib or the so-called

second-generation treatment dasatinib or nilotinib should be used
first line. International trials will help answer this question. Nearly all
have haematological remission, and a majority become Philadelphia
chromosome-negative and a good percentage have complete molecular
remission, particularly with the newer agents. Continued response is
monitored by specialized blood tests (BCR–ABL molecular levels).
* Due to the recent development of imatinib, dasatinib, and nilotinib,
many will enjoy long periods of remission, with good disease control.
A minority become resistant to first- and second-generation treatment,
and a bone marrow transplant is then considered.

Allogeneic stem cell transplantation
(➔ See Chapter 19, Allogeneic haematopoietic stem cell transplant.)
* The introduction of successful drug treatments in CML has now
dramatically reduced the use of bone marrow transplant for this
disease.
* The risks of transplantation are considered too high in the light of very
effective, non-toxic treatment. It is probably the case that patients need
to stay on medication long term to suppress CML. Transplants are still
performed, although these are in the few resistant patients.

Other treatment approaches
These include SC interferon (which still has a role for women who plan to
become pregnant) and hydroxycarbamide (for initial control of the white
cell count and spleen size).

Key nursing issues
Patients with CML are often fairly well at diagnosis and frequently respond
well to treatment. However, certain problems are unique to these patients:
* Patients can feel that their disease is a 'time bomb'. They know that they
are in the chronic phase but may transform to life-threatening acute
leukaemia at any time. This can cause considerable anxiety and concern
for the future and for dependent relatives.
* The arrival of imatinib and other TKIs is great news. Many will live in the
chronic phase for many years. This should always now be the first- and
second-line treatment options. A few do become resistant to treatment
and, without bone marrow transplantation, can progress to acute
leukaemia and die of this disease. Patients can generally be reassured
that, although they have a form of leukaemia that previously had a
relatively poor outcome, the new medications now available are likely
to work very well.

Chronic lymphocytic leukaemia

This is the most common leukaemia in adults. The incidence of CLL rises
with age, reaching a peak in men of 40 per 100,000. It is more common in
men and in developed countries. Diagnosis is made on lymph node core or
excision biopsy or by flow cytometry testing on a raised peripheral blood
lymphocyte count level. The disease remains incurable with standard treatment, but patients can enjoy long periods of remission and approximately
one-third of patients never need treatment during their lifetime.

Presentation
- On a routine blood test in a healthy patient (increasingly common).
- Lumps in the neck, axillae, and groin (enlarged lymph nodes).
- Bone marrow failure (anaemia, low platelets, low white cell count).
- Autoimmune haemolytic anaemia (AIHA) (jaundice, dark urine, and symptoms of anaemia) or immune-related thrombocytopenia (ITP).
- Weight loss, loss of appetite, and night sweats.

Staging
- Bone marrow biopsy (rarely routinely performed outside of clinical trials) ± a CT scan.
- Specialist tests, such as fluorescence *in situ* hybridization (FISH), looking for tumour suppressor gene (*p53*) deletion and *TP53* mutation status, are very important to guide treatment.
- Widespread lymph or organ involvement and bone marrow failure are poor prognostic factors.

Treatment options
'Watch and wait'
- Treatment is offered only if there is evidence of disease progression.
- Treatment is indicated if symptoms develop or when there is a rapidly rising white cell count.

Chemotherapy
Generally, the choice of chemotherapy is dependent on how fit the patient is. The main agents used are chlorambucil and bendamustine in the more elderly, and fludarabine in combination with cyclophosphamide and the monoclonal antibody rituximab in younger, fitter patients.

Novel agents in CLL
New treatment options include ibrutinib, idelalisib with rituximab, and venetoclax. These are licensed in relapsed CLL, and ibrutinib and idelalisib in first-line patients with *p53* mutation/deletion. These are novel agents that have revolutionized the management of CLL. Ibrutinib and idelalisib target the B-cell receptor signalling pathway (the pathway that helps CLL B-cells divide and grow), and venetoclax inhibits specifically BCL-2 [a protein designed to stop B-cells from dying (apoptosis)]. Each of these agents are approved for use in CLL and have therefore limited the number of patients requiring allogeneic stem cell transplantation, because each of these drugs are effective in patients with high-risk clinical and biological features.[1,2,3]

Supportive care
In the palliative care setting, radiotherapy may be used for specific sites of the disease that are causing symptoms. Blood product support may be required for more intensive chemotherapy regimens, and prompt treatment of infections is required. In the terminal stages of CLL, patients most commonly succumb to an infection such as pneumonia.

Nursing issues
With CLL, there is often no initial indication to treat, and patients may remain well for many years on no treatment. However, once diagnosed, patients often associate the word 'leukaemia' with intensive therapy, major

side effects, and immediate threat to life. It can be very difficult to accept if individuals are then not offered a specific treatment. Patients need specially tailored and accurate information regarding their own condition, and, in particular, the stage of their disease. General leukaemia information leaflets may be too broad and may lead to confusion or ↑ anxiety.

References

1 Byrd JC, Brown JR, O'Brien S, et al.; RESONATE Investigators. Ibrutinib versus ofatumumab in previusly treated chronic lymphoid leukemia. N Engl J Med 2014;371:213–23.
2 Furman RR, Sharman JP, Coutre SE, et al. Idelalisib and rituximab in relapsed chronic lymphocytic leukemia. N Engl J Med 2014;370:997–1007.
3 Roberts AW, Davids MS, Pagel JM, et al. Targeting BCL2 with venetoclax in relapsed chronic lymphocytic leukemia. N Engl J Med 2016;374:311–22.

Hodgkin lymphoma (previously Hodgkin disease)

This is a cancer of B-lymphocytes. It affects 1 in 100,000 people per year. In the majority of cases, the cause is unknown, although in a proportion, EBV is thought to be involved.

The peak age at diagnosis is 20–29 years, with another smaller peak in older age (over 60s). Patients diagnosed over the age of 45 have a poorer prognosis.

Presentation
- One or more visible lumps, representing enlarged lymph nodes.
- Breathlessness and cough due to enlarged lymph nodes in the chest (called mediastinal lymphadenopathy).
- Weight loss, fever, and drenching night sweats (called 'B symptoms').

Diagnosis
A biopsy of the affected region is taken. The hallmark of the disease is the Reed–Sternberg cell. The biopsy should distinguish between the two main types of Hodgkin lymphoma. Treatment and prognosis are very different for each type.

The two types of Hodgkin lymphoma are:
- Nodular lymphocyte-predominant Hodgkin lymphoma (NLPHL) (5% of Hodgkin lymphoma)
- Classical Hodgkin lymphoma (the most common variety—95% of cases).

Staging
- PET CT scan of the chest, abdomen, and pelvis is excellent at staging the disease, including bone marrow involvement, accurately.
- The Ann Arbor staging classification is used.[4]

Treatment
Nodular lymphocyte-predominant Hodgkin lymphoma
The vast majority of patients present early with lymph node enlargement in the neck or axilla. This disorder typically affects adolescents and young men. Options for treatment include watch and wait, radiotherapy, rituximab, or, in more advanced stage patients, combination chemotherapy (e.g. CVP, CHOP, ABVD). It is generally an indolent condition, and the prognosis is excellent.

Classical Hodgkin lymphoma
This is typically a more aggressive condition and requires aggressive treatment. Treatment varies according to staging:
- Early stage IA or IIA:
  - **With favourable features**: two cycles of chemotherapy (usually ABVD regimen), with radiotherapy to the affected regions
  - **With unfavourable features** (e.g. anaemia, high ESR, B symptoms): four cycles of ABVD with radiotherapy is a standard approach

- **Advanced stage (II with disease bulk, III, IV):** the standard of care is ABVD (doxorubicin, bleomycin, vinblastine, dacarbazine) combination chemotherapy or BEACOPP (bleomycin, etoposide, cytarabine, cyclophosphamide, procarbazine, and prednisolone).

Interim PET CT
- PET CT scans following two cycles of ABVD are now commonly performed in advanced- and limited-stage disease. There is evidence from large clinical trials that treatment can be safely escalated or de-escalated in patients, depending on how they respond to the initial two cycles of treatment.
- There is now very good evidence from a large trial that patients can safety drop bleomycin (known to cause lung toxicity) without any detrimental effects to the outcome with advanced-stage disease (stage II with bulk, stage III, stage IV) if an interim PET CT scan shows a complete metabolic response. This is now common practice.[5,6]
- There is good evidence for escalating the intensity of chemotherapy in patients with limited-stage disease who are not in complete metabolic remission.

Side effects
ABVD is an intensive regimen. Common side effects include bone marrow suppression, nausea, lung toxicity, cardiac toxicity, peripheral nerve damage, fatigue, and hair loss.
  Note: ABVD is often not tolerated well in elderly patients. Alternative regimens may then be considered.

Prognosis
With combination chemotherapy, long-term survival rates are around 75–80% overall. In early-stage, good-risk disease, this rises to >90%. Even in advanced-stage disease, this can be as high as 80%. In patients with poor-risk disease, long-term survival falls to around 50%.

Relapsed Hodgkin lymphoma
It is still possible to offer curative treatment. This normally involves two phases:
- **Salvage chemotherapy:** normally 2–3 courses of a platinum-based chemotherapy regimen, often with stem cell collection planned for after the second or third course.
- **HDT with autologous stem cell support:** BEAM (carmustine, etoposide, cytarabine, and melphalan) is the usual conditioning therapy. It is thought that around 50% of those who relapse after chemotherapy can be cured (➔ see Chapter 18, High-dose therapy (autologous transplant)).

Long-term toxicity
Due to the excellent cure rates, many patients live long enough to experience long-term toxicity from the treatment. The two major problems are:
- **Secondary cancers**—breast cancer and lung cancer for those who received chest radiotherapy. Acute leukaemia for patients treated with very aggressive chemotherapy regimens
- **Heart disease**—particularly for older patients treated with radiotherapy to the chest and those treated with anthracycline chemotherapy

- At around 15 years after treatment, the risk of dying from a complication of the treatment becomes greater than the risk of dying from relapse of Hodgkin lymphoma. Efforts are being made to reduce the treatment intensity, whilst maintaining cure rates and ensuring close monitoring and long-term follow-up.

The future

New agents, such as brentuximab vedotin, an anti-CD30 monoclonal antibody with a linked toxin, and PD-1 inhibitors nivolumab and pembrolizumab, have shown excellent responses in large trials of relapsed and refractory Hodgkin lymphoma patients.

Nursing issues

Hodgkin lymphoma frequently affects young people. Particular concerns include the following.

Fertility

Standard ABVD chemotherapy does not generally render the patient infertile (♂ or ♀), although many men are offered sperm storage as a precaution.

Long-term toxicity

It should be emphasized that heart disease and secondary cancers are by no means inevitable later in life—although the risk is ↑. The patient should be encouraged to participate in any screening programmes offered after therapy (such as for breast cancer) and to optimize a healthy style of living (giving up smoking, taking regular exercise, eating a balanced diet).

Transfusion-associated graft-versus-host disease

It is important to remember that **any** patient who has had Hodgkin lymphoma in the past should receive only irradiated blood products, due to an ↑ risk of this very rare, but fatal, complication of blood product transfusion.

Age-related issues

Because the peak incidence falls in late adolescence, when young people have left home and are independent, there may be family conflicts and issues centred around the parents' need for control and to care for their child. This occurs whilst the patient still needs to maintain their newly developed sense of self and maintain control and independence. Families should be encouraged and supported to discuss the issues that are arising.

References

4 Cheson BD, Fisher RI, Barrington SF, et al. Recommendations for initial evaluation, staging, and response assessment of Hodgkin and Non-Hodgkin lymphoma: The Lugano Classification. *J Clin Oncol* 2014;32:3059–67.

5 Johnson P, Federico M, Kirkwood A, et al. Adapted treatment guided by interim PET-CT scan in advanced Hodgkin lymphoma. *N Engl J Med* 2016;374:2419–29.

6 Andre MPE, Girinsky T, Federico M, et al. Early positron emission tomography response-adapted treatment of stage I and II Hodgkin lymphoma: final results of the randomized EORTC/LYSA/FIL H10 Trial. *J Clin Oncol* 2017;35:1786–94.

Non-Hodgkin lymphoma

NHL is a broad term, which covers a number of very different conditions, all of which are cancers of lymphocytes.

The classification of NHL is a confusing and changing area. The most clinically relevant way of categorizing NHL is in terms of high-grade or low-grade disease (see Table 30.2).

Presentation

- Enlarged lymph node, commonly in the neck, axillae, and groin.
- Symptoms of NHL are due to extranodal disease, so presentation depends on the site of the disease. NHL can occur anywhere in the body, e.g. brain, eye, bone, kidney, bowel, and can present with quite severe complications, e.g. bowel obstruction, renal failure, seizures.
- Cough, breathlessness, tracheal deviation, SVCO due to mediastinal lymphadenopathy.
- 'B' symptoms—weight loss, fever, drenching night sweats.

Diagnosis and staging

- Core or excision biopsy of the lymph node or extranodal disease.
- It is important to establish the exact subtype of lymphoma, as the treatment depends on this.
- CT scan of the chest, abdomen, and pelvis. CT of the brain is sometimes required.
- Bone marrow trephine biopsy.
- The staging system is the Ann Arbor staging system for Hodgkin lymphoma.

Prognostic factors

Patients are categorized into risk groups, depending on the number of poor prognostic factors with which they present.

Table 30.2 Classification of NHL into high- or low-grade disease

High grade	Low grade	
• Diffuse large B-cell lymphoma	• Follicular lymphoma	
• Burkitt's lymphoma	• Small lymphocytic lymphoma	
• Lymphoblastic lymphoma	• Marginal zone lymphoma	
	• Lymphoplasmacytoid lymphoma	
Grade	High grade	Low grade
Speed of progression	Rapid	Indolent
Usual stage at presentation	More commonly early stage	More commonly late stage
Sensitivity to chemotherapy	Very sensitive	Less sensitive
Risk of TLS	High	Low
Potential for cure	40–50% chance of cure	Usually incurable

- Poor prognostic factors include age >60 years, high serum LDH, poor performance status, stage III or IV disease, and the existence of extranodal disease.

High-grade lymphoma
- For low-risk patients: 5-year survival is around 80%.
- For high-risk patients: 5-year survival rates are nearer 35–50% (these statistics apply to diffuse large B-cell lymphoma, the most common high-grade lymphoma).

Low-grade lymphoma
- For low-risk patients: 5-year survival is around 90%.
- For high-risk patients: 5-year survival rates are nearer 50%.

Note: although low-grade disease is not curable, the 5-year survival rates are better than for high-grade disease. However, survival rates continue to fall with time, due to the disease continuing to relapse and/or transform into high-grade disease.

Treatment

Treatment depends on the exact subtype, stage, and perceived aggressiveness of the disease, age, and general fitness of the patient.

High-grade lymphoma
Chemotherapy
Combination chemotherapy is standard therapy for high-grade lymphoma. For diffuse large B-cell lymphoma, the standard treatment is CHOP-R (cyclophosphamide, doxorubicin, vincristine, and prednisolone in combination with the monoclonal antibody rituximab). (For further information on monoclonal antibodies, ➲ see Monoclonal Antibodies, p. 235.)

This treatment is generally well tolerated. It will cause predictable neutropenia, and rituximab can cause an infusional hypersensitivity reaction, most common on the first dose (➲ see Anaphylaxis, p. 633). Other side effects include mucositis and cardiac and peripheral nerve toxicity.

Other forms of high-grade lymphoma may be treated differently.
For example:
- Burkitt's lymphoma regimens contain high doses of methotrexate and IT chemotherapy, so as to prevent CNS relapses. Multiple sequential doses of cyclophosphamide are also thought to be important.
- Lymphoblastic lymphoma is treated as per ALL (➲ see Acute leukaemia, p. 400).

Radiotherapy
Radiotherapy can be used in combination with a reduced number of chemotherapy courses or to target sites of bulky disease after chemotherapy has been given, in order to prevent relapse.

Relapsed disease
For patients who relapse after treatment, the aim is normally to get the patient into another remission by using different forms of chemotherapy, and then HDT in order to consolidate the remission (➲ see Chapter 18, High-dose therapy with autologous stem cell support).

Low-grade lymphoma

Low-grade lymphoma is often not treated actively until it causes one of the following:

• Generalized symptoms such as weight loss, night sweats, and fevers
• Falling blood counts due to bone marrow infiltration
• Progressive enlargement of the liver or spleen
• Symptoms such as painfully enlarged lymph nodes due to local disease
• Evidence of high-grade transformation such as asymmetrically, rapidly enlarging lymph nodes, rising LDH levels, or high calcium levels.

Once treatment is indicated, it can take a number of different forms:

• Oral chemotherapy: rarely curative but is well tolerated and may induce a remission
• IV combination chemotherapy: several regimes are used in combination with the monoclonal antibody rituximab
• Radiotherapy may be used to treat symptoms caused by local deposits of disease
• HDT with autologous stem cell support (➲ see Chapter 18, High-dose therapy with autologous stem cell support)
• Allogeneic stem cell transplantation for younger, fit patients, generally with relapsed disease (➲ see Chapter 19, Allogeneic haemopoietic stem cell transplantation).

Nursing issues

Patients with high-grade lymphoma pose similar challenges to patients with acute leukaemia (➲ see Acute leukaemia, p. 400). It can be hard to adjust to a diagnosis of a rapidly progressive, life-threatening lymphoma, and bewildering when treatment is started within a few days of diagnosis. The intense treatment regimens bring a range of severe and potentially life-threatening side effects. For the very high-grade lymphomas such as Burkitt's lymphoma, there is also a high risk of TLS (➲ see Tumour lysis syndrome, pp. 649–50).

Patients with low-grade NHL, on the other hand, face similar issues to CLL patients. They may find it confusing to be given a diagnosis of cancer, but not to be offered specific treatment straightaway. If the patient is young, then to be told they have a life expectancy of 10 years is potentially devastating.

Myeloma

Myeloma is a cancer of plasma cells—the antibody-producing cells which represent the final step in the development of a B-lymphocyte. In myeloma, the cancerous cells secrete a single type of antibody into the bloodstream called a paraprotein. As well as being a marker of myeloma, the paraprotein may lead to clinical problems. These include thinning bones, high calcium levels, high blood viscosity, reduced immunity, and obstruction of the renal tubules.

The incidence of myeloma increases with age. Presentation before the age of 50 is unusual. Incidence is around 5 per 100,000 in the UK. For unknown reasons, myeloma is more common in the African-Caribbean population.

Presentation

- Bone pain: predominantly due to bone thinning, causing fractures in any part of the body. This may also result in spinal cord compression.
- Hypercalcaemia: presenting with confusion or alteration in mental status, dehydration, and renal impairment (**➔** see Malignancy-induced hypercalcaemia, pp. 637–40).
- Anaemia due to bone marrow involvement or renal failure.
- Infections: the most common infection is pneumonia. There is a 10% mortality rate in the first 60 days after diagnosis related to infection alone.
- Acute renal failure: associated with a 30% mortality rate at 60 days.

Diagnosing myeloma

The main tests required for a diagnosis of myeloma are:
- Blood tests to find the paraprotein
- Urine tests to find the paraprotein—when present in the urine, the antibody is called the 'Bence–Jones protein'
- Skeletal survey: multiple X-rays to find any 'lytic lesions' where the myeloma is eroding bone away
- Bone marrow aspirate and trephine.

Note: if a patient presents with any symptoms suggesting compression of the spinal cord, then an urgent MRI of the spine is indicated (**➔** see Metastatic spinal cord compression, pp. 641–4).

Treatment

Myeloma is generally considered to be incurable; median survival is around 4–5 years. Symptom control is therefore an important part of treatment. Treatment options have improved over recent years, with the introduction of so-called the 'novel agents' thalidomide, bortezomib, and lenalidomide.

Single-agent oral chemotherapy

This offers around 50% response rate. Generally only used first line in more elderly patients.

Combination chemotherapy

The main aim of this is to debulk the disease, making it more amenable to HDT. First-line treatment is commonly with cyclophosphamide, thalidomide, and dexamethasone (CTD) in the UK in those under 70 years old. Thalidomide does have its problems. It can cause sedation, constipation, nerve damage, and thrombosis, as well recognized side effects.

High-dose therapy with autologous stem cell support
Available evidence suggests that this can probably prolong life expectancy by about 1 year. That extra year is often treatment-free and therefore of reasonable quality (➔ see Chapter 18, High-dose therapy (autologous transplant)). This is now debated in the era of novel therapies.

Thalidomide and the risk of pregnancy
Women of child-bearing age must be counselled to use at least two forms of contraception (one being a barrier method), due to the well-known toxic effects of thalidomide on a developing fetus. Men must also be told to wear a condom during sexual intercourse, as thalidomide is excreted into semen.

Bortezomib-based regimens
Bortezomib is a novel agent, which targets enzymes involved in controlling cell growth. It has shown good activity in relapsed patients when used with dexamethasone.

IV treatment with bortezomib can cause marked nerve damage; however, this has been improved with the new SC formulation. Bortezomib does also cause diarrhoea and nausea, which is sometimes severe and dose-limiting.

Bisphosphonates
Adding bisphosphonates to myeloma treatment reduces pathological fractures and pain. A recent UK trial has also shown improved survival using zoledronic acid.

Solitary plasmacytoma
- These are rare single-site plasma cell tumours. They account for <10% of all plasma cell tumours.
- Can occur in bone [solitary bone plasmacytoma (SBP)] or soft tissue [extramedullary plasmacytoma (EMP)].

Solitary bone plasmacytoma
- Commonly presents in spine, pelvis, or femur. Pain is the most common presenting symptom.
- Diagnosis is through histological examination and ruling out other sites of disease.
- Treatment is with fractionated radiotherapy and curative in 50% of cases. If there is evidence of dissemination (the majority of patients will relapse with myeloma), treat with myeloma regimens.

Extramedullary plasmacytoma
- Commonly presents in upper airways but can occur at almost any site.
- Treatment is with radical radiotherapy, possibly including regional lymph nodes.
- Progression to myeloma can occur, but less commonly than SPB. The cure rates are higher than SPB.

Nursing issues

Myeloma can cause a variety of problems, which frequently require specialist input. An important role for a specialist myeloma nurse is to coordinate this care and to help the patient assimilate all the information.

Key problems faced by patients include the following:

- Bone pain: radiotherapy, opioids, and bisphosphonates all have a major role in managing this. In selected cases, surgery or vertebroplasty can also be used to manage collapsed vertebral bodies (➔ see Metastatic bone disease, pp. 287–9)
- Spinal cord compression (➔ see Metastatic spinal cord compression, pp. 641–4)
- Immunosuppression: although myeloma patients may not be neutropenic, they should be considered very immunosuppressed, and prompt antibiotic treatment should be given for proven or likely episodes of infection
- Acute renal failure: dialysis may be required for patients who present with acute renal failure, and this may be needed long term if their kidneys fail to recover.

Further reading

Browne M, Cutler T. *Haematology Nursing*. Chichester: Wiley-Blackwell; 2012.
Hoffbrand AV, Moss PAH. *Essential Haematology*, 6th ed. Oxford: Blackwell Science; 2011.
National Institute for Clinical Excellence. *Guidance on Cancer Services: Improving Outcomes in Haematological Cancers: The Manual*. London: National Institute for Clinical Excellence; 2003.

Chapter 31

Head and neck cancers

Introduction

- H&N cancer is the eighth most common cancer worldwide. It describes a group of solid tumours of the upper aero-digestive tract, often arising from the surface mucosa. The most common type of tumour is SCC.
- There are over 30 specific sites in the H&N where cancer can occur, including the oral cavity (the most common site), pharynx, hypopharynx, and larynx. Rarer sites include the saliva glands, post-nasal space and sinuses, and middle ear.
- Oral cancer incidence has ↑ in the UK by around 83% since the 1970s, with a 34% increase in the last decade. It is thought that this ↑ incidence may be linked to the ↑ prevalence of HPV in the younger population.
- Conversely, the incidence of laryngeal cancers has ↓ by around 5% in the last decade, most likely linked to a reduction in smoking. Metastatic spread is common in most H&N cancers, and the lymph glands in the neck tend to be the first area where deposits occur.
- Mortality in H&N cancers has generally ↓ over the last two decades, with improved treatment and reduction in smoking being possible causes. The exception to this is oral cancer which has shown ↑ mortality, almost certainly due to higher incidence.

Risk factors

Smoking and alcohol

- Around 75% of H&N cancers are associated with smoking and alcohol use.
- Combined cigarette and alcohol use has a potentiating effect.
- The risk of oral cancer in this group is over 35 times higher than for non-smokers and non-drinkers. For those who smoke but do not drink, the risk of developing H&N cancer is ten times higher than for non-smokers.
- Nurses can help the patient to manage their alcohol and tobacco use, in order to optimize treatment outcomes (**➲** see Nursing management of people who are alcohol-dependent, p. 602; **➲** Smoking cessation, p. 61).

Sexual behaviour

- Recent research would suggest that the large increase in oral cancers, particularly in a previously unaffected younger age group, is due to infection with HPV.
- Oropharyngeal, tonsil, and base of the tongue cancer risk is higher in people with multiple sexual partners, particularly oral sex partners.
- It is thought that between 8% and 14% of all oral and oropharyngeal cancers could be due to infection with HPV.

Diet

- People who drink and smoke heavily may have a poor diet and be malnourished, which exacerbates the risk of H&N cancer.
- Low risk associated with a well-balanced diet rich in vegetables and fruit.
- It is estimated that around 45% of laryngeal cancers and 56% of oral cancers may be linked to a diet low in fruit and vegetables.
- ↑ risk with a poor diet, particularly deficient in vitamins A and C.

Presentation

Depending on the site of the tumour, H&N malignancies may present with:

• Hoarseness
• Difficulty in swallowing
• Local or referred pain.

Some tumours are detected during a dental examination.

Diagnosis and staging

• Clinical examination.
• Panendoscopy and biopsy.
• FNA for cytology is useful in patients presenting with neck lumps.
• PET/CT or MRI scan.
• Staging is carried out using the TNM staging system.
• Most tumours invade locally; bone and vascular involvement can occur in advanced disease.

Prognostic factors

Metastatic nodal involvement is more important prognostically than the size of the primary tumour, i.e. smaller tumours and extensive nodal involvement have a worse prognosis than a large tumour and no nodal involvement. Other prognostic factors include age and the histopathology of the tumour.

Websites

The following charitable organizations can play an important role in supporting the patient and their family:

British Red Cross Camouflage Service. Available at: ℘ http://www.redcross.org.uk

Changing Faces. Available at: ℘ http://www.changingfaces.org.uk

National Association of Laryngectomee Clubs. Available at: ℘ https://www.laryngectomy.org.uk

Further reading

British Association of Head and Neck Oncology Nurses (BAHNON). Available at: ℘ https:// bahnon.org.uk (provides guidelines and protocols for health professionals).

Dempsey L, Orr S, Lane S, Scott A. The clinical nurse specialist's role in head and neck cancer care: United Kingdom National Multidisciplinary Guidelines. *J Laryngol Otol* 2016;**130**(Suppl S2):S212–15.

Foulkes M. Oral cancer: risk factors, treatment and nursing care. *Nurs Stand* 2013;28:49–57.

Treatment of head and neck cancer

The main treatment approaches for H&N cancer are radiotherapy and surgery. Chemotherapy is occasionally used in combination with radiotherapy or as a palliative treatment.

Treatment of early-stage disease (30–40% of presentations)

The main options are surgery, radiotherapy, or a combination of both. Post-operative chemo-irradiation is also an option for specific high-risk, fit patients.

- Cure rates with primary radiotherapy appear to be equivalent to surgery for early-stage disease of many H&N tumours.
- The specific cancer site, patient health, and their own preference will be major factors in which the treatment option is chosen.

Surgery alone

Potential advantages of surgery alone include:

- It provides complete staging of the disease and quick local clearance
- It avoids radiotherapy toxicities, including the risk of radiotherapy-induced second malignancies.

Radiotherapy alone

Options are EBRT ± a boost to the tumour site, either with further EBRT. EBRT is given in divided doses (20–30 fractions) for solid tumours (commonly SCC). The continued development of IMRT has reduced some of the side effects of radiotherapy, most notably radiotherapy-induced xerostomia (dry mouth), which can be a debilitating and long-term problem for patients.

Potential advantages of primary radiotherapy include:

- Avoidance of operative mortality in patients who have significant comorbidities
- Organ conservation is more likely, including preservation of the voice and swallowing
- Radiotherapy treats clinically occult regional lymph node disease with relatively little extra morbidity
- Surgery remains an option as treatment after radiotherapy if that is unsuccessful, though this is associated with greater morbidity
- It allows the treatment of multiple primary tumours.

Combined surgery and radiotherapy

- Bulky tumours are generally best treated by a combination of surgery and radiotherapy to minimize the risk of locally advanced disease recurrence.
- Risk factors for recurrence include large tumour size, positive resection margins, vascular invasion, and lymph node spreads.

Post-operative chemo-radiotherapy

- Radiotherapy with concurrent cisplatin in oropharyngeal cancers shows fewer local and regional relapses and improvements in disease-free survival.
- An improvement in overall survival has not been consistently demonstrated.

- Toxicity is significantly ↑ in patients receiving both cisplatin and radiotherapy.
- May be considered for selected high-risk, fit patients with resected H&N SCCs.

Management of involved neck nodes

Options include: therapeutic neck dissection, radiotherapy, or surgery for any relapsed disease after radiotherapy.

Neck dissection

Neck dissection involves removing the affected lymph glands, along with the other glands in the lymphovascular chain.

H&N surgery is complex, with associated complications and a potentially huge impact on a patient's long-term QoL.

Treatment of locally advanced unresectable disease

Chemo-irradiation

- The majority of H&N SCCs have locally advanced unresectable disease at presentation.
- Surgery is often not technically possible or may produce unacceptable morbidity.
- Primary radiotherapy offers 5-year survival of only 10–30%.
- The addition of cisplatin offers a modest survival advantage over treatment with radiotherapy alone (4–8% increase in 5-year survival).
- This is associated with ↑ toxicity, in particular mucositis. It is most appropriate for patients with a good performance status and relatively few comorbidities.

Biological therapies

- Cetuximab (➔ see Introduction to targeted and biological therapies, p. 227).

In the UK, cetuximab has been approved for use, alongside radiotherapy, in patients with locally advanced SCCs of the H&N who cannot receive any platinum-based chemotherapy. It can only be used in patients with a good performance status. It has been shown to be of limited benefit in patients with advanced or metastatic disease.

Treatment of metastatic disease

Chemotherapy/systemic anti-cancer therapy

Certain agents, e.g. cisplatin, 5FU, capecitabine, methotrexate, and docetaxel, have been shown to be effective in advanced SCC. Highest response rates appear to be achieved by combination regimes. The risk versus potential benefits have to be carefully considered for each patient.

Radiotherapy

Radiotherapy is used in metastatic disease to give short-term local control and to palliate symptoms such as bleeding and pain.

Palliative procedures

The use of palliative surgical procedures in H&N cancer has gradually declined since the 1980s, but there is still a place for invasive procedures to help maintain quality of life in the face of problems such as:

- Airway maintenance (tracheostomy, stents)
- Nutritional support (e.g. gastrostomy or other feeding tubes)
- Tumour debulking
- Fistula repair
- Tumour ablation
- Arresting or preventing haemorrhage
- Pain control (nerve ablation).

It is important that decisions around these kinds of procedures involve the patient, the carers, and the full MDT. A good guiding principle is that the extension of life should not be carried out at the expense of the quality of life.

Further reading

National Institute for Health and Care Excellence. *Upper Aerodigestive Tract Cancer Overview.* Available at: ⅆ https://pathways.nice.org.uk/pathways/upper-aerodigestive-tract-cancer/upper-aerodigestive-tract-cancer-overview

Roland NJ, Bradley PN. The role of surgery in the palliation of head and neck cancer. *Curr Opin Otolaryngol Head Neck Surg* 2014;22:101–8.

Laryngectomy and tracheostomy

Anatomy and physiology of the airway

The upper respiratory tract (URT) consists of the nasal airway, naso-pharynx, oral cavity, oropharynx, hypopharynx, larynx, and trachea. The nose has an important role in humidifying, warming, and filtering the air. The whole URT is lined with mucus-secreting columnar ciliated epithelium. This prevents debris and microorganisms from entering the respiratory tract.

If the airway is altered due to tracheostomy or laryngectomy, it is exposed to cold air, large quantities of particulate matter, and bacteria, pathogens, and debris, and there is a rapid increase in the production of mucus.

Laryngectomy care

Stoma care is aimed at maintaining the patient's airway, preventing infection, including secondary chest infection and tracheitis, and promoting healing.

The main priority of post-operative support for laryngectomy patients is self-care and independence, through individualized teaching plans. Family members or carers should be included.

Basic information needs to be provided, and individual coping strategies developed for dealing with the following: loss of normal speech, loss of smell, inability to sniff or blow one's nose, loss of sphincteric function of the larynx (affecting lifting and ability to 'push' during defecation), using bronchodilator inhalers, and avoiding water entering the stoma when showering or swimming. A number of devices are available to help with this.

Tracheostomy

A surgeon will perform a tracheostomy when the airway is obstructed by a tumour or post-operative oedema. A tube is inserted into the tracheostomy, and a tract develops after 4 days—a tube change should not be attempted before this, unless in the case of emergency.

A tracheostomy can be temporary or permanent:

- Temporary: to protect the airway from oedema and swelling, following surgery or radiotherapy
- Permanent: following laryngectomy, airway obstruction caused by an inoperable tumour or the effects of a tumour, e.g. when there is a fixed vocal cord.

Nursing management of tracheostomy

Preoperative counselling

Counselling should be given to the patient and their family, if possible. A permanent tracheostomy can have life-long effects on speech, swallowing, and respiration. Input from a CNS, speech and language therapist (SALT), dietician, and physiotherapist is essential if the patient is to achieve optimum rehabilitation.

For patients undergoing laryngectomy, a meeting with a patient who has already had a laryngectomy (a laryngectomee) can help the process of adjustment. Some areas operate a 'buddy' system of support.

Patients with tracheostomy will produce higher levels of pulmonary secretions. These are difficult to remove with coughing and can block breathing. Patients will need suction to help to clear them.

Neck dressings and securing tapes should be changed daily, or more frequently if required. This should only be undertaken by two practitioners, as there is a risk of the tracheostomy tube being coughed out when the neck tapes are removed. The condition of the peri-stomal skin should be monitored, and any concerns raised with the surgical team.

When the patient is capable, the nurse should support the patient in becoming independent with care of the stoma and change of tube. Give the patient a pen and paper or a magnetic writing board to facilitate patient communication.

Complications of tracheostomy

- Obstruction of the tube: a blocked tube can be fatal. Warning signs of tube occlusion include ↑ respiratory rate and ↓ oxygen saturation. If a tube without an inner cannula becomes blocked, then the tube must be changed immediately to prevent cardiopulmonary arrest.
- Haemorrhage: erosion of the tracheal wall is possible by excessive tube or cuff pressure, causing a haemorrhage from the innominate or right common carotid arteries—this can be fatal. Surgical repair of the damaged vessel is undertaken if the patient survives long enough.
- Infection: as tracheostomies bypass the immune system provided by the upper airways, chest infections can be a problem. Tracheitis can be due to infection or irritation. Fungal infection is not common but can be seen with signs of fungal growth on the tracheostomy tube.
- Other complications include tracheo-oesophageal fistula, tube displacement, excessive granulation tissue, and pressure sore formation inferior to the stoma.

Nursing management issues

H&N cancers can have a profound effect on a person's quality of life, as they affect the most visible parts of the body and the critical functions of eating, drinking, breathing, and speaking. A large MDT is needed to manage the complex nature of the disease and the side effects of treatment.

The patient's journey through the health-care system can be complex, so continuity of care is important. The H&N cancer nurse specialist has an important role in providing continuity; other professionals may take a key worker role at different points. Developing effective links with community services, i.e. GP, district nurse, and/or community palliative care teams, is essential in providing long-term support of these patients.

Effective nursing care involves supporting the patient through a complex series of treatments and helping them manage the side effects and complications of treatment and changes to their self-image.

Impact of radiotherapy

Side effects

The upper aero-digestive tract is extremely sensitive to radiotherapy. It can have a profound, long-term impact on the QoL of the H&N cancer patient. Common side effects include:

- Mucositis, causing severe pain, taste loss, dysphagia, and sleep disturbance
- Xerostomia: mouth pain, loss of appetite, chewing difficulties, taste changes, halitosis
- Fatigue
- Skin damage
- Loss of hair.

For management of each of these side effects, see the appropriate chapter under ⮊ Section 7 Symptom management.

Impact of surgery

Preoperative management

Counselling is essential to prepare patients for the possible long-term side effects of neck dissection, e.g. body image, swallowing, nutrition, communication (⮊ see Speech and language therapy, p. 426). In addition, the nurse should discuss post-operative pain and how to deal with numb skin on the neck. A physiotherapy referral enables a baseline assessment to be undertaken and post-operative management to be discussed. A nutritional assessment is also required.

Post-operative management

For standard post-operative care, ⮊ see Chapter 15, Surgery. Specific issues in H&N surgery include management of skin flaps and grafts, meticulous oral hygiene, pain, swallowing, and speech therapy. Laryngectomy and tracheostomy have been explored earlier in this chapter.

Potential emergencies

Carotid haemorrhage

Bleeding from the neck is uncommon, but it can occur following neck dissection, particularly if the tumour has involved a main artery or vein. This is an emergency situation. Very firm pressure should be applied to the bleeding point; the resuscitation team and the surgeon should be alerted for immediate return to theatre, if possible, and the patient resuscitated with fluids (➡ see Bleeding, p. 483).

Chylous fistula

A rare side effect of surgery to the neck is damage to the thoracic duct. The thoracic duct is the main portal for lymph and dietary fat to reach the venous circulation, and any damage may result in a major leak of lymphatic fluid. Leakage into a surgical drain which appears milky may be a chylous fistula, and failure to note the problem can result in the patient suffering major electrolyte and immune system disruption.

The patient should have a pressure dressing applied and be commenced on a totally fat-free diet for up to 6 weeks, to allow the fistula to heal. Surgical repair of the thoracic duct may be required.

Later complications include lymphoedema and subcutaneous fibrosis. This is more frequent with combined surgery and radiotherapy.

Nutritional support for head and neck cancer

Many patients with H&N cancer are nutritionally compromised prior to treatment. A full dietician assessment is essential prior to their treatment, to plan appropriate nutritional support (➡ see Nutritional support, pp. 542–5).

Enteral support

H&N cancer and its treatment may compromise or obstruct the GI tract. In these situations, short- or long-term enteral support is required such as an NG feeding tube or a gastrostomy tube (➡ see Nutritional support, pp. 542–5).

Psychological support for head and neck cancer

Over time, the cumulative effects of disease and multiple treatments can result in 'patient burnout'. This is a severe state of mental and physical exhaustion and demoralization. Referral to a psycho-oncology team may be required (➡ see Psychological support, p. 580).

Speech and language therapy

Patients should be referred to a SALT as early as possible, so that baseline assessments can be made. Potential problems include the following.

Difficulty in swallowing

This may be caused by anatomical changes in any part of the oral cavity, pharynx, or oesophagus. New swallowing techniques may need to be mastered in the post-operative period.

Speech

Most centres use tracheo-oesophageal puncture and prosthetic valves to facilitate speech, following laryngectomy. Many patients are taught how to change their own speech valve, following the surgery. Some patients are not eligible for prosthetic valves and will need an alternative method of communication, e.g. an electrolarynx (a vibration device that is placed on the neck).

HIV-related malignancies

HIV-related malignancies

Epidemiology

HIV represented the worst epidemic of the late twentieth and early twenty-first centuries. There are ~36.9 million cases worldwide. The highest prevalence is in Eastern and Southern Africa, with around 19 million people living with HIV in 2015. Western Europe and North America combined has around 2.4 million people living with HIV infection. Since 2005, there has been a worldwide reduction in the number of deaths from AIDS and HIV-related causes due to major increases in the number of patients receiving retroviral therapy. Standard antiretroviral therapy (ART) is made up of a combination of antiretroviral drugs which suppress HIV, stopping the progression of HIV disease. The therapy also reduces the transmission of HIV.

Aetiology

Transmission is through direct contact with blood or body fluid of infected individuals. It is usually spread through:
- Unprotected sex or sharing needles for drug use
- Mothers if they are infected, from whom infants can get HIV.

ART has ↑ survival for many people with HIV infection. However, the rate of malignant disease in HIV-infected patients remains much higher than in the general population.

AIDS and cancer

AIDS stands for acquired immune deficiency syndrome. When HIV infection becomes advanced, it often is referred to as AIDS. It is characterized by the appearance of opportunistic infections, such as *Pneumocystis carinii* pneumonia, and malignancies such as KS, NHL, and invasive cervical cancer. These malignancies can be termed 'AIDS-defining'. Since the widespread availability of ART, the incidence of AIDS-defining cancers has ↓, but there has been an accompanying relative increase in the incidence of other malignancies (non-AIDS-defining), compared to the general population.

Management

Management of cancer in HIV is complex, involving the management of the cancer, of the underlying immune deficiency, and of the complex psychological and social issues which usually coexist. Where possible, patients with HIV and a cancer diagnosis should be treated in specialist centres.

Specific AIDS-defining cancers

Kaposi's sarcoma

Despite its falling incidence, this incurable, multifocal soft tissue sarcoma remains the most common HIV or AIDS-related malignancy. Cutaneous involvement of multiple red-purple lesions affecting the upper body, face, and legs is characteristic. Disease progression is usually slow, although it can behave aggressively, causing significant morbidity.

Treatment
- Is usually palliative in intent.
- Local therapy options (for local control and cosmesis) include cryotherapy and laser therapy.
- Intralesional chemotherapy or radiotherapy can produce short-term regression in ~75% of cases.
- Systemic therapy—with ART ± chemotherapy are front-line treatments for systemic disease.

Supportive care
- Camouflage with cosmetics.
- Psychosocial support.
- Palliation of symptoms.

Systemic non-Hodgkin lymphoma
NHL is the second most common malignancy to affect those with AIDS.

Treatment
- Systemic chemotherapy with concomitant ART is the usual approach (➋ see Non-Hodgkin lymphoma, Treatment, p. 412).
- Response rates to treatment are worse than in patients with non-AIDS-related lymphoma.

Primary CNS lymphoma
Primary CNS lymphoma (PCNSL) is usually a late manifestation of AIDS. Patients presents with a range of CNS symptoms and also lymphoma 'B' symptoms (➋ see Non-Hodgkin lymphoma, presentation, p. 411).

Treatment
- Whole brain radiotherapy, with corticosteroids and methotrexate-containing chemotherapy, combined with appropriate ART.
- Overall survival remains poor with 5-year survival of 9%.

Cervical cancer in HIV-positive females
The prevalence of CIN is four times more common in HIV-infected women. It is important to screen patients frequently, e.g. every 6–12 months, as effective ART is associated with regression of CIN (➋ see Cervical cancer screening, pp. 54–6).

Non-AIDS-defining cancers
As people living with HIV survive longer on ART, there is increasing evidence that this population has a significantly higher incidence of non-AIDS-defining cancers[1] and up to sevenfold greater mortality from these malignancies[2] than those in the non-HIV-infected population.

Those cancers which have both a higher incidence and ↑ mortality include:
- Anal cancer
- Lung cancer
- Primary liver cancer
- Hodgkin's disease

In order to address these issues, patients with HIV infection should be monitored for these malignancies, e.g. being added to screening programmes for lung cancer. Patients with HIV who have any malignancy should also be referred to a specialist treatment centre (→ see Nursing management, pp. 431–2).

References

1 Patel P, Hanson DL, Sullivan PS, *et al.* Incidence of types of cancer among HIV-infected persons compared with the general population in the United States, 1992–2003 *Ann Intern Med* 2008;148:728–36.

2 Zucchetto A, Virdone S, Taborelli M, *et al.* (2016) Non-AIDS defining cancer mortality: emerging patterns in the late HAART era. *J Acquir Immune Defic Syndr* 2016;73:190–6.

Nursing management issues

People with HIV disease continue to face social isolation for a number of reasons, including homophobia, prejudice against drug users, lack of family acceptance, or discrimination. They may therefore already be feeling vulnerable, and this can make the additional diagnosis of cancer very hard to deal with. Nurses are in an important position to support patients with their symptoms, the side effects of treatment, and the social and psychological impact of both illnesses.

Patient education

After a diagnosis of HIV, it is important to reduce exposure to general infections, as these may precipitate the development of some malignancies. In addition to this, advice should be given to prevent the transmission of HIV to others.

Topics for patient education include:
- Safer sex techniques
- Use of clean drug equipment
- Perinatal transmission risks
- Advice about rest, nutrition, and stress reduction, to reduce the risk of opportunistic infections
- Education about the signs and symptoms of specific cancers such as KS or NHL, and the importance of early treatment.

Support can come from specialist HIV counsellors. Contact your local sexually transmitted infections (STI) unit for a list of appropriate services that may be helpful. Useful information may also be obtained from support organizations such as the Terrence Higgins Trust.[3]

Treatment decisions

Many patients are very immunosuppressed and may not tolerate full-dose chemotherapy or radiotherapy regimens. It is therefore advisable that patients are managed in specialist centres with experience of these different, and sometimes competing, treatment aims. The British HIV Association recommends that all patients with HIV and malignancy should be referred to centres that have developed expertise in the management of these diseases.[4] Dose reductions and modifications are more common when treating patients with HIV due to levels of immunosuppression. Chemotherapy may leave patients exposed to infection and other side effects. In some cases, the risks of further treatments might have to be weighed up against the prevention of tumour progression. Patients need advice and explanations about the reasons for these difficult decisions.

The risk of life-threatening infections can be high with immunosuppression, due to both HIV and systemic chemotherapy. Good patient education is required on both the early signs of infections and the need to contact their treatment unit immediately with any suspected signs.

Body image disturbance

This is common due to KS lesions and severe weight loss. In addition, hair loss or steroid effects can add to body image disturbance (➜ see Body image, p. 607).

Palliative care

Early access to palliative care services is important, as most patients will already have treatable symptoms and psychosocial problems at diagnosis. The combination of physical symptoms and psychosocial problems, including depression and spiritual distress, means that the patient is ripe for patient-centred palliative care. This includes multidimensional assessment, an integrated approach to management, and, where necessary, referral to specialist palliative care services (➔ see Palliative care, pp. 148–9). Loss of this opportunity may result in the patient withdrawing from care until the disease is advanced.

Websites

Medscape. *HIV/AIDS.* Available at: ℘ https://www.medscape.com/hiv (website of educational articles).

National AIDS Manual (NAM) aidsmap. Available at: ℘ http://www.aidsmap.com (excellent website with up-to date treatment news).

Further reading

Bower M, Palfreeman A, Alfa-Wali M, *et al*. British HIV Association guidelines for HIV-associated malignancies 2014. *HIV Med* 2014;**15**(Suppl 2):1–92.

National Institute for Health and Care Excellence. *Guidance on Cancer Services—Improving Outcomes in Haematological Cancers: The Manual.* London: National Institute for Health and Care Excellence; 2003.

Simms VM, Higginson IJ, Harding R Palliative. Care-related problems do patients experience at HIV diagnosis? A systematic review of the evidence. *J Pain Symptom Manag* 2011;42:34–753.

References

3 Terrence Higgins Trust. Available at: ℘ https://www.tht.org.uk

4 Bower M, Palfreeman A, Alfa-Wali M, *et al*. British HIV Association guidelines for HIV-associated malignancies 2014. *HIV Med* 2014;**15**(Suppl 2):1–92.

Lung cancer

Introduction

Despite lung cancer being a relatively rare disease until the twentieth century, it is now a modern epidemic as the most common cancer worldwide. It accounts for around 8 million deaths per year, with over 35,000 deaths in the UK from the 45,500 diagnosed.

The 5-year survival remains poor, despite changes in treatment modalities, diagnostic procedures, and recent falling smoking rates amongst many sectors of society. Lung cancer is a mainly preventable disease, the main cause being cigarette smoking. A higher incidence of lung cancer has been linked to social deprivation, reflecting the higher smoking incidence in deprived groups. The link between smoking and lung cancer has led to the significant public perception as it being a disease of smokers, and therefore a self-inflicted disease.

Much criticism has been levelled at the lack of attention and research funding given to lung cancer, relative to other cancers. Recent government policy in the UK has emphasized the importance of smoking cessation clinics. The 'Smoke Free Law' was introduced in July 2007, which introduced legislation banning smoking in all public places in the UK. This has resulted in only a modest reduction in smoking rates but has significantly reduced the impact of passive smoking. The key to reducing deaths from lung cancer remains smoking prevention and cessation work (➔ see Smoking cessation, pp. 61–62) and earlier detection.

The impact of a diagnosis of any lung cancer is devastating, with a poor overall prognosis for most individuals. Coupled with complex symptom management issues, nursing these patients is particularly challenging. The following section covers the key treatment approaches for the two main types of lung cancer and mesothelioma. Key nursing issues are highlighted at the end of the chapter.

Epidemiology

- Third most common cancer in the UK, comprising 13% of all cancers.
- It is the most frequent cause of cancer deaths in the UK in men and women.
- Incidence strongly related to age, with 61% of cases diagnosed in people aged 70 and over.
- Incidence and mortality rates are falling in men but rising in women in the UK.
- The most common cancer worldwide and its incidence is continuing to rise.
- Most people (77%) are diagnosed at an advanced stage (stage III or IV).
- Survival rates have slowly improved but remain dismal, with 5-year survival at 9–16% in the UK.

Risk factors

- 80–90% of lung cancers are due to smoking.
- Risk relates to the number of cigarettes smoked and the number of years of smoking.
- Passive smoking.
- Residential radon.
- Occupational exposure to industrial carcinogens, particularly to asbestos.

Common presenting symptoms and signs

Presentation is often late, as lung cancer is often asymptomatic until it is at an advanced stage, and symptoms such as persistent cough and dyspnoea are attributed to smoking.

- Persistent cough, haemoptysis, dyspnoea
- Recurrent chest infections
- Chest or shoulder pain (constant, progressive)
- Hoarse voice (vocal cord palsy)
- Anorexia, weight loss
- SVCO
- Finger clubbing
- Symptoms from metastatic disease
- Fatigue.

Investigations

After a physical examination and CXR, patients with suspected lung cancer require further imaging with a CT scan of their chest, abdomen, and pelvis, and a tissue diagnosis obtained by the least invasive route, e.g.:

- Sputum cytology
- Bronchoscopy with biopsy
- Mediastinoscopy
- Video-assisted thoracoscopic surgery (VATS)
- Bronchial brushings and washings
- CT-guided biopsy
- Endobronchial and endoscopic ultrasound.

Other important assessments include performance status, pulmonary function tests, FBC, and a biochemical profile. Patients with symptoms suggestive of metastatic disease may require a bone scan or CT of the brain.

Pathology

For the purposes of management, lung cancers are grouped as non-small cell lung cancer (NSCLC) and small cell lung cancer (SCLC). Staging is via the TNM system (see the latest TNM staging manuals).

Common sites of metastatic spread

- Regional lymph nodes
- Bone
- Liver
- Adrenal glands
- Lung
- CNS
- Skin.

In SCLC, it is estimated that >90% of patients have either overt or occult metastases at presentation.

Mesothelioma arises from the serosal lining of the chest. Metastatic spread is normally to the peritoneum (➲ see Mesothelioma, pp. 440–1).

Management of non-small cell lung cancer

Surgery

Complete surgical removal of NSCLC offers the best possibility of a cure. This is appropriate for patients with stage I–II disease who are fit for surgery with adequate lung function. Advanced stage of the disease and significant comorbidity reduce the number of people who are offered surgical resection.

Major lung resection carries significant risks of morbidity and mortality. Post-operative mortality rate should be <3% following lobectomy, and <5% following pneumonectomy (see Table 33.1).

Surgical resection

The aim is to resect the primary tumour with clear margins and regional draining nodes. This may require lobectomy, bi-lobectomy, or pneumonectomy. Lung parenchyma-sparing operations (segmentectomy or wedge resection) are not recommended, because of the risk of incomplete resection, but may be appropriate occasionally in patients with small tumours and poor lung function. The operation should include regional lymph node sampling.

Post-operative management

Patients should be nursed in an intensive care or a high-dependency unit. Excellent pain control, oxygen therapy, and regular chest physiotherapy are essential.

Results of lung resection

Overall 5-year survival for patients undergoing resection may be as high as 40%, approaching 70% in cases without nodal involvement (N0). When mediastinal nodes are involved (N2), only 15% of patients will survive 5 years.

Multidisciplinary team meetings

The MDT discussion of each case is key to the optimal management of lung cancer, with input from radiologists and pathologists, as well as chest physicians, thoracic surgeons, clinical and medical oncologists, CNS, and specialist palliative care teams.

Non-surgical treatment for non-small cell lung cancer

Chemotherapy

NSCLC is not as sensitive to chemotherapy as SCLC. However, regimens with a platinum agent, in combination with newer chemotherapy agents, have shown improved success in recent years. Chemotherapy has a developing role prior to surgery to downstage tumours and also as adjuvant therapy for stages I–II.

In advanced disease, chemotherapy offers modest survival benefit, but improved symptom relief and QoL in >50% of people:
• Cough, haemoptysis, and pain are relieved in 70%
• Anorexia in 40%
• Dyspnoea in 30%.

Table 33.1 5-year survival after surgery for NSCLC by stage

Stage	5-year survival (%)
I	60–80
II	25–40
IIIa	10–30
IIIb and IV	<5

There is little evidence to justify >4 cycles of chemotherapy. Patients with poor performance status 2 or worse (➔ see Clinical performance status, p. 177) may be treated with single-agent chemotherapy such as gemcitabine or vinorelbine.

Targeted therapies

The introduction of oral targeted therapies for locally advanced or metastatic NSCLC has offered significant improvements in survival and quality of life for those with identifiable genetic mutations within the tumour. Epidermal growth factor receptor tyrosine kinase (EGFR-TK) mutation and anaplastic lymphoma kinase (ALK) fusion gene testing is recommended in all patients with advanced NSCLC of a non-squamous subtype.

Patients testing positive for an EGFR-TK mutation should be offered a EGFR-TK inhibitor such as erlotinib or afatinib as first-line therapy. Crizotinib should be considered as second-line treatment in those with an ALK re-arrangement. These agents cause less toxicities than standard chemotherapies and can be offered to patients with a performance status 2–4.

Radiotherapy

EBRT is used as local treatment for thoracic disease in many NSCLC patients. Radical radiotherapy can be offered to selected stage I–II patients who are unfit for surgery and can produce a cure in some of this group.

- SABR is the choice of treatment for peripherally located stage I NSCLC.
- For tumours of >5cm and/or centrally located, the UK's recommended approach is continuous hyperfractionated radiotherapy (CHART): 54Gy in 36 fractions over 12 days (this is not yet offered in all centres).
- Difficulties of this treatment include inconvenience for patients and staff and ↑ acute toxicity.

For many patients with advanced NSCLC, palliative radiotherapy is a key component in alleviating symptoms from thoracic disease, in particular:
- Haemoptysis
- Chest pain
- Cough
- Large airway obstruction or stridor
- SVCO (➔ see Superior vena cava obstruction, pp. 645–6)
- It also produces useful palliation for many metastatic sites, including lymph nodes, bone, brain, and soft tissue (➔ see Chapter 16, Radiotherapy).

Chemo-irradiation

Combination chemo-radiotherapy should be considered for those with stage II or III NSCLC. Additional toxicities, in particular oesophagitis, remain a major problem and should be balanced with the potential benefit in survival.

Management of small cell lung cancer

SCLC accounts for 15–20% of all lung cancers. Staging and management of SCLC are quite distinct from NSCLC because:
• SCLC demonstrates rapid growth and early dissemination, with >90% of individuals having systemic disease at presentation
• Chemotherapy is the key primary treatment and has an important impact on survival.

Staging and prognostic factors

A two-stage system applies.

Limited-stage disease

The tumour is confined to one hemithorax and regional lymph node, and can be covered by tolerable radiotherapy fields.

Extensive-stage disease

The disease is beyond the bounds stated for limited disease.

Treatment

Surgery

In general, surgical resection is not recommended for SCLC. If SCLC is treated by primary surgery, the systemic relapse rate is high, and adjuvant chemotherapy is recommended.

Chemotherapy

Without treatment, median survival is:
• 6 weeks for patients with extensive disease
• 3 months for those with limited disease.

Combination chemotherapy leads to a response in the majority, with improved survival times, and is now the standard primary treatment for both stages of the disease (see Table 33.2).

Principles of treatment

Four to six courses of etoposide plus cisplatin or carboplatin has been established as the best first-line treatment.
    The response rate is around 80% of all patients. Complete responses in:
• 30–40% patients with limited-stage disease
• 10–20% with extensive disease.

Table 33.2 Outcome of chemotherapy for SCLC

Stage of disease	Median survival (months)	1-year survival (%)	3-year survival (%)
Limited	18–24	50–70	10–20
Extensive	8–10	20	
Relapsed*	6		

* Limited to patients who remain fit to receive chemotherapy for relapsed disease.

Almost all patients relapse after chemotherapy only. There is a high risk of CNS relapse after chemotherapy, and this can be reduced by prophylactic cranial irradiation. This is given at the end of chemotherapy in an effort to minimize CNS toxicity.

Note: chemotherapy can be considered for elderly patients and those with poor WHO performance status (2–3) (⊃ see Clinical performance status, p. 177). Careful selection is required, and mortality rates may be high during chemotherapy treatment.

Second-line chemotherapy

SCLC can remain chemosensitive at relapse after primary chemotherapy. If the patient is fit enough, second-line regimens can be considered.

Radiotherapy

SCLC is a highly radiosensitive disease.

- For those with limited-stage disease, thoracic irradiation, in addition to chemotherapy, can improve survival. Dose: 40–50Gy in 15–25 fractions.
- Concurrent radiotherapy appears to be most effective, but toxicity, especially severe oesophagitis, may prevent its use.
- Prophylactic cranial irradiation reduces the risk of brain metastases.
- Palliative radiotherapy is an effective treatment in patients relapsing after, resistant to, unfit for, or refusing chemotherapy.

Mesothelioma

Malignant pleural mesothelioma (MPM) is an aggressive tumour arising from the serosal lining of the chest. It often leads to encasement of the lung by a solid tumour and has a poor survival rate.

Epidemiology
- Rare, around 2500 cases each year in the UK.
- The median age is 75 years.
- ♂:♀ ratio is 5:1

Aetiology
- Most mesothelioma is caused by asbestos exposure. All types of asbestos fibre are implicated.
- 90% have an occupational history of exposure, e.g. builders and shipyard workers have a high risk. The use of asbestos in schools and hospitals has led to an increasing incidence of mesothelioma attributed to environmental exposure.
- Clinical presentation is often 30–40 years later.

Clinical presentation
Late presentation is common. Classic symptoms are:
- Non-pleuritic chest pain
- Dyspnoea
- Systemic symptoms of fatigue, weight loss, sweating, and fever.

Spread
- Mainly local invasion into the mediastinum and chest wall.
- Peritoneal involvement through direct spread.
- Advanced spread to other organs such as the liver.

Investigations
- CXR: pleural effusion/thickening.
- CT/MRI scan: extent of pleural mass and effusion, and encasement of the lung.
- Histological diagnosis should be obtained in the majority of cases, using the least invasive technique.
  - Aspiration cytology (30% positive)
  - Thoracoscopy and biopsy (80% positive).

Note: there is a high incidence of false-negative biopsies, leading to the need to repeat it. There is a risk of seeding the tumour along biopsy tracts.

Staging

Patients should be staged by the TNM classification, although this is not commonly done. Staging is vital if patients are considered for surgery.

Treatment
Without treatment, the average patient with MPM survives <1 year from the time of diagnosis.

Surgery

Radical surgery for mesothelioma has no proven survival benefit but may offer improved control of the thoracic disease. For patients with a good performance status and early-stage disease, palliative pleurectomy/decortication (removal of the pleura without removing the whole lung) can provide relief from effusions, dyspnoea, and pain from the tumour. Surgery should ideally be done as part of a clinical trial.

Radiotherapy

Prophylactic irradiation of the chest drain, biopsy, and wound sites to prevent the development of chest wall tumours can be considered, although the evidence for the efficacy of this remains uncertain. Short-course palliative radiotherapy can be used for painful chest disease/masses.

Chemotherapy

Treatment with pemetrexed and a platinum agent should be offered to those with a good performance status. This can offer a modest improvement in survival but importantly can palliate symptoms of pain, fatigue, anorexia and cough.

Palliative care

Symptom control is often difficult, in particular pain and dyspnoea; early involvement of specialist palliative care services is strongly recommended.

Compensation and notification

Patients may be entitled to claim compensation in two ways:
- A claim for Industrial Injuries Disablement Benefit and/or The 2008 Diffuse Mesothelioma Scheme from the Department of Social Security (via the Benefits Agency)
- A Common Law claim for damages from the firm/firms where exposure to asbestos occurred.

It is important that patients and their family are aware of their right to pursue a compensation claim.

All deaths of patients with mesothelioma must be notified to the coroner (procurator fiscal in Scotland), as in law, they are seen as 'unnatural'. Even where there is confirmed tissue diagnosis in life, the coroner may still request a post-mortem. Every effort should be made to ensure the family are aware of the coroner's involvement before the death to minimize distress this may cause.

Nursing management issues

The poor prognosis of all types of lung cancer can make nursing these patients extremely challenging. The approach is often for palliative support from diagnosis. Comorbidity due to smoking may prevent access to effective surgical or pharmacological treatments. Patients and their families often have little time to come to terms with the diagnosis before facing the reality of dying from their disease. MDT involvement, including surgeons, oncologists, site-specific CNS, palliative care specialists, dieticians, and social workers, is crucial to the effective management of these patients.

Treatment issues

Lung cancer treatment raises a number of important nursing support issues. Patients will require high levels of support in making decisions about different treatment options. The success rates of many of these treatments are low. The balance between toxicity and potential benefit means that choices are not straightforward. The lung cancer CNS is a very useful support at this time.

Particular treatment issues include the following.

Surgery
- Fear due to high surgical mortality and morbidity rates.
- Respiratory problems: breathlessness, pneumonia, acute respiratory distress syndrome (ARDS).
- Cardiac arrhythmias and myocardial infarction.
- Chronic post-thoracotomy pain can last for many months.
- Longer-term patients may need to make lifestyle changes and cope with reduced activity.
- Thoracic radiotherapy: fatigue, oesophagitis, pneumonitis.
- Chemotherapy: has a wide range of side effects, including fatigue, risk of infection, fatigue, mucositis, nausea, and vomiting.

Psychosocial issues

- The poor prognosis of lung cancer means that patients and families often have little time to come to terms with the diagnosis. Because of its link with smoking, patients and their families can also have feelings of an attribution of blame. These require skilled and sensitive nursing support.
- The highest incidence of lung cancer is in people from lower social classes, and there can be difficult social and financial support issues to be resolved. A specialist cancer or palliative care social worker and specialist benefits advisors can be an invaluable support in these circumstances.
- Pain and breathlessness often cause panic and anxiety. Patients may need to use anxiolytics. Nurses can support patients to develop effective relaxation techniques (➔ see Anxiety management, pp. 588–9).
- Cerebral metastases can lead to altered behaviour and personality, as well as difficulties with communication. This can be extremely distressing for patients and relatives (➔ see Acute confusional state or delirium, pp. 594–5).

• This group of patients may particularly benefit from ↑ community support, and referral to palliative care services would be essential to provide this.

Breathlessness

This is common in all lung cancers. It can be particularly severe in mesothelioma, due to pleural involvement limiting lung capacity. Treatments such as chemotherapy and radiotherapy may be effective in SCLC but are less likely to work for mesothelioma or NSCLC (➔ see Chapter 41, Cancer-related breathlessness).

Fatigue

Fatigue will be experienced almost universally to some degree, due to treatments or to some facet of the disease itself. Fatigue negatively impacts on physical, social, and emotional functioning and overall QoL (➔ see Chapter 42, Cancer-related fatigue).

Weight loss/anorexia

Poor appetite is common and may be caused by the cancer itself or a secondary effect from other symptoms such as breathlessness and pain or anti-cancer treatments such as chemotherapy and radiotherapy. Weight loss is a poor prognostic indicator for both lung cancer and mesothelioma. It can cause significant emotional distress for the patient and their carer.

Pain

Many lung cancer patients present with chest pain. This can be a major problem. Specific pain issues include:
• Pleuritic pain: which often responds well to NSAIDs
• Bone pain: from bone metastases
• Nerve pain: caused by mesothelioma and also Pancoast's tumour—a tumour high in the lung apex, causing classic shoulder pain radiating down the ulnar nerve distribution (➔ see Chapter 46, Pain management).

Cough

This often exacerbates pain and breathlessness and causes sleeplessness, which can be extremely debilitating. Codeine linctus or morphine may be helpful (➔ see Chapter 41, Cancer-related breathlessness).

Superior vena cava obstruction

Due to regional tumour spread, this can be extremely frightening, with severe breathlessness and a feeling of drowning. It is also potentially life-threatening (➔ see Superior vena cava obstruction, pp. 645–6).

Haemoptysis

This can be distressing and is often a symptom that makes patients see their GP prior to diagnosis. Palliative radiotherapy and tranexamic acid can both be helpful. There is also a real, though rare, potential risk of catastrophic bleed (➔ see Bleeding, pp. 483–5).

Further reading

Detterbeck FC, Lewis SZ, Diekemper R, Addrizzo-Harris DJ, Alberts M. Diagnosis and management of lung cancer, 3rd ed: American College of Chest Physicians evidence-based clinical practice guidelines. 2013; *Chest* **143**(Suppl):7S–37S (complete volume of articles focusing on lung cancer management).

Eaby-Sandy B. Lung cancer. In: Yarbro CH, Gobel BH, Wujcik D (eds). *Cancer Nursing, Principles and Practice*, 7th edn. Sudbury, MA: Jones and Bartlett; 2010. pp. 1424–57.

Leary A. *Lung Cancer: A Multidisciplinary Approach*. Oxford: Wiley-Blackwell; 2012.

National Institute for Health and Care Excellence (2011). *Lung Cancer: Diagnosis and Management*. Clinical Guideline [CG121]. Available at: ℞ https://www.nice.org.uk/guidance/cg121

Tobias J, Hochhauser D. Tumours of the lung and mediastinum. In: Tobias J, Hochhauser D. *Cancer and Its Management*, 7th ed. Oxford: Wiley-Blackwell; 2014. pp. 209–36.

Skin cancer

Malignant melanoma

Epidemiology

- Malignant melanomas arise from melanocytes, mainly found in the basal layer of the skin. These cells produce melanin and are responsible for the tanning response after exposure to UV radiation.
- A few melanocytes exist elsewhere in the body—this explains the rare melanomas that can occur elsewhere, e.g. intra-ocular, mucosal.
- Incidence rates are rising faster than for any other cancer worldwide. In some countries (Australia, New Zealand, USA, and Norway), the rate is beginning to slow and stabilize, but in most European counties, it continues to climb.

Risk factors

- Sunlight is the greatest risk factor, in particular, excess exposure in early life.
- Caucasians have the highest risk (>1:80).
- There is a genetic risk. ~10% of people affected will have a strong family history of melanoma.
- Benign pigmented moles.
- Atypical mole syndrome, which is hereditary.

Screening and prevention

(➔ See Skin cancer prevention, p. 63.)

Clinical presentation

- Alteration in a pre-existing pigmented mole on the skin: irregular pigmentation, irregular border, or new asymmetry of a lesion oozing, crusting, itching, or bleeding.
- A new pigmented lesion—particularly relevant if ≥40 years.
- Less commonly, signs of metastatic disease.

Diagnosis

- Use of dermoscopy for lesion identification.
- Excision biopsy—complete excision with normal skin margins is optimal.
- Further imaging, depending on anatomical location and thickness of primary melanoma, e.g. staging CT head, neck, chest, abdomen, and pelvis.
- Other imaging, such as US or MRI, guided by symptoms of metastatic spread or thickness of primary melanoma.
- Core biopsy or FNA if presents with palpable lymphadenopathy. Core biopsies are more commonly carried out, as they enable further diagnostic genetic testing and results from such tests can guide further treatment management. These tests are not always possible with the cells provided in an FNA.
- Full body examination/skin check to identify primary and to look for any evidence of metastatic spread.

Prognostic indicators
- Tumour thickness (Breslow thickness), any invasion of dermal blood vessels or lymphatic invasion, ulceration, and the rate of cell division (mitosis) are key factors.
- Sentinel lymph node biopsy is a useful tool in determining melanoma behaviour for some sizes and sites of lesion and supports staging.
- Genetics of the melanoma.
- Other factors:
  - Women seem have better survival rates due to hormonal factors.
  - Head, neck, and trunk melanomas tend to fare worse than those on the extremities.

Surgical treatment

Surgery at the primary site
- Complete excision of the tumour with a 2mm margin.
- Followed by a wider surgical excision to reduce the risk of local recurrence—the margin varies according to tumour thickness. From *in situ* disease only: 0.5mm to ≥4mm = 3cm margin.
- Excision must be adequate laterally and in depth.
- Sites such as foot soles require tailored surgical techniques.
- A minority may require either a flap or a graft to achieve closure.

Surgery for regional lymph nodes/lymph node dissection
This is indicated when there is clinical evidence of lymph node involvement, reducing the risk of local disease. Sometimes, solitary nodes may be removed for local control. Often, following a positive sentinel lymph node biopsy, a complete lymph node dissection is performed. This is because any spread to other lymph nodes is unknown, until they have been removed and examined under the microscope. Information gained from the lymph node dissection results provides accurate staging information. Surgery also helps to gain local disease control. Short-term complications of surgery may include infection and seroma or lymphoedema in the longer term.

Prognosis and risk of relapse

In the early stage of the disease, surgery is curative in 70–90% of cases. Relapse rates rapidly increase if the disease has a higher stage at diagnosis, with involvement of lymph nodes and bloodborne disease.

More than half of melanomas diagnosed are stage I. Survival for stage I melanoma is 100%, meaning that no one with stage I would be expected to have a shorter life expectancy than the general population.[1] In 2007, median survival with stage IV (metastatic disease) was typically <9 months.

Median survival has significantly ↑ in recent years, because of advances in drug treatments. There are limited accurate survival data for metastatic melanoma at present, because constant changes in treatments in the last few years mean that median survival is difficult to quantify.

Chemotherapy, biological therapy, immunotherapy, and adiotherapy

At the time of writing, systemic treatment of melanoma is a rapidly developing area, with very regular changes made to treatment recommendations at international, national, and local levels. This has been brought about by the revolutionary use of immunological and targeted therapies in the field. With this in mind, relevant updated treatment guidelines should always be checked before communicating with patients.

Adjuvant therapy

There is little current evidence to support the widespread use of adjuvant therapies in melanoma. The use of adjuvant interferon may improve overall survival in patients with resected stage III disease, and this should be offered to this group of patients if they are able to tolerate it. Trials are ongoing to evaluate the use of monoclonal antibodies in an adjuvant setting, but these drugs can have significant side effects, and therefore, the benefits need to be clearly indicated.

Loco-regional disease

- If there is no evidence of disseminated disease, further resection should be undertaken.
- Radiotherapy should be considered to establish local control.
- Alternative approaches may include 'regional' chemotherapy treatment via hyperthermic isolated limb perfusion. This is only offered in specialist centres and, in some patients, can provide regional control with limited systemic side effects.

Treatment of metastatic disease

There is no curative treatment for stage IV disease, but longer-term survival in this group of patients has been radically improved with the use of biological therapy and immunotherapy. The aim of treatment is to palliate symptoms and maximize QoL.

Surgery in metastatic disease

Where biological therapy and immunotherapy are being employed, with some evidence of local control, surgery to single distant metastases should be considered on a patient-to-patient basis by the MDT (e.g. in single cerebral metastases). Tumour debulking may occasionally be appropriate.

Biological therapy and immunotherapy

Treatment of high-risk or metastatic melanoma has benefitted from the continued development of targeted therapies. A number of therapies have been developed in recent years, which have improved the outlook for patients with metastatic melanoma.

BRAF (V600) mutations

The identification of *BRAF (V600)* mutations is increasingly important when optimizing treatment decisions and outcomes for patients with high-risk melanoma. Adults who have *BRAF* mutation-positive, unresectable, or metastatic melanoma can be offered treatment with a specific range of drugs known as BRAF inhibitors. Examples of these types of drug used in current treatment are dabrafenib and trametinib. (Some of these drugs, such as trametinib, work by inhibiting a protein pathway known as 'MEK' and can also be termed MEK1 inhibitors.)

Immunotherapy

PD-1 inhibitors

PD-1 is a receptor which has a key role in downregulating the immune system response and allows tumour cells to grow uncontrolled, with no check on their proliferation. Specific monoclonal antibodies which inhibit the action of PD-1 have shown efficacy in treating metastatic melanoma. Examples of PD-1 inhibitors in current usage would be pembrolizumab and nivolumab.

CTLA-4 inhibitors

CTLA-4 is a receptor which tumour cells utilize to prevent tumour cells from being attacked and destroyed by T-cells. Ipilimumab is a monoclonal antibody which inhibits the action of these receptors and thus stimulates the body's immune system response against cancer cells.

Combination therapy

Recent trials have led to the adoption of combination therapy, using a PD-1 inhibitor and a CTLA-4 inhibitor in metastatic melanoma. The combination of nivolumab and ipilimumab in current usage has been shown to be very effective in controlling disease and extending survival. The toxicities of this regime can be significant but is largely tolerable in patients with a good performance status prior to treatment.

Side effects of immunotherapy

There is a risk of severe immune-mediated inflammation of the lungs, colon, liver, or kidneys and the endocrine system, which can be fatal. Patients need intensive courses of corticosteroids if symptoms occur. Effective management of these side effects is dependent upon good levels of education of staff likely to meet the patients across a range of settings and effective local protocols for managing side effects of immunotherapies.

Chemotherapy

Chemotherapy offers limited benefit in the treatment of melanoma and is now seldom used since recent breakthroughs using immunotherapies and targeted therapies. These have been shown to be more effective than chemotherapy. There are some trials exploring the use of chemotherapy in combination with immuno- or targeted therapies, but, even so, the novel drugs are tending to show longer-term survival benefit without the use of chemotherapy alongside them.

Radiotherapy

- Can be used for pain from bone metastases or in the emergency treatment of metastatic spinal cord compression from melanoma.
- Cerebral metastases are relatively common. Total cranial irradiation can be considered if symptomatic, or referrals may be made for stereotactic radiotherapy in specialist centres for solitary cerebral metastasis.
- Symptom management for pain/bleeding/fungating wounds.
- Can be considered to treat nodal basins if nodal involvement is beyond the lymph node capsule.

References

1 Office for National Statistics (2016). *Cancer Survival by Stage at Diagnosis for England: Adults Diagnosed in 2015 and Followed up to 2016 (Experimental Statistics)*. Available at: ℴ https:// www.ons.gov.uk/peoplepopulationandcommunity/healthandsocialcare/conditionsanddiseases/ bulletins/cancersurvivalinengland/adultstageatdiagnosisandchildhoodpatientsfollowedupto201 6#cancer-survival-by-stage-at-diagnosis-for-england-adults-diagnosed-in-2015-and-followed-up-to-2016-experimental-statistics

Non-melanoma skin cancer

The two main forms are squamous cell cancer (SCC) and basal cell cancer (BCC). Malignant skin lesions may also represent metastases, e.g. from breast, lung, or GI primaries.

Epidemiology and aetiology

- These are the most common malignancies in western populations.
- The main risk factors for development include:
  - Excess UV radiation exposure—the main environmental cause
  - Easily burnt, fair-skinned individuals
  - Outdoor work, outdoor recreational activities
  - Psoralen ultraviolet A (PUVA) treatment
  - Immunosuppression, e.g. post-organ transplant.

Presentation

BCC—75% of non-melanoma skin cancers

- Lesions arise on sun-exposed areas, normally hair-bearing skin.
- Slow-growing, pink papule with telangiectasia.
- Typically indolent, can be locally invasive, metastases are rare (0.1%).

SCC—20% of non-melanoma skin cancers

- Arise on sun-exposed sites or at sites of chronic inflammation.
- Rapidly growing, red papule, or non-healing skin lesion.
- Ulceration and bleeding may occur.
- 5–10% metastasize; commonly initial spread is to regional lymph nodes—poor prognosis for disseminated disease.

Management

- **Surgical excision**: allows assessment of histological features and adequacy of resection margin; ≥90% cure for primary disease.
- **Mohs**: allows a surgical technique carried out in some cancer centres to remove as little tissue as possible with clear surgical margins for BCCs. This can offer the best chance of cure, with minimal normal skin removed and reduced scarring. It is generally used on areas such as the face, so that the cosmetic outcome is as good as possible whilst still achieving cure.
- **Radiotherapy**: may be useful for poor surgical candidates, such as frail or elderly people, or where surgical excision is difficult, e.g. eyelids, nose, and lips, and the cosmetic result is likely to be superior to surgery.
- **Chemotherapy**: topical 5FU can be used for low-risk BCCs. Otherwise not as successful as other therapies.
- **Immunotherapy**: imiquimod cream can be used for small, non-nodular BCCs and can be used where surgery is not desirable.
  - Vismodegib is an oral antagonist in the 'hedgehog signalling pathway', which plays a critical role in the development and homeostasis of many organs and tissues. It is currently under appraisal by NICE for use where surgery is not possible for locally advanced or metastatic BCC.
- **Cryotherapy**: occasionally, cryotherapy may be used to treat clinically diagnosed low-risk small BCCs; it is not appropriate treatment for any other type of skin cancer.

- Photodynamic therapy (PDT): topical application of a tumour-localizing photosensitizing agent, which may require metabolic synthesis, followed by activation of the agent by light of a specific wavelength, used for BCCs.
- Ongoing surveillance: most recurrences will occur within the first 5 years.
  - Patients are also at risk of developing other non-melanoma skin malignancies.
  - Advise patients with a non-melanoma skin cancer about the importance of sun avoidance to minimize future risk.

Further reading

Erdmann F, Lortet-Tieulent J, Schüz J, et al. International trends in the incidence of malignant melanoma 1953–2008: are recent generations at higher or lower risk? *Int J Cancer* 2013;132:385–400.
Rotte A, Bhandaru M. *Immunotherapy of Melanoma*. Basingstoke: Springer; 2016.

Teenage and young adult cancer

Teenage and young adult cancer

Introduction
There is increasing recognition that teenagers and young adults (TYAs) are a distinct group from children and older adults and have their own unique needs. In order to provide best practice to these individuals, expert medical management, alongside expert, age-appropriate psychosocial management, is required.

Adolescence and young adulthood are a phase of rapid development, including changes in physical, cognitive, physiological, and social behaviour. These individuals are developing a sense of identity and moving towards independence; they are making the transition from childhood to adulthood.

TYAs refer to the age range of 16–24 year olds inclusively, as determined in the Improving Outcome Guidance for Children and Young Adults with cancer (NICE 2005).[1]

Epidemiology
- Cancer is relatively rare in TYAs, accounting for <1% of cancers in all ages. However, cancer is the leading natural cause of death in TYAs.
- ~2200 TYAs are diagnosed with cancer each year in the UK.
- The incidence of all cancers in 15–24 year olds increases with age, with the majority being diagnosed in the 20- to 24-year-old group.
- Lymphomas are the most common group of cancers in TYAs.
- Around 310 TYAs die from cancer each year in the UK; brain, other CNS, and intracranial tumours are the most common cause of death in TYAs.
- Survival for TYA cancer is improving, and >80% of TYAs diagnosed with cancer in the UK survive for at least 5 years.

Risk factors
- TYAs' risk of developing cancer depends on factors including age, genetics, and a range of other factors.
- Lifestyle factors probably have less impact on TYA cancer risk than adults, because they have had less time exposed to these factors.
- UV light: melanoma risk is increasing amongst young adults and is disproportionately high in younger people.
- Infection:
  - HPV—cervical cancer
  - EBV—Hodgkin lymphoma, some forms of nasopharyngeal carcinomas.
- Previous cancer: TYAs who have undergone treatment for a previous cancer have a higher risk of developing a second cancer later in life.
- Height: osteosarcoma is linked with rapid adolescent growth spurt.
- Genes and family history: Li-Fraumeni syndrome is a rare genetic condition that carries a high risk of multiple primary tumours in childhood and young adulthood.

Cancer types affecting TYAs
Broadly divided into three categories:
- Late paediatric, i.e. Wilms' tumours, neuroblastoma
- True TYA, i.e. Hodgkin lymphoma, osteosarcoma, germ cell tumours
- Early-onset adult tumours, i.e. melanoma, nasopharyngeal.

Table 35.1 highlights the most common cancers affecting TYAs.

Table 35.1 Most common cancers affecting teenagers and young adults

Rank	Diagnosis	Comments
1	Lymphomas	Cases slighter higher in ♂
2	Carcinomas	For example, thyroid, cervix, bowel
3	Germ cell tumours (GCTs)	Testicular GCTs make up the majority of this group
4	Brain, other CNS, and intracranial tumours	Comprises a range of tumours such as astrocytoma and pituitary adenoma
5	Malignant melanoma	Number of cases are twice as high in ♀ than in ♂
6	Leukaemias	Three main types: ALL (most common), AML, and CML
7	Bone tumours	Osteosarcomas and Ewing's sarcoma make up the majority of this group. Cases are higher in ♂
8	Soft tissue sarcomas	Comprises a range of tumours such as synovial sarcoma and rhabdomyosarcoma

Presentation/delays in diagnosis

Common presentations are either as an emergency, following a routine GP referral, or via a '2-week wait' GP referral.

As with adults, early diagnosis is crucial. However, diagnostic delay is a significant problem in the 16- to 24-year-old age group, with more delays in this population than in younger children or older adults. Patients therefore often present with advanced disease which can impact on their outcome. Causes of delay include: TYA patients not thinking about going to their GP, not understanding the seriousness of their symptoms, or embarrassment about discussing them. For GPs, it is rare for them to see young people with cancer; also the symptoms can be non-specific and can be attributed to more usual problems such as sporting injuries, general fatigue, and stress.

Treatment

The mainstay treatments for most cancers in TYAs are various combinations of surgery, chemotherapy, and radiotherapy. TYA patients are generally more able to tolerate intensive therapies, as they are less likely to have other medical problems and have healthy organs. However, there can be many long-term consequences of cancer therapies, including secondary malignancies, fertility issues, and other organ comorbidities, including cardiovascular and pulmonary toxicities (➔ see Late effects, pp. 457–8).

An important function of the TYA MDT, whose core members include paediatric and adult oncologists/haematologists, is to recommend, discuss, and plan the best available treatment option for the patient. Some TYA cancers, e.g. ALL, will be better treated with paediatric protocols.

For general information on treatment modalities, ➔ see Chapter 16, Radiotherapy and ➔ Chapter 17, Systemic anti-cancer therapy.

Place of care

In 2005, NICE published the Improving Outcomes Guidance (IOG) for children and young people with cancer in England and Wales. This document outlined key recommendations for the delivery of cancer services for 16–24 year olds.

- TYA patients should be treated in an age-appropriate place of care in a designated principal treatment centre (PTC) for TYAs. Cancer care should be provided by both a site-specific MDT and a specialist TYA MDT. Clear communication, collaboration, and joint decision-making between TYA MDTs and site-specific MDTs are essential. Core members of the TYA MDT, such as the youth worker, social worker, clinical psychologist, and specialist nurse, have the skills and experience to meet the age-related needs of the young person, and the site-specific MDT have the expertise in the young person's cancer and treatment.
- The 16–18 year olds must be referred to the PTC for initiation of treatment; the 19–24 year olds must be given the choice of receiving care at their local designated hospital or at the PTC, but always to have unhindered access to age-appropriate support.
- The development of clinical trials that include TYAs should be encouraged.

Impact of cancer diagnosis on TYAs

Cancer diagnosis and its treatment will affect all aspects of the young person's life—practically, socially, physically, and emotionally:

- Loss of education (an average of a year's education can be missed)
- Loss of employment
- Change in relationships
- Interruption to 'normal' routine/life of a TYA
- Isolation from their peer group: their peer groups will continue to meet up and evolve, and the TYA will feel they are being left behind
- Change in appearance/body image
- Loss of independence
- Loss of fertility—the importance of this can often be underestimated. It needs to be acknowledged and addressed. Discussions around fertility may need revisiting a number of times, and appropriate referrals must be made to reproductive specialists
- Loss of identity
- Depression/anxiety
- Loss of control
- Loss of future prospects.

Family support issues

Cancer affects not only the TYA, but also the whole family, and their needs must also be considered and met. There are substantial costs associated with a cancer diagnosis and all it entails; travel costs can be significant, as some families will have to travel long distances, and parents may also need to give up work for a while, putting them under huge financial pressure. Access to benefits advisors at the hospital and to a CLIC Sargent Social Worker is essential.

It is also very important to consider the impact on siblings when their brother or sister is diagnosed with cancer. Staff should provide space and time for the siblings to talk to them and also provide them with opportunities to meet with other siblings going through similar experiences.

Nursing support

It is important to remember that a cancer diagnosis and the complex challenges that both the diagnosis and the treatment present to the TYA have to be faced alongside the normal difficulties of adolescence. In order to offer the most appropriate support, staff need a comprehensive understanding of the young person's development and behaviour.

For a lot of TYAs, their treatment schedules will require frequent hospitalization, with hard-to-tolerate side effects, and adherence and compliance can become an issue.

A friendly, age-appropriate approach by staff is required, but professional boundaries must be maintained.

The preservation of a therapeutic relationship between staff and patients can be threatened if professional boundaries are crossed.

Staff working with young people have an ↑ risk of crossing boundaries for a number of reasons:
- Some staff will be the same age as some of the patients
- The TYA environment is intentionally very informal, promoting a home-from-home feel
- Patients are often treated for long periods, increasing the patient/ professional interactions
- TYA patients can be emotionally demanding
- They are at a vulnerable age (dependence can be an issue)
- Use of social networking
- More relaxed communication style.

Helpful hints
- See the TYA as a young person first and as a cancer patient second; take time to get to know them, and find out about their interests and hopes for the future.
- Offer the TYA time alone, to enable them to discuss issues they may not have felt comfortable discussing with the family present.
- Allow the amount of information and depth of any discussions to be led and guided by the young person.
- Adopt a flexible approach in planning their care (e.g. with treatment dates and clinic appointments).
- Keep them informed at all times, empowering them to make their own decisions where possible.
- Facilitate young people to maintain a sense of 'normality'.
- Give them time.
- Make sure appropriate referrals to other health professionals are made in a timely manner, i.e. psychologist, social worker, and teacher/learning mentor.

Late effects

Treatment completion does not signal the end of the cancer experience; some TYAs will have health problems associated with their treatment, so an understanding of the individual's risks of late effects is important. Health problems can include impairment of endocrine function (including infertility and abnormal growth and development), cardiac and neurological impairment, cognitive decline and psychological effects, and an ↑ risk of developing a second cancer.

The model of care required by TYAs at the end of treatment is evolving nationally, as part of the National Cancer Survivorship Initiative (NCSI). This model of care risk-stratifies the patient's need for long-term follow-up. The frequency, type of follow-up, and level of intervention are linked to the disease type, treatment received, and therefore likely late effects of that treatment. The QS55 standard (NICE 2014)[2] has stipulated that young people should have a care plan at the end of treatment and that this should be reviewed 5 years later in order to assess any ongoing late effects.

End of life

Palliative care for TYAs is a very difficult and challenging area of practice.

Young people facing death prematurely, when most people their age are looking towards the future and deciding on personal goals, is very distressing.

Supporting young people to die in a place of their choice is very important. This may be the hospital, home, or in a hospice. Young people may choose to die on specialist Teenage Cancer Trust units where staff are experienced and confident in caring for them. However, these units can be far from home, which will limit access to family and friends.

They may wish to die at home, but their parents may feel very anxious about this, with the expectations and responsibility placed on them and also concern about the effects on other family members.

Access to adolescent hospices is limited; therefore, hospice care for a lot of young people is delivered in an adult or a children's hospice.

It is essential that early, honest, and open discussions are had with the young person and their family about what support is available in their area and what can be delivered safely. Multidisciplinary teamwork, involving the GP, local palliative care teams, and community nurses, is required when planning care.

When a young person dies, the psychological impact involves many people; well-developed bereavement support for the immediate family, significant others, and peers is essential. Staff should be given the opportunity to access formal support, i.e. counselling/clinical supervision. Organizing a staff debrief is also usual to enable staff to share their thoughts and feelings.

Further reading

Cancer Research UK. Available at: 🔗 http://www.cancerresearchuk.org/home/

Kelly D, Gibson F. *Cancer Care for Adolescents and Young Adults*, 1st ed. Oxford: Blackwell Publishing; 2008.

National Cancer Intelligence Network (now National Cancer Registration and Analysis Service, NCRAS). Available at: 🔗 http://www.ncin.org.uk

National Cancer Survivorship Initiative (2010). (now National Cancer Registration and Analysis Service, NCRAS). Available at: 🔗 http://www.ncin.org.uk

Smith S, Cable M, Cargill J, et al. *A Blueprint of Care for Teenagers and Young Adults with Cancer*. London: Teenage Cancer Trust; 2012 2nd ed. 2016.

References

1 National Institute for Health and Care Excellence (2005). *Improving Outcomes in Children and Young People with Cancer*. Cancer Service Guideline [CSG7]. Available at: 🔗 https://www.nice.org.uk/guidance/csg7

2 National Institute for Health and Care Excellence (2014). *Cancer Services for Children and Young People*. Quality standard [QS55]. Available at: 🔗 https://www.nice.org.uk/guidance/qs55

Section 7

Symptom Management

Assessment

Introduction to assessment

Assessment is one of the most complex nursing activities. It involves inter-personal and communication skills and decision-making skills.

Assessment has a number of purposes. It aims to:
- Establish a working relationship with the patient
- Understand the patient's preferences and priorities
- Identify their needs and match them with the services available
- Record the patient's needs for the benefit of teamwork
- Enable effective care planning and symptom management to take place
- Assess risk.

Assessment tools can be used, but assessment is also a matter of clinical judgement. Although it is one of the most common activities in nursing, assessment is not always undertaken in a systematic or effective way.

The purpose of assessment can be related to the **diagnosis** of specific conditions, in order to ensure that the necessary treatment is given. However, assessment is often focused on the assessment of **needs** or health-related goals (➋ see Quality of life, p. 470). This enables needs to be matched with the appropriate care and services.

It is important to be aware that the patient and the nurse may view their needs differently. The subjective experience of a problem is not the same as the assessment of a need for care. For example, a patient may experience pain but not want to accept the pain relief that is being offered.

The following factors will influence an assessment:
- The purpose of assessment
- The skills of the nurse
- The time and facilities available
- The condition of the patient, including their level of consciousness and capacity to understand information given and make decisions
- The patient's personal preferences and priorities regarding their care.

Context of assessment

An assessment is influenced by the context in which it takes place.

The patient's context

It is very important to understand the patient's context—their current life circumstances, concerns, and priorities. Without this, key elements of the patient's experience may be missed or misunderstood by the nurse. For example, a nurse may assess the patient's main need as symptom relief, when their most pressing concern may be their relationship with their family. It is important to always identify the patient's key concerns, as part of the assessment process. There are assessment tools that can be used to structure the process of identifying concerns (➋ see Assessment tools, p. 467).

The family

Involving the family in the assessment process ensures a common understanding about problems, and information and decision-making can be shared. At times, however, a patient may feel more comfortable being seen on their own, so that they can be open about how they feel, without worrying about the reaction of family members. It is good practice to ask the patient if they give their permission for family members or significant others to be present.

Purpose of assessment

Assessment is initiated at the start of a process of care, but it is an ongoing activity that should happen regularly. Assessment should be interactive, a negotiation and information exchange between the nurse and patient, an opportunity for both to get to know each other and identify personal and health-care priorities. It is important that assessment is a deliberate process. Information gathered incidentally may not be complete. It is important to share information and focus on concerns that are raised by patients in this way.

Amount of time available

Detailed assessment cannot always be undertaken at busy times. If time is limited, focus on the key information that you need to know. Be clear with the patient what you need to know and how much time you have, and gain their consent for this.

Space and privacy

The ideal context for assessment is one where the patient is comfortable and privacy is assured, e.g. in a room that is separate from other people. If it is not possible to find a room, make the context as private as possible, ensuring the patient's confidentiality is respected. In hospital, this could involve drawing curtains around a bed and talking quietly.

Timing of assessment

Assessment is an ongoing process and should take place regularly across the patient's journey. Key points for assessment have been identified in the NICE Guidance on Supportive and Palliative Care for Adults with Cancer:[1]

- Diagnosis
- Prior to and during treatment
- End of treatment—often a very difficult time when support is less available
- Recurrence
- Entering the terminal phase of illness.

It is also essential to be aware of the wider personal context of the patient's life when undertaking an assessment (➲ see Cancer survivorship, pp. 72–4).

References

1 National Institute for Health and Care Excellence (2004). *Improving Supportive and Palliative Care for Adults with Cancer*. Cancer service guideline [CSG4]. Available at: ℜ https://www.nice.org.uk/guidance/csg4

Process of assessment

Assessment as a process involves both non-verbal observation and verbal exchange of information, or conversation.
- **Observation:** includes the patient's behaviour (e.g. restlessness), posture, facial expression and eye contact, skin colour, and temperature.
- **Conversation:** a two-way process, involving eliciting information by asking questions and listening, clarifying, and responding.

The most important aspect of the assessment process for the nurse is to listen. Each patient (and carer) will have their own priorities and expect-ations, their own understanding of events, and their personal story to tell (➔ see Cancer stories or narratives, p. 77). Assessment is an opportunity for them to tell the nurse about these. This must be balanced with the clinical imperatives that drive care and treatment. The process of each as-sessment will vary according to circumstances, but the following are offered as guidelines:
- Be clear about why the assessment is being done.
- Introduce yourself and explain the reason for the assessment, how long it will take, and what it will involve.
- Establish mutual expectations of the purpose of the assessment, i.e. what are the patient's understanding of the purpose and likely outcome of the assessment?
- Ask specific questions about the things you need to know.
- Check that your questions are understood.
- Give the patient the opportunity to respond to your questions in their own terms.
- Discuss the available care and treatment options, and what actions you or your team will take to deal with any problems.
- Care planning should be done collaboratively with the patient and their family as far as this is possible.
- Does the patient (or their family) have any questions?
- Combine data from different sources—clinical notes, other informants, and colleagues.
- Ensure that the assessment and its outcome are documented in a way that is accessible to colleagues

Self-awareness and assessment

Assessment can be influenced by the perceptions or attitudes of the nurse. For this reason, it is important to develop self-awareness:
- Note your own responses to the patient.
- Do not make assumptions about the patient on the basis of their age, gender, diagnosis, or other personal characteristics.
- Develop sensitivity to your reaction to the needs of individuals from minority groups (e.g. ethnic minority, sexual orientation, socio-economic status).

Reflection points

- Can you recall an occasion on which you felt your attitudes or feelings towards a patient made the assessment more difficult for you or the patient?
- Is there anything that you would do differently if this happened again?

Holistic needs assessment and care planning

Many wards or units have a proforma for assessment, which guides the questions asked. A holistic assessment will cover the different dimensions of a patient's experience of illness, treatment, and life. Holistic needs assessment (HNA) and care planning is an important aspect of care, particularly as patients rebuild their lives after treatment.

Holistic assessment should cover the following:

- Physical concerns:
  - Fatigue, pain, concentration, effects of treatment, sexuality
- Practical concerns:
  - Family responsibilities, accommodation, finances, education, work, insurance
- Family and relationship concerns:
  - Partner, children, relatives, friends, other sources of support
- Emotional and spiritual concerns:
  - Anxiety and depression, loneliness, spiritual or religious concerns
- Lifestyle and information needs:
  - Activity and exercise, diet, support groups, smoking, alcohol.

The UK charity Macmillan Cancer Support promotes HNA and care planning, with the following aims:[2]

- To provide a holistic assessment of patients' concerns, through treatment and beyond
- To provide insight into patients' coping skills and to enable patients to access services
- To identify strategies of self-care that the patient can use to manage their concerns
- Aims of care and support planning:
  - To document the patient's concerns
  - To summarize the actions of both the professional and patient
  - To resolve anxiety about the concerns raised.

HNA can be enhanced by using a structured approach, including, for example, the Concerns Checklist, Distress Thermometer, and the Sheffield Profile for Assessment and Referral to Care (SPARC). Whatever format is used, the interaction between the professional and the patient is a central aspect of the assessment. This builds the working relationship, alongside the collection of information and care planning.

One option that promotes collaborative assessment and care planning involves the use of an electronic device (tablet) that the patient uses to complete the assessment, and the resulting care plan is emailed to the patient and can be shared with other health-care professionals[3]. The collection of data in this way enables the professional to build a picture of the patient's concerns and progress and to work with them to resolve their concerns over time.

The assessment of pain and sexual problems are dealt with in other sections of the book (→ see Pain management, p. 550; → Sexuality and cancer, Assessment, pp. 611–12).

Further reading

Macmillan Cancer Support. *Holistic Needs Assessment (HNA) Care and Support Planning*. Available at: ℘ https://be.macmillan.org.uk/be/p-23400-holistic-needs-assessment-hna-care-and-support-planning.aspx

National Cancer Action Team (2012) *Holistic Needs Assessment for People with Cancer*. NHS: Available at: ℘ http://webarchive.nationalarchives.gov.uk/20130513211237/http://www.ncat.nhs.uk/sites/default/files/work-docs/HNA_practical%20guide_web.pdf

References

2 Macmillan Cancer Support. *Holistic Needs Assessment. Care and Support Planning*. Available at: ℘ http://be.macmillan.org.uk/Downloads/CancerInformation/ResourcesForHSCP/InformationResources/MAC16266HNAHowtoguide2016A4DIGITALAW.pdf

3 Macmillan Cancer Support. *Electronic holistic needs assessment (eHNA)*. Available at: ℘ http://www.macmillan.org.uk/Aboutus/Healthandsocialcareprofessionals/Macmillansprogrammesandservices/RecoveryPackage/ElectronicHollisticNeedsAssessment.aspx

Assessment tools

Assessment tools are a means of ensuring consistency across assessments or across different team members. They also serve as a guide or checklist, so that the nurse enquires about specific problems or symptoms. These tools will only be used if they are seen to have value within clinical practice, and their use varies considerably. Some assessment tools rely on patient self-assessment, an important way of ensuring that outcomes of care meet patients' needs.

Patient-Reported Outcome Measures

In any assessment, it is necessary to achieve a balance between objective evaluation of the patient's problems (e.g. whether they need a specific form of care) and their subjective experience of illness or symptoms. PROMs measure outcomes of treatment or care, as they are reported by the patients themselves, thus achieving an objective measure based on patient experience. PROMs may assess health and health-care needs and monitor patient progress, or they can also be used to evaluate the effectiveness of a service. They are usually in the form of a questionnaire that can be completed by the patient or on their behalf, and express outcome as a score or number. They may be disease-specific or generic assessment tools.

- An example of a cancer-specific PROMs is:
  - Functional Assessment of Cancer Therapy (FACT)—assesses four dimensions of physical, social, emotional, and functional well-being. There are versions that are specific to different cancers, e.g. breast, lung. Available at: ℘ http://www.facit.org/FACITOrg/Questionnaires
- An example of a generic PROM that can be used in cancer is:
  - EQ-5D (EuroQol survey of five dimensions of QoL: mobility, self-care, usual activities, pain/discomfort, anxiety/depression). Available at: ℘ https://euroqol.org

When used in clinical practice, PROMs need to be combined with other information and clinical judgement, to make a full assessment of the patient's health-care needs or QoL.

Examples of assessment tools used in cancer care

Cancer Care Monitor (CCM)
- Screening and assessment tool for symptoms and QoL in cancer patients.[4]

Cancer Rehabilitation Evaluation System (CARES)
- Measure of rehabilitation needs and QoL.[5]

Symptoms and concerns checklist
- Measure of prevalence and severity of symptoms and concerns in practice.[6]

Problems checklist
- Measure of the frequency and severity of psychosocial problems in cancer.[7]

Further reading

Department of Health – Quality Health (2012). *Quality of Life of Cancer Survivors in England. Report on a Pilot Survey Using Patient Reported Outcome Measures (PROMS)*. Available at: ℘ https://www.gov.uk/government/uploads/system/uploads/attachment_data/file/267042/9284-TSO-2900701-PROMS-1.pdf

Patient Reported Outcome Measurement Group. *Instrument Selection*. Available at: ℘ http://phi.uhce.ox.ac.uk/instruments.php

Richardson A, Sitzia J, Brown V, Medina J, Richardson A. *Patient's Needs Assessment Tools in Cancer Care: Principles and Practice*. London: King's College; 2005.

References

4 Fortner B, Okon T, Schwartzberg L, Tauer K, Houts AC. The Cancer Care Monitor: psychometric content evaluation and pilot testing of a computer administered system for symptom screening and quality of life in adult cancer patients. *J Pain Symptom Manage* 2003;26:1077–92.

5 UCLA Jonsson Comprehensive Cancer Center. *Cancer Rehabilitation Evaluation System (CARES)*. Available at: ℜ https://cancer.ucla.edu/patient-care/survivorship/for-healthcare-providers/cancer-rehabilitation-evaluation-system-cares

6 Lidstone V, Butters E, Seed PT, Sinnott C, Beynon T, Richards M. Symptoms and concerns amongst cancer outpatients: identifying the need for specialist palliative care. *Palliat Med* 2003;17:588–95.

7 Bonevski B, Sanson-Fisher R, Girgis A, Burton L, Cook P, Boyes A (2000). Evaluation of an instrument to assess the needs of patients with cancer. *Cancer* 2000;88:217–25.

Quality of life

- QoL is a key element of assessment. It is a complex, multifactoral concept in the context of cancer and involves the individual's appraisal of their position in life, relative to their expectations.
- QoL can involve both positive and negative appraisals—there can be good features of life, like a sense of well-being, and bad effects of the illness, like symptoms, and these can occur together.
- QoL is subjective—only an individual can judge what their QoL is, but objective measures can also be used, e.g. to assess levels of physical functioning.
- QoL is dynamic, and ideas about what it means have changed over time, e.g. from treatment outcome to subjective feeling of well-being.

Concepts related to QoL

The following are terms you will come across in the literature on QoL:

- **Need:** a need is a complex concept that can be viewed differently from the patient's or the professional's point of view, e.g. a patient may perceive a need to be well, whilst a nurse may perceive a patient's need for care. It can have the following meanings:
  - A health-related goal, e.g. to be free of a distressing symptom
  - A measurable deficiency from a health-related goal
  - A means of achieving a health-related goal, e.g. a treatment
- **Outcome:** the achievement or failure to achieve defined health-related goals
- **Health-related QoL:** QoL conceptualized as involving a complex range of factors, including, for example, subjective feelings of social and psychological well-being
- **Disease-related QoL:** QoL relating primarily to the effects of illness and treatment
- **Health status:** can mean either:
  - Absence of illness, or
  - Presence of physical, psychological, social, and spiritual well-being
- **Functional status:** ability to perform usual activities or roles within limitations imposed by illness
- **Symptom distress:** the degree of physical or mental distress or suffering experienced from a symptom.

Dimensions of quality of life

QoL is multidimensional; it affects different aspects of the person's life. Dimensions of QoL include:

- **Physical well-being:** this includes features such as fatigue, pain, other symptoms, and side effects of treatment
- **Functional well-being:** this refers to the activities of living, including basic functions of eating, sleeping, washing, and also activities that support occupation and relationships
- **Emotional well-being:** emotional reactions to cancer can be both positive and negative. Emotional well-being can be enhanced by the support of family and friends, or patients may experience distress or low mood
- **Social well-being:** this is complex and can include social support, family relationships, intimacy, and sexuality
- **Spiritual well-being:** this includes religion and cultural aspects of life, as well as a personal sense of meaning and purpose in life, and attitudes to death and dying.

There is considerable overlap between these dimensions, and improvement or decline in one area may or may not affect the others. For example, fatigue may not stop a person going out with friends, but it may be bad enough to reduce their enjoyment.

QoL measurement has a number of uses in health care, and this can lead to confusion. Within the context of cancer nursing, its meaning is primarily concerned with the assessment of needs and care planning, but it can also be used for:

- Research and clinical trials
- Audit
- Treatment planning and evaluation of treatment outcomes.

QoL measurement tools should be approached with caution for this reason. Measures designed for research purposes may not be suitable for care planning.

Quality of life in practice

In day-to-day cancer nursing practice, QoL provides a means of focusing on the priorities of the patient and their family. QoL can be viewed as a global measure of how the patient feels about their life at that point. This can provide the patient with a means of monitoring their progress, in their own terms, and act as a balance to care or treatment outcomes. The simplest way to establish this is to ask the patient to rate their QoL today on a scale of 1–10.

Other strategies that you can use to monitor and enhance QoL are:

- Help patients and their family to identify what makes their QoL better or worse by reflecting on their progress
- Encourage patients to participate in activities that improve their QoL
- Monitor the effects of cancer treatments on the patient's and their families' QoL
- Address the negative impact of cancer treatments on QoL
- Evaluate symptoms within the framework of QoL
- Intervene to provide adequate symptom management.

Further reading

Bowling A. *Measuring Health. A Review of Quality of Life Measurement Scales*, 3rd ed. Maidenhead: Open University Press; 2005.

Chapter 37

Bone marrow suppression

Bone marrow function

The bone marrow makes all of the cellular elements of blood. These are:
• Red blood cells—carry oxygen around the body
• White blood cells—fight infection
• Platelets—assist in blood clotting.

The bone marrow is an extremely active organ, producing over a million red blood cells per second. It is also very adaptive, being able to selectively increase the production of cells in response to depletion in the peripheral blood. This ↑ production of red cells occurs in bleeding and haemolytic (red cell destruction) anaemia.

Active blood-forming (haematopoietic) bone marrow is not found in every bone in an adult. It is concentrated in the axial skeleton—the pelvis, vertebrae, ribs, shoulder girdle, and skull.

Bone marrow suppression results in a reduced number of blood cells in the circulation. This can produce a number of different problems, depending on which cell type is mainly affected (see Table 37.1). Frequently, patients display features caused by a reduction in >1 type of blood cell; when all three cell types are low, the patient is said to have pancytopenia.

Table 37.1 Impact of bone marrow suppression

Condition	Definition	Symptoms	Other complications
Anaemia	Low red blood cell count (Hb level <13.5g/dL for men, <11.5g/dL for women)	Fatigue, breathlessness, headache, dizziness, palpitations, angina (cancer patients commonly are anaemic but are rarely symptomatic if above 10g/dL)	Dependence on blood transfusions to correct anaemia—results in iron overload, which can be difficult to treat Anaemia can worsen pre-existing symptoms from other disorders, e.g. angina with ischaemic heart disease, or dizziness with Parkinson's disease
Neutropenia	Low neutrophil count (<1 × 10⁹/L)	Bacterial or fungal infections: fever, rigors, local signs (cough, chest pain, diarrhoea, pain on passing urine, pain around central venous line). May be no specific signs	Overwhelming sepsis Mouth ulceration Note: pus and normal inflammatory processes may not be present
Thrombocytopenia	Low platelet count (high risk of bleeding when count below 10 × 10⁹/L)	Petechial rash, nosebleeds, gum bleeds, haematuria, heavy menstruation, GI bleeds, retinal bleed, intracranial bleed (rare)	Dependence on repeated platelet transfusions to correct thrombocytopenia may result in formation of antibodies, which make further platelet transfusions less effective

Anaemia

Anaemia is defined as a reduction in the oxygen-carrying capacity of blood. It occurs when the Hb concentration falls to <13.5g/dL in a man and <11.5g/dL in a woman.

Causes

Anaemia in cancer patients has a number of causes:

- Bone marrow suppression due to chemotherapy, radiotherapy, or infiltration by malignancy
- Chronic blood loss
- Iron deficiency
- Anaemia of chronic disease—caused by persistent inflammation, infection, or malignancy
- Haemolysis—premature destruction of red blood cells
- Inherited disease such as thalassaemia and sickle-cell disease.

Consequences

Common symptoms include:

- Fatigue (⟴ see Nature and assessment of cancer- related fatigue, p. 520,)
- Shortness of breath on exertion
- Headache
- Dizziness
- Palpitations
- Angina.

Severe anaemia itself can cause heart failure, resulting in peripheral oedema and breathlessness on lying flat. Although uncommon in the UK, a typical cause of this worldwide is untreated thalassaemia in children.

Treatment

Assessment

It is useful to carry out a pre-cancer treatment risk assessment for anaemia:

- FBC, anaemia-related symptoms, e.g. cardiac, pulmonary
- Risk factors: advanced age; low starting Hb; lung, gynaecological, and haematological malignancy; prior myelosuppressive therapy.

Treatment of underlying cause

- Correct underlying cause, if possible, e.g. iron, folate, vitamin B12 supplementation.
- Treatment of haemolytic causes.
- Prevention or stopping chronic/acute blood loss.
- Treat infective, inflammatory, or malignant processes
- Blood product support.

For correction of anaemia via blood transfusions and use of erythropoiesis-stimulating proteins, ⟴ see Blood product support, p. 488.

Neutropenia

A normal neutrophil count for an adult is $2.5–7.5 \times 10^9/L$. Neutropenia can be defined as any neutrophil count less than the lower limit. In practice, it generally does not cause great concern until it has fallen to $<1.0 \times 10^9/L$, and infections remain uncommon until the count is $<0.5 \times 10^9/L$.

Causes

There are many causes of neutropenia; in a cancer patient, the main ones are related to bone marrow suppression. These include:

- Chemotherapy
- Radiotherapy
- Infiltration of the bone marrow by cancer cells, most commonly:
  - Haematological cancers—leukaemia, myeloma, lymphoma
  - Prostate cancer
  - Breast cancer
  - Lung cancer
  - Thyroid cancer
  - RCC.

Infection risks

Neutropenia is expected and reversible when caused by chemotherapy or radiotherapy. Most infections come from the patient themselves, rather than from relatives or friends with whom they come into contact whilst neutropenic. Infections are common in neutropenic patients, largely because mucosal barriers, such as those lining the GI tract, are broken down. This allows bacteria, which are normally resident there, to enter the bloodstream (bacterial translocation). Damage to skin integrity through treatment or siting of a central venous line is another major source of bacterial translocation.

Those most vulnerable to serious infection are patients with haematological malignancy, neutropenia of >7 days, age >60 years, CVCs, and mucositis.

> ### Bone marrow infiltration
> - Neutropenia caused by bone marrow infiltration is often progressive and is only reversible if the underlying cancer is effectively treated.
> - Death often occurs from an overwhelming infection such as pneumonia or a line infection.

Prevention of infection in the neutropenic patient

A number of measures are taken to reduce infection in the neutropenic patient, although evidence for the effectiveness of many of them is limited.

Essential practices are:

- Scrupulous handwashing by the patient and those with whom they come into contact, e.g. health professionals, family, and friends (see Box 37.1).

Box 37.1 Hand hygiene
- The only sure way to reduce infection is scrupulous hand hygiene. Studies conclusively support reduced infection rates in many hospital settings due to the high level of hand hygiene.
- Use of alcohol gel rubs has been effective in reducing hand microbial colonization and infection rates.
- Easy access to hand cleansing equipment is an essential part of ensuring a high level of adherence to hygiene. Many hospitals have alcohol gel rubs available at the entry to wards and patient rooms, and staff may carry small bottles clipped onto their uniform.
- Alcohol gels strip away the outer layer of oil on the skin, destroying any transient microorganisms present. They combine a high level of immediate antimicrobial effect with ease of use. However, on visibly soiled hands, frictional rubbing with soap and water is still the recommended approach.
- Hand hygiene guidelines:
  • When hands are visibly dirty or contaminated, they should be washed with soap and water.
  • Decontaminate hands with an alcohol rub:
    — Before and after having any direct contact with a patient
    — After contact with inanimate objects in the immediate vicinity of the patient
    — Before and after manipulating any invasive devices
    — After removing gloves.
- If an alcohol rub is not available, wash hands with an antimicrobial soap and water.

Note: alcohol is less effective than soap and water against *Clostridium difficile* toxin.

- Meticulous care of indwelling venous catheters, with scrupulous aseptic/non-touch technique when accessing these.
- Other commonly used practices include:
  • Isolation: many neutropenic patients are put in a side room when on a ward. Some units restrict the number of visitors. In some bone marrow transplant settings, protective laminar airflow and/or high-efficiency particulate air (HEPA) filter environments are used to nurse patients.

Note: there is limited evidence to suggest that different isolation procedures impact on patient long-term survival.

- Avoidance of crowded places and individuals who obviously have an infection such as a respiratory tract infection.
- Neutropenic diet—the rationale is to minimize the intake of bacteria in food. This includes avoiding unpasteurized milk products, blue cheeses, uncooked vegetables, salads, uncooked herbs and spices, raw nuts, and raw or undercooked meat and fish. However, there is limited evidence to support this practice, and not all centres will recommend this approach.

- Take care when handling pets, washing hands after contact. If possible, ask the carer to clean up after pets.
- Good dental hygiene—including brushing with a soft toothbrush (➔ see Oral mucositis: managing the process and symptoms, p. 620).

Prophylactic antibiotics

National guidance by NICE (2012) suggested using prophylaxis with a fluoroquinolone, e.g. ciprofloxacin, for patients with acute leukaemia, stem cell transplants, or solid tumours when a neutrophil count of 0.5×10^9/L or lower is expected. Prophylaxis should only be used during the expected period of neutropenia.

Many units do not routinely prescribe antibiotics due to concerns that regular use may lead to the emergence of resistant organisms. The local antibiotic resistance patterns often guide these decisions.

- **G-CSF injections**: these have been shown to reduce the length of the neutropenic period in patients treated with high-dose chemotherapy regimens, to reduce the incidence of infections in these patients and to allow full dosage and schedule of drugs to be given in a number of standard chemotherapy regimens[1] (➔ see Targeted and biological therapies, p. 227).

Patient education

Many patients will spend a period of time at home when they may be neutropenic and at risk of infection. It is essential to educate the patient and their family about why they are at risk of infection, how they might get an infection, and measures to try and prevent infection (➔ see Prevention of infection in the neutropenic patient, p. 479).

- Patients should know about potential signs and symptoms of an infection, the potential dangers, and the need to respond quickly to any such signs, regardless of the time of the day or night.
- Although a temperature (>37.5°C) is the most common and important sign of infection in the neutropenic patient, other symptoms or feeling unwell, even without a temperature, should be reported.
- The patient and their family should be supplied with clear instructions on what to do and who to contact if they develop new or worsening symptoms, cough, sweats, feeling cold, diarrhoea, fever, or feel unwell.
- Give patients clear instructions on how to take their temperature and guidance on how frequently they should do this. The most important time to take their temperature is when they feel unwell.

Note: it must always be remembered that some patients may be septic without having a temperature. Ensure that patients know the temperature-masking effects of paracetamol and aspirin, which can give false reassurance and potentially delay seeking advice or admission to hospital. Patients taking steroids can have infections masked, as they often may not mount a fever, compared to other patients

Acute oncology and neutropenic sepsis

Every year, patients die because they do not seek advice quickly enough.
- Patients and their carers must have written and oral information,
  on: neutropenic sepsis, how and when to contact 24-hour specialist
  oncology advice, and emergency care.
- All patients should carry an emergency card with the appropriate
  contact numbers on it.
- All patients should have 24/7 access to an Acute Oncology Service,
  experienced in managing side effects of anti-cancer treatments
  (➔ see Acute Oncology Services, p. 651).
- UK Oncology Nursing Society: provide 24-hour triage, rapid
  assessment, and access tool kit which is now widely used in the UK
  ('traffic light' assessment system).
- This provides a safe and understandable guideline for both staff
  and patients dealing with the emergency side effects of anti-cancer
  treatment, including neutropenic sepsis.

Patient anxiety and information giving

Many cancer patients find the idea of being susceptible to infection
frightening. Discussions need to emphasize the potential risks and the
need to respond rapidly to any signs of infection and the consequences
of delay in accessing health-care advice. Information giving needs to be
accurate and balanced, and support should respond to the individual's
concerns and anxiety.

References

1 Dolan S, Crombez P, Munoz M. Neutropenia management with granulocyte colony stimulating factors: from guidelines to nursing practice protocols. *Eur J Oncol Nurs* 2005;9:s14–23.

Treatment of neutropenic sepsis

Definition
Diagnose neutropenic sepsis in patients having anti-cancer treatment whose neutrophil count is 0.5×10^9/L or lower and who have either a temperature higher than 38°C or other signs or symptoms consistent with clinically significant sepsis.

Confirmed neutropenic sepsis is a medical emergency
NICE guidance suggests a 'door-to-needle time' of <1 hour for patients arriving in an acute setting and receiving their first course of IV antibiotics.

Offer empiric antibiotic therapy immediately
- Patients with neutropenic sepsis may become very ill rapidly, with a risk of developing septic shock and multi-organ failure, leading to death. The mortality rate of septic shock is high (over 40%).
- Such patients may require cardiovascular support with inotropic medications, such as dobutamine, and support by the intensive care unit (ICU). The ICU should be informed if any neutropenic patient with an infection has hypotension that is resistant to initial fluid resuscitation.

Physiology of sepsis
Sepsis and the resulting endotoxin release from bacteria stimulate a systemic inflammatory/immune response, causing:
- Damaged pulmonary and systemic vasculature, vasodilatation, and ↑ permeability of vessels
- Further delay in bone marrow function recovery
- Systemic activation of clotting cascades and coagulation abnormalities.
- These lead to:
  • Hypovolaemia
  • Pulmonary oedema
  • Thrombocytopenia, bleeding, and low clotting factors
  • Disseminated intravascular coagulation (DIC)
  • Cardiac and renal dysfunction
  • Ongoing pancytopenia
  • Multi-organ failure.

Management of sepsis
- Identify and treat sources of infection. Often the source is unclear, and broad-spectrum empirical antibiotics are required.
- Support the patient symptomatically.
- Detect any onset of organ/multi-organ failure.

Nursing management
This includes:
- Ensuring the patient's safety regarding line management and administration of drugs and blood products
- Close constant observation and monitoring

- Careful fluid balance documentation, which is very important in these patients. They may require a urinary catheter to assist with this
- Maintaining comfort
- Hydrating and maintaining nutritional needs
- Supporting the patients symptomatically
- Supporting the patient and family psychologically (see box for specific nursing measures).

Nursing management of neutropenic sepsis

- Take routine observations: temperature, pulse, blood pressure, oxygen saturations, and respiratory rate, and reassess at frequent intervals.
- Ensure that an urgent CXR is taken.
- Take the following blood tests: blood cultures (from any indwelling lines and from peripheral blood), full blood count, clotting screen, biochemistry (including kidney and liver function), C-reactive protein (CRP).
- If symptoms are present, send urine cultures, sputum cultures, and a specimen of diarrhoea (requesting microscopy, culture, and sensitivity and *Clostridium difficile* toxin).
- The patient should be assessed by medical staff for any obvious source of infection.
- Administer prescribed antibiotics urgently—usually with two broad-spectrum IV antibiotics. The most common combination of broad-spectrum antibiotics used is piperacillin with tazobactam and gentamicin.
- Perform regular observations: temperature, pulse, blood pressure, oxygen saturations, and urine output. If the patient is clinically dehydrated, tachycardic, hypotensive, or oliguric, then:
  - Administer any prescribed IV fluids or oxygen, as required
  - Increase the frequency of observations, up to every 15 minutes.
- These patients are at high risk of pulmonary oedema (➔ see Physiology of sepsis, p. 481). Maintain accurate fluid balance and central venous pressure (CVP) readings. Observe breathing sounds and lungs for signs of fluid overload.
- Any deterioration should prompt an urgent medical review.
- Assess the skin, mucosal membranes, orifices, and body fluids for signs of bleeding—patients with sepsis are at risk of clotting abnormalities and DIC (➔ see Disseminated intravascular coagulation, p. 635). If there is bleeding, administer prescribed blood products and drugs, e.g. vitamin K.
- Maintain the patient's comfort throughout. Assist with personal hygiene, including regular mouth and skin care. Assist with all activities to help the patient reserve energy.
- Keep the patient and their family fully informed. They may be extremely frightened by the situation, particularly in cases of rapid deterioration or if the patient requires intensive care admission.
  - Ensure that you offer calm and reassuring nursing management, despite the emergency nature of treatment.

Bleeding

Bleeding occurs in many patients with cancer, ranging from minor bleeds, which may be part of the initial diagnosis, to potentially life-threatening haemorrhage, e.g. haemoptysis or carotid artery rupture.

Signs of bleeding

Bleeding can be obvious, e.g. nosebleeds, oral mucosa, haemoptysis, haematemesis. It can also be hidden:

- GI: melaena, anaemia
- Pulmonary: breathlessness, pleural effusion
- GU: haematuria
- Cerebral: headaches, visual disturbances, other neurological disturbances.

Causes

Altered platelet count/function

- Tumour: mainly haematological cancers, but also secondary spread into the bone marrow, e.g. lung, breast, prostate cancers.
- Treatment:
  - Many chemotherapy agents
  - Radiotherapy: dependent on the volume of bone marrow in the treatment field.
- Enlarged spleen.
- Immune-mediated damage, e.g. idiopathic thrombocytopenia purpura.
- Altered coagulation mechanisms, e.g. acute pro-myelocytic leukaemia causing DIC (➔ see Disseminated intravascular coagulation, p. 635).
- Liver primary or secondary cancer.

Direct tumour impact

- Invasion into the bone marrow, causing altered platelet count.
- Tumour erosion into blood vessels:
  - Can be minor and part of initial presentation, e.g. gynaecological, lung, bowel, GU
  - Can be extreme, e.g. lung cancer—haemoptysis, H&N cancer—carotid artery erosion.

Cancer treatment

- Chemotherapy/radiotherapy: causing thrombocytopenia.
- Surgery: carotid artery rupture.

Other drugs

- Heparin, aspirin, NSAIDs.

Infections

- Septic shock, causing DIC.

Assessment

- Risk factors, e.g. the tumour, cancer treatment, other drugs such as NSAIDs.
- Past medical history.
- Signs and symptoms of anaemia (➔ see Anaemia, p. 476).

- Physical examination: being aware of both obvious and less obvious signs of bleeding (➔ see Signs of bleeding, p. 483).
- Screening tests: platelet count, clotting screen [prothrombin time (PT), activated partial thromboplastin time (APTT), fibrinogen], bone marrow aspirate, international normalized ratio (INR) if on warfarin.

Thrombocytopenia (low platelets)

The normal adult platelet count is 150–400 × 10^9/L. Thrombocytopenia can be defined as any count less than this. However, patients rarely bleed spontaneously, unless the count falls to <20 × 10^9/L, and most invasive procedures can be performed with a count of >50 × 10^9/L.

Causes of thrombocytopenia

As with neutropenia, there are many potential causes of thrombocytopenia. The most common causes in a cancer patient are:

- Bone marrow suppression
- Drugs, e.g. high-dose co-trimoxazole treatment for *Pneumocystis jiroveci* pneumonia
- Severe infection alone which can cause thrombocytopenia
- Enlarged spleen (splenomegaly) which results in pooling and destruction of platelets.

Consequences of thrombocytopenia

The major types of bleeding associated with thrombocytopenia are:

- Nosebleeds
- Gum bleeding and blood blistering in the mouth
- GI bleeds, rectal bleeding, blood in stool, or black-coloured stool (melaena)
- GU bleeds, dark-coloured, or blood in the urine
- Petechial rash (small, purple spots which do not blanch on pressure, often prominently seen around the ankle).

Bleeding into the brain is the most severe complication, but this is uncommon.

The bleeding risk is ↑ in the following situations:

- Concurrent infections
- Concurrent coagulation abnormalities, e.g. if the patient is on warfarin
- Administration of antiplatelet medications such as aspirin
- Recent history of a bleeding episode
- Invasive procedure.

Prevention of bleeding

- Avoid antiplatelet medication, e.g. aspirin, clopidogrel, NSAIDs (ibuprofen, diclofenac, etc.).
- Avoid IM injections—these can result in a very painful intramuscular haematoma.
- Administer a therapeutic adult dose of platelets if the count falls to <10 × 10^9/L (or <20 × 10^9/L in the presence of another risk factor for bleeding; most commonly infection).
- Ensure the platelet count is adequate to cover any planned invasive procedure.

Treatment of bleeding due to thrombocytopenia
- Administer a pool of platelets.
- Correct any reversible factors contributing to the bleeding risk, e.g. treat underlying infection, stop antiplatelet medication.
- In the case of nosebleeds, pressure and ice packs may help.
- Tranexamic acid treatment can help in long-standing low platelet counts to prevent mucosal bleeding.

Nursing management

Patients require accurate advice if they are thrombocytopenic. They may also be anxious about the risk of a serious bleed. Ensure that they are aware of potential risks, preventative measures, and action to take if they are bleeding. Reassure them that most bleeds are short-lived and can be effectively managed with platelet transfusions (➔ see Blood product support, p. 488).

Patient education
Educate patients about:
- The reason that they are at risk of bleeding
- The first signs of a low platelet count (➔ see Consequences of thrombocytopenia, p. 484)
- Bleeding risk with drugs such as aspirin or NSAIDs—give advice to use paracetamol for headache.

Preventative measures
- Do not use dental floss.
- Use a soft toothbrush or sponge.
- Maintain moist mouth and lips.
- Do not use tampons if menstruating.
- Avoid straining at stool. Use a stool softener or laxative if prone to constipation.
- Do not perform rectal examination or use rectal thermometers, suppositories, or enemas.
- Use an electric razor for shaving.
- Use a water-based lubricant, and avoid vigorous thrusting during sexual intercourse.

What to do if any signs of bleeding
- Patients should contact their cancer unit or centre immediately. They will normally require an immediate FBC to assess their platelet count. They may need to be admitted for a platelet transfusion.
- If there is a major bleed or injury, the patient should immediately go to their local hospital emergency unit and inform them that they are at risk of thrombocytopenia.

Bleeding in advanced cancer

Localized bleeding caused by cancer may be treated by radiotherapy. Examples of its use include ulcerating skin tumours, haemoptysis caused by lung cancer, vaginal bleeding caused by gynaecological cancers, and haematuria caused by bladder/prostate cancer.

Massive terminal haemorrhage

- Occurs as a result of a major arterial bleed and causes death, usually in minutes. The most common cause is tumour erosion into the:
  - Aorta or pulmonary artery: leads to haematemesis or haemoptysis, or
  - Carotid artery: external bleeding, or
  - Femoral artery: external bleeding.
- May be preceded by smaller minor bleeds, allowing some warning or awareness of the risk. Invasive fungal infections can also cause erosion into pulmonary arteries and massive fatal pulmonary haemorrhage. Thankfully, this is uncommon.

Management

- The aim of management is to rapidly sedate the patient in order to relieve any distress. If the bleed is anticipated, then it may be appropriate to discuss this with the patient and family members.
- For anticipated bleeds, it is useful to have the drugs available at the bedside, already drawn up—many wards have patient medication lockers, which can enable this to be done safely.
- Red, blue, or green towels mask the colour of blood and should be available to control the spread of blood.

Pharmacological

IV is the preferable route due to the quicker onset of action of the drugs.
- Midazolam: 10mg SC/IV or buccally.
- Ketamine: 150–250mg IV. Provides rapid sedation. For IM route, the dose needs to be ↑ to 500mg.
- Opioids: these are less recommended, as they cannot be left at the patient's bedside; they take time to draw up, and titration of the appropriate dose is more difficult.

Further reading

Browne M, Cutler T. *Haematology Nursing*. Chichester: Wiley-Blackwell; 2012.
National Institute for Health and Care Excellence (2012). *Neutropenic Sepsis: Prevention and Management in People with Cancer.* Clinical guideline [CG151]. Available at: ℜ http://www.nice.org.uk/CG151
UK Oncology Nursing Society (UKONS). *Central West Chemotherapy Group. Oncology/Haematology 24 HOUR TRIAGE Rapid Assessment and Access Tool Kit.* Available at: ℜ http://www.ukons.org

Blood product support

Blood products

The introduction of safe, reliable blood products has enabled the development of intensive chemotherapy programmes for a variety of malignancies. This has led to significantly improved remission rates.

It must be remembered, however, that blood product use is not without risks and that these are a very expensive resource. The pool of acceptable donors is also diminishing because of more stringent screening. Blood products should only be used in appropriate situations, in consultation with national and local guidelines [see British Committee for Standards in Haematology (BCSH)].[1] The advent of erythropoiesis-stimulating proteins (EPS), such as EPO, has started to change the management of cancer-related anaemia.

Erythropoietin

Recombinant human EPO has been shown to reduce transfusion requirements and potentially can improve QoL by reducing fatigue and other anaemia-related symptoms in some cancer patients receiving chemotherapy or radiotherapy. However, only around 50% of patients respond and it is expensive. EPO is administered as a regular SC injection, which is not always popular with patients. There is an ↑ risk of thrombosis using EPO, though this is rare.

Guidelines on the use of EPO

Recent guidelines from NICE support the use of EPO to reduce the symptomatic period of anaemia in patients receiving SACT when Hb concentrations are 100g/L or lower. The aim is to maintain the Hb concentration high enough to avoid transfusion, but not to increase it to >120g/L (see ℛ https://www.nice.org.uk/guidance/ta323/chapter/1-Guidance)

Blood transfusion

Whole blood is almost never currently used in the UK. When a unit of blood is donated, it is separated into the following fractions:
- Red cells
- Platelets
- Plasma.

Plasma is frozen and is subsequently used as fresh frozen plasma (FFP). It is most frequently used to correct problems with blood clotting in patients.

Red cells

Packed red cells are frequently administered to cancer patients who are anaemic. Most oncology and haematology units have a protocol whereby red cells are administered if the Hb concentration falls below a particular cutoff, e.g. 80 or 90g/L. The threshold may be higher with patients receiving radiotherapy. The disadvantage with this policy is that it leads to high use of blood products, with attendant cost and risks. Some patients cannot tolerate such a low level of Hb, e.g. those with symptomatic ischaemic heart disease. The Hb threshold for transfusion may be raised accordingly, based on their symptoms.

Complications of red cell transfusions

Acute haemolytic transfusion reaction

This is the most severe complication of a red cell transfusion and is due to ABO-mismatched blood being administered. This can cause:

- Fever
- Shortness of breath
- Hypotension
- Oliguria
- Abdominal or flank pain
- Jaundice
- A general feeling of 'impending doom'
- Renal failure
- DIC (➜ see Disseminated intravascular coagulation, pp. 635–6)
- Death.

The most common cause for this is clerical error, e.g. blood samples being mislabelled or patient checks being incorrectly carried out. It is therefore vital that local protocols for blood transfusion are strictly adhered to.

If an acute haemolytic transfusion reaction (AHTR) is suspected, urgent medical attention should be sought. Treatment is supportive, involving careful fluid balance, IV fluids, treatment of DIC, and renal support.

Febrile non-haemolytic reaction

This is much less common since the introduction of universal white cell depletion during processing of blood donations. Management includes:

- Assessment of the patient, including pulse, blood pressure, temperature, and oxygen saturations
- Considering slowing or stopping the transfusion for a short period if the patient is unwell, and continuing to monitor vital signs
- Administering paracetamol 1g orally, chlorphenamine 10mg IV/4mg orally, and/or hydrocortisone 100–200 mg IV.
- Stopping the transfusion and seeking medical advice if the patient feels unwell or their observations are unstable. They should be investigated for an AHTR (➜ see Acute haemolytic transfusion reaction, p. 489).

Delayed haemolytic transfusion reaction

The patient becomes anaemic and jaundiced a few days after a transfusion.

- Management is largely supportive. Blood tests should be sent to the transfusion laboratory to determine the type of antibody causing the reaction.
- If the patient requires further transfusions, any blood that they receive should be negative for the protein molecule that the antibody recognizes.

Note: any patient with an antibody that reacts against certain types of red blood cells and has caused a reaction in the past should carry a card stating the antibody type.

Transfusion reaction notification

Any complication of transfusion from any blood product should be notified to the blood transfusion department, so that the product can be screened and further complications for other patients prevented.

Other complications of red cell transfusion
These include:
• Bacterial contamination of blood
• Transmission of viral infection—this is extremely rare. The risk is in
  the order of 1/350,000 for hepatitis B, 1 in 8 million for HIV, and 1 in
  30 million for hepatitis C
• Variant Creutzfeldt–Jakob disease (vCJD). The true risk is unknown but
  is likely to be extremely low. Four cases of vCJD transmission via blood
  transfusion have been described in the last 20 years. Leucodepletion
  was introduced in order to minimize this risk as much as possible
• Transfusion-associated GvHD (TAGvHD)—this is extremely rare, but
  nearly always fatal (➔ see Irradiated blood products, p. 492). It is likely
  that leucodepletion has lessened this risk too
• Iron overload—this commonly occurs after 25–30U of blood and
  results in iron deposition within the liver, heart, and endocrine glands.
  It is potentially very serious and is treated by an arduous regime of long
  SC infusions of desferrioxamine treatment. Newer oral iron chelators
  are now available
• Cardiac overload due to fluid overload/rapid transfusion.

Compatibility of red cell transfusions
Red cells of one ABO blood group should preferably be given to a patient
of the same blood group. The main exceptions to this rule are:
• Group O (so-called 'universal blood') can be given to any patient in an
  emergency, but it is still preferable to match the ABO group, if at all
  possible
• A patient who has had an allogeneic stem cell transplant may change their
  blood group, receiving different blood from their original type (➔ see
  Allogeneic haematopoietic stem cell transplantation, pp. 258–60).

The rhesus D (RhD) group is also important. A woman of childbearing
age who is RhD-negative and does not have any RhD antibodies should
not be given RhD-positive red cells, if at all possible. This is to avoid the
production of antibodies that can subsequently cause haemolytic disease
of the fetus or newborn. RhD-negative men and women who are beyond
childbearing age can receive RhD-positive red cells, as the formation of
antibodies will not have deleterious effects. Once RhD antibodies have
formed, however, only RhD-negative products should be given, to avoid
a delayed haemolytic transfusion reaction. Certain patients should receive
irradiated and/or CMV-negative products only (➔ see CMV-negative
blood products, p. 492).

Platelets

The most common indication for a transfusion of platelets is the prevention of bleeding for patients receiving chemotherapy and/or radiotherapy
affecting the haematopoietic system. Most units have a 'cutoff' point below
which prophylactic platelets are administered. This is commonly 10×10^9/L
but may be higher if the patient has other risk factors for bleeding such as
severe sepsis.

Note: results of the recently published TOPPS trial support the need for continued use of prophylaxis with platelet transfusion and show the benefit of such prophylaxis for reducing bleeding, as compared with no prophylaxis. A significant number of patients undergoing stem cell transplant or chemotherapy had bleeding despite prophylaxis.[2]

Unlike blood, a platelet transfusion is given rapidly to avoid aggregates forming in the bag and IV line. There are two main sources of platelets:
- Those obtained from a process called apheresis where a single donor can give enough platelets for a transfusion. This is the source of ~90% of UK platelets
- Those obtained by pooling together the platelets from four individual blood donors—~10%.

If platelets of a particular type are required, e.g. HLA-matched, they must be collected by apheresis (➔ see Chapter 19, Allogeneic haematopoietic stem cell transplantation). Platelet donations from apheresis donors reduce the exposure of patients to numerous donors. This reduces the risk of infection to the recipient, as well as the risk of antibody formation.

Complications of platelet transfusions
- Febrile reaction: this is less common since the widespread introduction of white cell depletion during donation processing. It may be accompanied by rigors and urticaria (hives). Management includes:
  - Stopping transfusion (if not already completed)
  - Administering hydrocortisone 100–200mg IV and chlorphenamine 10mg IV (or 4mg orally)
  - Considering pethidine 25mg IV for persistent rigors
  - Pre-medicating the patient with hydrocortisone and chlorphenamine for further platelet transfusions
  - Occasionally, patients who react badly to platelet transfusions may require HLA-matched or washed platelets.
- Bacterial contamination: this is more common than with red cells, because platelets must be stored at room temperature. Every bag of platelets should be visually checked for discoloration or cloudiness prior to administration.

Viral transmission
- As with red blood cells (➔ see Other complications of red cell transfusion, p. 490).
- Development of anti-HLA antibodies: this can lead to platelet refractoriness whereby further platelet transfusions are ineffective and specially HLA-matched platelets are required.
- Transfusion-related acute lung injury (TRALI): this is a serious condition resulting in respiratory failure and possibly death. It is usually due to antibodies in donor plasma. Treatment is supportive, e.g. mechanical ventilation.

Compatibility of platelets

Where possible, ABO-matched platelets are given. It is perfectly acceptable to administer ABO-mismatched platelets, but the patient's platelet count may not rise as much as expected. RhD-negative platelets should be administered to RhD-negative women of childbearing age who do not have RhD antibodies already. As with red cells, certain patients should receive irradiated and/or CMV-negative platelets (➔ see CMV-negative blood products, p. 492).

Irradiated blood products

Packed red cells and platelets contain a small number of contaminating white blood cells. Normally, if these cells are transfused with the blood product, the host's immune system would rapidly clear them. In immuno-suppressed patients, however, these white cells can grow, divide, and attack the recipient's tissues. This can lead to a very serious condition called TAGvHD.

Transfusion-associated graft-versus-host disease

This condition is characterized by bone marrow failure, severe rash, diarrhoea, and liver failure. It is nearly always fatal but is extremely rare. TAGvHD can be prevented by exposing the blood product to γ radiation. The product is then said to be irradiated. Irradiated products should be used in the following situations:

- From the start of conditioning therapy in all patients receiving a stem cell transplant. For autologous transplants, this should continue for at least 3 months after the transplant; for allogeneic transplants, at least 6 months and some would argue lifelong (➔ see Allogeneic haematopoietic stem cell transplantation, pp. 258–60)
- Indefinitely for patients who have received a purine analogue in the past, e.g. fludarabine, cladribine
- Indefinitely for those who have received bendamustine or Campath®
- Patients with Hodgkin lymphoma
- All HLA-matched platelet transfusions.

CMV-negative blood products

CMV is a common virus that can theoretically be transmitted by a blood transfusion. It is harmless in most cases, but it can lead to serious disease in patients who are immunosuppressed. A number of blood products are assessed for the presence of CMV, and many haematology units will administer only CMV-negative products to the following groups of patients:

- Any patient who may be given a stem cell transplant in the near future, e.g. a fit patient with acute leukaemia and who is either CMV-seronegative or who has not yet been tested
- Any CMV-seronegative patient who is undergoing an autologous or allogeneic transplant from a seronegative donor.

If a patient is CMV-seropositive, they will harbour the virus already, and so there is no need to only give CMV-negative products.

Note: there is much debate nationally about the need for CMV testing in transfusion practice and the approach outlined above. Some centres in the UK feel that universal leucodepletion reduces the risk of cellular-based viruses such as CMV, so much so that the risk of transfusion-related transmission is almost completely eliminated.

TAGvHD guidelines card system

To ensure adherence to these guidelines, the blood bank should be informed of any patient fulfilling one of the criteria described previously, and a note should be made on the computer system. The patient should be informed and given a card stating their need to have blood products irradiated. A card should also be attached to their medical notes. The patient should be assured that even if they were to receive non-irradiated blood products, the risk of TAGvHD is still low.

References

1 British Committee for Standards in Haematology (BCSH) website. Available at: ℘ http://www. bcshguidelines.com/

2 Stanworth SJ, Estcourt LJ, Powter G, *et al.*; TOPPS Investigators. A no-prophylaxis platelet-transfusion strategy for hematologic cancers. *N Engl J Med* 2013;368:1771–80.

The nurse's role in blood product transfusions

Educating the patient

Patients should be informed of the reasons for their blood product transfusion and consented for the transfusion. They should also be made aware of any risks and benefits and any potential alternatives, including autologous transfusion. Some patients may be anxious about receiving blood products, for fear of contracting infections such as hepatitis or for fear of transfusion reactions. Misconceptions need to be corrected and any particular fears dealt with sensitively.

Administration errors

Errors at the time of administration of blood or blood components are the most common cause of transfusing the wrong blood. It is essential to follow hospital blood administration policies when administering any blood product.

Checking blood products

- The bedside check is a vital step in preventing transfusion error. The nurse must be vigilant in ensuring that the patient is positively identified and that the patient's identification details on their wristband match those on the blood transfusion report form, and the compatibility label is attached to the blood pack.
- Further checks must include the blood unit number, blood group, and special requirements such as CMV-negative or irradiated.
- Checks should be made between the following:
  - Patient's identification wristband and blood transfusion compatibility report form
  - Compatibility label attached to the blood pack
  - Prescription chart
  - Medical notes.

Full national guidelines are available on the BCSH website (➲ see Further reading, p. 495)

Administration

- Blood should be transfused through a sterile blood administration set.
- Platelet concentrates should be transfused through a sterile blood or platelet administration set.
- Electronic infusion pumps should not be used for the administration of red cells, unless they are verified safe according to the manufacturer's instructions.
- Giving sets should be changed every 12 hours to prevent bacterial growth.

Monitoring patients

- Visual observation is probably the most effective check. Patients having transfusions should be in areas where they are easily visible and accessible. There should also be quick and easy access to emergency resuscitation equipment, if appropriate. Patients should be advised to report a rash, temperature, shivering, feeling unwell, feeling cold, or pain at the site of the infusion.
- Patients should be monitored for signs of potential complications of transfusion. They should be observed most closely during the first 15 minutes of the start of each unit, when severe reactions are most likely to occur.
- Temperature, pulse, and blood pressure should be measured and recorded before the start and at the end of each transfusion episode.
- Temperature and pulse should be measured 15 minutes after the start of each unit.
- Vital signs should be clearly dated and recorded separately from routine observations.

The use of further observations is at the discretion of each clinical area.

Further reading

British Committee for Standards in Haematology (BCSH). Available at: ℘ http://www.bcshguidelines.com/

Contreras M. *ABC of Transfusion*, 4th ed. London: BMJ Books; 2009.

National Institute for Health and Care Excellence (2014). *Erythropoiesis-stimulating Agents (Epoetin and Darbepoetin) for Treating Anaemia in People with Cancer Having Chemotherapy*. Technology Appraisal Guidance [TA323]. Available at: ℘ https://www.nice.org.uk/guidance/ta323

Stanworth SJ, Estcourt LJ, Powter G, *et al.*; TOPPS Investigators. A no-prophylaxis platelet-transfusion strategy for hematologic cancers. *N Engl J Med* 2013;368:1771–80.

Thrombosis

Venous thrombosis

Venous thromboembolism (VTE) includes thrombosis of superficial and deep veins (DVT), usually of the leg, thigh, and pelvis, pulmonary embolus (PE), and thrombosis associated with CVCs.

Venous thrombosis can have a profound impact on a cancer patient's QoL. It is a well-recognized, major complication of cancer and the second leading cause of death in hospitalized patients with cancer. It remains an underdiagnosed and undertreated condition.

Aetiology

- Tumoural production of a range of procoagulant factors.
- Cancer treatments, including surgery, hormonal therapy, chemotherapy, and more recently anti-angiogenesis drugs, e.g. bevacizumab.
- Use of CVCs.
- Venous thrombosis may be the first sign of malignancy, and the development of VTE in patients with cancer is often associated with a poor prognosis (see Box 39.1).

Signs and symptoms

- DVT: unilateral swelling of an extremity, with oedema, erythema, and pain.
- PE: tachypnoea, tachycardia, dyspnoea, chest pain aggravated by inspiration, and unexplained haemoptysis.

Diagnosis

- Thorough patient history.
- Assessment of risk factors.
- Physical examination.
- Contrast venography or venous ultrasonography, for diagnosing DVT.
- Ventilation/perfusion scan or pulmonary angiography, used for diagnosing PE.

Management

Prophylaxis

Primary prophylaxis should be considered for patients with cancer in the presence of additional risk factors (see Box 39.2).

Box 39.1 Venous thrombosis and malignancy

Around 60% of occult cancers are actually discovered after an episode of 'unprovoked VTE' (i.e. with no other transient risk factors), and around 10% of people with a newly diagnosed VTE event will turn out to have cancer within the following year. Formal screening programmes have been proposed and investigated, but currently there is no strong evidence that this would be an effective cancer screening tool.[1]

However, health professionals should consider at least a brief cancer health check in any patient with an unprovoked VTE.

Box 39.2 Risk factors for VTE in patients with cancer

- Primary site: stomach, pancreas, lung, gynaecological, stomach
- Metastatic disease
- High BMI (>35)
- Comorbidities: infection, chronic obstructive pulmonary disease (COPD)
- Recent surgery
- Current hospitalization
- CVC
- Hormonal therapy or chemotherapy
- Anti-angiogenesis therapy

Use of low-molecular-weight heparin (LMWH) reduces the risk by 40–80% and is used pre-surgery for many acute medical admissions and can be considered for high-risk ambulatory patients. Compression stockings are also indicated pre-surgery and for acute medical admissions.

Central venous catheters for administration of chemotherapy
Long-term indwelling CVCs increase the risk of thromboembolic complications, leading to significant morbidity, catheter malfunction, and treatment delays. Recent analyses of studies suggest that though there may be some reduction in DVTs, there is no clear overall benefit in patients given prophylactic heparin.[2]

Results of recent large trials have shown low-dose warfarin and LMWHs to be of no apparent benefit. VTE prophylaxis with low-dose warfarin or LMWHs is therefore currently not recommended for thromboprophylaxis.

Treatment of VTE

The management of DVT and PE are similar, with initial administration of weight-adjusted doses of LMWH by SC injection. Combined use with warfarin oral anticoagulation may be difficult in patients with cancer, due to drug interactions, deranged LFTs, and a higher rate of VTE recurrences and bleeding, compared with non-cancer patients. As there is a significant risk of recurrent thrombosis, guidelines now recommend the use of LMWH, instead of warfarin, for long-term treatment of acute VTE for 3–6 months. All patients admitted to an acute hospital should have a VTE assessment carried out within 24 hours of admission.

Contraindications
A number of cancer patients will have contraindications to anticoagulation use, e.g. active bleeding, high risk of bleeding, peptic ulcer, some primary CNS tumours, thrombocytopenia, or clotting dysfunction.

Vena cava filters may be considered if anticoagulation is contraindicated or in patients with recurrent VTE, despite the use of LMWH.

New oral anticoagulants

In recent years, a number of new oral anticoagulant drugs have been developed that specifically target either factor Xa or thrombin. Advantages over warfarin include fewer drug interactions and fixed dosing, reducing the need for INR testing. However, they are not yet recommended for use in patients outside trial settings.

Overview of nursing care

For those patients who survive a VTE, there is often reduced limb function (with DVT) or low respiratory function (with PE), resulting in immobilization, hospitalization, interruption of lifesaving treatments (with CVC-related DVT), and heightened anxiety. The treatment puts patients at high risk of injury from bleeding. Identification of patients at high risk of thrombosis is crucial. Nurses first have to raise awareness of thrombosis with patients through counselling about the risk of VTE, followed by risk assessment. Active or passive exercise should be encouraged to support venous circulation, and pharmacologic and non-pharmacologic measures to reduce anxiety, pain, or dyspnoea. Managing the complications of anticoagulant therapies and overall coordination of the patient pathway are crucial to optimal support for the patient and carer.

Further reading

Lyman GH, Bohlke K, Khorana AA, *et al*.; American Society of Clinical Oncology. Venous thrombo-embolism prophylaxis and treatment in patients with cancer: American Society of Clinical Oncology clinical practice guideline update. *J Clin Oncol* 2015;33:654–6.

References

1 Carrier M, Langner A, Shivakumar S, *et al*. Screening for occult cancer in unprovoked venous thromboembolism. *N Engl J Med* 2015;373:697–704.
2 Akl EA, Vasireddi SR, Gunukula S, *et al*. Anticoagulation for patients with cancer and central venous catheters. *Cochrane Database Syst Rev* 2011;4:CD006468.

Altered bowel function

Diarrhoea

Diarrhoea is an unpleasant and potentially embarrassing symptom for patients. There is no uniformly accepted definition, but a stool or liquid stool frequency of >3 times per day is generally the accepted norm.

It can have a major impact on an individual's QoL, potentially causing:

- Faecal incontinence
- Social isolation
- Malnutrition and dehydration
- Stopping or reducing the dose of anti-cancer therapy
- Fatigue, exhaustion.

Diarrhoea may also be associated with abdominal pain, cramps, urgency, and tenesmus. Nausea and vomiting may be present if the upper gut is involved.

Causes

- Diet, e.g. high-fibre diet, spicy food, alcohol.
- Drugs: chemotherapy, TKIs, laxatives, antibiotics, antacids, NSAIDs, and iron preparations.
- Surgery, e.g. bowel resection, gastrectomy.
- Radiotherapy to pelvic area or gut.
- Bowel obstruction: faecal overflow.
- Malabsorption: particularly in pancreatic cancer and bowel cancer.
- Infection, e.g. *Clostridium difficile*.
- Disease, e.g. colorectal cancer, pancreatic cancer, NETs.
- Faecal impaction; overflow diarrhoea.
- GvHD (➔ see Graft-versus-host disease, pp. 261–2).
- Non-cancer-related, e.g. inflammatory bowel disease, coeliac disease.
- Anxiety.

Assessment

- Assessment needs to be carried out sensitively. Patients may be embarrassed and reluctant to talk about their bowel habits, and diarrhoea may be seen as dirty.
- It is important to clarify both the range of potential causes and the patient's individual perception and interpretation of the term diarrhoea.
- Without a detailed assessment, it can be difficult to plan appropriate treatment and support. Early management can prevent related consequences such as dehydration and exhaustion (see Table 40.1).

Management of diarrhoea

Accurate assessment

Where the cause of diarrhoea is not explicit, further investigations may be required, e.g. physical observation, abdominal palpation, stool specimens to rule out infection, and barium studies or endoscopy.

- Fluid and electrolyte replacement.
- Identification and treatment or removal of the cause.
- Symptomatic relief.
- A proactive approach to skin care and hygiene is essential to prevent burning and breakdown of skin. Consider using a barrier cream when diarrhoea persists for longer than 24 hours.

Table 40.1 Assessment of diarrhoea

Question	Rationale
• What is the patient's normal bowel habit? • When was the last normal bowel action? • What is the patient's perception of normal?	• Provides a baseline and determines when the problem started • It may help in establishing a new 'norm' for the patient, particularly if the cancer or its treatment has affected the bowel
• What is the patient's perception of the cause and the impact on their QoL? • How frequently does it occur? What does it smell like? • What does it look like (colour, consistency, and amount)? • Is there obvious blood in the stool?	• It is important to establish the extent of the problem and impact on the patient's QoL • This provides a benchmark to monitor and record improvement or worsening of the symptom • Dark stool may suggest the need for FOBT. Pale or greasy stool may suggest malabsorption
• Is the diarrhoea a side effect of treatment?	• Consideration of the cause of diarrhoea may affect how the diarrhoea is managed
• Is the patient currently taking laxatives?	• Diarrhoea caused by an increase in laxatives to treat constipation will normally resolve within 24–48 hours if the laxatives are reduced or stopped • Care should be taken not to re-induce constipation

Note: stopping anti-cancer treatment may reduce persistent and unbearable diarrhoea, but it can have major consequences for the patient. The risk and benefit of stopping these treatments needs to be discussed with the patient and the health-care team.

Further information on drug management of diarrhoea can be found in the *British National Formulary* (available at: ℗ http://www.bnf.org).

Management of cancer treatment-induced diarrhoea
(See Table 40.2.)

Cytotoxic drugs
Cells within the GI tract have a high rate of reproduction. Effects of cytotoxic drugs on the mucosal stem cells can be seen within days of treatment. Post-chemotherapy-induced diarrhoea occurs during or immediately post-treatment until the gut settles. Immunosuppression from treatment can increase the risk of *C. difficile* gut infection.

Note: diarrhoea from capecitabine (used to treat colorectal cancer) can be prolific and requires careful monitoring. It has the potential of causing severe dehydration, if left untreated.

Table 40.2 Drug management for symptomatic relief

Drug	Action
Antimotility drugs: 1. Loperamide Starting dose of 4mg, then 2mg 4-hourly or after each bowel action. Maximum 16mg in 24 hours	To reduce the motility of the gut in uncomplicated acute diarrhoea in adults, e.g. diarrhoea of known cause, and where there is a need to improve faecal consistency.
2. Codeine 10–60mg four times daily. Maximum 240mg daily	
3. Octreotide Starting dose 250–500 micrograms daily. Maximum 750 micrograms	Reduces motility, enhances fluid absorption, reduces secretions. Used in GvHD (➲ see Chapter 19, Allogeneic haematopoietic stem cell transplantation) and chemotherapy-related diarrhoea. Useful in carcinoid syndrome-related diarrhoea
Antispasmodic drugs Hyoscine butylbromide: 10–20mg four times daily. Maximum 80mg daily	Used to treat abdominal cramps but should not be used as a primary treatment of diarrhoea
Antibacterial drugs Antibacterial drugs should be prescribed following the result of a stool sample and on the advice of the microbiologist	Used to treat systemic bacterial infections, e.g. *Campylobacter* enteritis, shigellosis, and salmonellosis

Management
- Most chemotherapy-induced diarrhoea can be managed with loperamide or codeine.

Immunotherapies
Some of the recently introduced therapies, such as ipilimumab and pembrolizumab, can cause severe colitis. Patients with diarrhoea that does not immediately respond to loperamide need to be assessed for colitis as a cause. Treatment includes high-dose corticosteroids and, in refractory cases, may require treatment with infliximab (used to treat autoimmune diseases).

Radiotherapy
High-dose radiotherapy to the abdomen or pelvis increases peristaltic activity by damaging the intestinal mucosa (acute radiation enteritis). Symptoms may be immediate but can occur several weeks into the course of treatment or after the radiotherapy has stopped.

Initial damage is due to immediate mucosal cell death. Progressive loss of cells, atrophy, and fibrosis of the bowel lining can occur in the following weeks. Patients suffering from acute enteritis may complain of nausea, vomiting, abdominal cramping, tenesmus, and watery diarrhoea.

Management

Generally as for cytotoxic drug-induced diarrhoea, plus:

- Aspirin: can be helpful because of its effect in blocking prostaglandins
- Colestyramine: can also help in late chronic diarrhoea where there is evidence of bile salt malabsorption
- If pain relief is required, opioids have the benefit of being constipating.

Stoma management

For bowel cancer patients who have a colostomy or an ileostomy, management of diarrhoea follows similar guidance; however, consideration should be given to the following:

- Is there adequate adherence and comfort of stoma appliances?
- Does the patient have good skin protection?
- Is the stoma overactive?
- Could diet be used to manage overactivity?
- Is fluid and electrolyte support required?

For patients with an overactive ileostomy, loperamide (melts or tablets) could be considered 45 minutes prior to meals (➜ see Stoma care, p. 329).

Non-pharmacological management

There is limited research evidence base to support one particular approach.

- Spend time with the patient assessing possible exacerbating factors, e.g. anxiety, diet, and alcohol, and discuss behavioural modification.
- Diet: for many patients, a high-fibre diet, alcohol, spicy food, milk products, and caffeine all exacerbate diarrhoea. Getting patients to keep a diary of food intake and their pattern of diarrhoea can help to identify causal factors. Dietician advice on dietary modification is a useful strategy.
- Use of prophylactic probiotics, such as *Lactobacillus rhamnosus* GG, may have some benefit in radiation-induced diarrhoea and is the subject of an ongoing Cochrane systematic review.

Websites

British National Formulary. Available at: ℘ http://www.bnf.org
Palliative Drugs.com. Available at: ℘ http://www.palliativedrugs.com

Further reading

Royal College of Nursing. *The Management of Diarrhoea in Adults: RCN Guidance for Nursing Staff.* London: Royal College of Nursing; 2013.

Constipation

Constipation is a commonly occurring symptom, often exacerbated by cancer and its treatment and management.

It is defined as the infrequent passage of small, hard faeces with difficulty and less frequently than the individual's normal pattern. If untreated, constipation can lead to further symptoms: nausea, vomiting, poor appetite, weight loss, overflow diarrhoea, rectal bleeding, faecal incontinence, urinary incontinence, pain, tenesmus (an urgent and painful desire to defecate), bowel obstruction, and confusion.

Nursing management should be proactive and anticipate the potential for constipation before it occurs as a problem. Potential causes of constipation in cancer patients are highlighted in Table 40.3.

Regular assessment for constipation is important and should include the following.

Accurate patient history

- Identification and possible removal of the potential cause of constipation, identifying how long the problem has existed and establishing the normal pattern. A patient diary is useful.
- Stool frequency, stool consistency, discomfort on passing stool, smell of faecal leakage. A stool chart may be helpful.
- Assessment of diet, including fluid intake.
- Use of laxatives.

Examination

- Physical observation, including abdominal palpation.
- Plain X-ray of the abdomen is helpful if an inconsistent clinical picture.
- Digital rectal examination can assess for the presence of stool, haemorrhoids, and anal tone.

Table 40.3 Potential causes of constipation in cancer patients

Cancer-related	Treatment-related	Cancer impact
• Hypercalcaemia • Abdominal or pelvic disease • Cord compression • Cauda equina syndrome	• Chemotherapy (vinca alkaloids, particularly vincristine) • Radiotherapy (long-term bowel fibrosis) • Opioids • Anti-emetics (cyclizine and ondansetron) • Anticholinergics • Antispasmodics • Antidepressants • Neuroleptics • NSAIDs	• Weakness • Inactivity or bed rest • Poor nutrition • Dehydration/poor fluid intake • Confusion • Inability to reach toilet • Embarrassment due to lack of privacy

Note: multiple causes of constipation are common, particularly in advanced cancer.

Record of potentially associated symptoms
- Nausea; vomiting; abdominal pain; abdominal distension; malodorous breath.

Mobility
- Access to toilet; lack of privacy; need for assistance/mobility aids.
- Constipation can cause faecal leakage or watery faecal-stained fluid to be passed. The fluid can contain small, hard faeces and have a stale smell. This should not be confused with diarrhoea, which is more likely to have a soft consistency. If in doubt, abdominal palpation or an abdominal X-ray should be undertaken to determine the correct management.

Management of constipation
- Identify and remove the cause where possible.
- Set goals based on the patient's normal bowel habits and established management regimen, taking into consideration the cancer treatment plan.
- Explore the potential for increasing fluid intake and adjusting the diet.
- Consider measures to improve privacy.
- Appropriate encouragement to exercise.
- Consider prophylactic use of laxatives.

Diet and other non-pharmacological measures
Diet
- Dietary advice is complementary to the prescription of laxatives. Advice should be realistic and given with consideration to the patient's disease status, treatment plan, and individual needs.
- Try to maintain a fluid intake of at least 2L a day.
- Where possible, inclusion of fibre in the diet should be encouraged. This should not, however, be introduced too quickly or in excess, to avoid flatulence and bloating. In dehydrated patients, fibre may exacerbate constipation.
- Consider referral to a dietician, particularly for patients where constipation is an ongoing problem.

Other measures
- Assist with other symptom control, e.g. patients with pain and/or nausea are unlikely to maintain adequate oral intake.
- Maintain good oral care, and ensure that patients are comfortably positioned at mealtimes.
- Assist with maintaining mobility, if appropriate.

Pharmacological management
Where the patient already has a management regime for their constipation, it may be necessary to increase laxatives or intervene to achieve a bowel evacuation pattern which is normal for the patient. The evidence base supporting the management of constipation in cancer patients is limited. General guidelines on the use of laxatives based on best available evidence are covered in Table 40.4.

Table 40.4 Guidance for use of laxatives

Classification	Action	Indication for use	Examples of drugs
Bulk-forming drugs	Increases faecal mass (**Note**: need high fluid intake)	Of value in patients where fibre in diet cannot be ↑ Useful in patients who have a colostomy or an ileostomy, to add bulk to stool. Effect NOT immediate	Ispaghula husk (e.g. Fybogel Regular®) Methylcellulose Sterculia (e.g. Normacoll®)
Osmotic laxatives	Draws water into the large bowel	Discourages proliferation of ammonia-producing organisms Useful in the treatment of **hepatic encephalopathy** (**Note**: cautious use in patients with low fluid intake or vomiting, as can increase dehydration and volume of vomiting)	Lactulose syrup Macrogol (Movicol®), magnesium hydroxide suspension (milk of magnesia) Phosphate enema Micro enema
Faecal softener/ lubricants	Lubricate and soften impacted faeces to promote bowel action	Patients who have hard stools and difficulty passing stool	Liquid paraffin/mineral oil (**Note**: causes anal skin irritation) Sodium docusate Arachis oil enema Glycerol suppositories
Contact (stimulant) laxatives	Increase intestinal motility	For patients who may be taking opioids or other drugs which slow the action of the gut May cause abdominal cramp (**Note**: should be avoided in bowel obstruction) Prolonged use can cause diarrhoea and symptoms associated with diarrhoea	Bisacodyl Dantron (Danthron) Senna Sodium picosulfate (mild irritant to bowel, acting as a rectal stimulant)

The use of oral laxatives should be considered for patients who may not be able to achieve regular bowel evacuation by diet, ↑ fluid intake, and exercise alone. Treatment should be preventative, if possible, e.g. patients on opioids or vincristine should be on regular laxatives. Enemas or suppositories can be undignified and painful and are generally not the first treatment option. They are useful in cases of faecal impaction and spinal cord compression.

Further information on laxatives and dosages can be found in the *British National Formulary* (available at: ℰ http://www.bnf.org).

Bowel obstruction

Obstruction occurs when digested food is unable to pass through the intestine due to tumour, impacted faeces, oedema, or motility disorders. It is commonly associated with intestinal and gynaecological cancers.

Causes
- Oedema caused by tumour.
- Faecal impaction.
- Intestinal muscle paralysis.
- Lumen occlusion—due to primary tumour enlargement, recurrence of abdominal mass, fibrosis, or adhesions.
- Carcinomatosis with concurrent infiltration of the mesentery or bowel muscles and nerves by the tumour. Small bowel NETs also often infiltrate the mesentery.

Symptoms
The obstruction can be partial or complete. Presenting symptoms commonly include:
- Nausea and vomiting, including occasionally faecal vomiting
- Central severe abdominal pain and distension. Colicky in nature
- Initial ↑ bowel sounds but can be absent or high-pitched.

Note: in the case of partial obstruction, presenting symptoms may be inconsistent and resolve for short periods of time.

Investigations
- If bowel obstruction is suspected, an abdominal X-ray to determine air, fluid, and stool levels may be helpful.
- CT scan is indicated if the diagnosis is not clear—usually confirms the underlying cause.

Management
- The approach taken to manage bowel obstruction should be considered in collaboration with the patient and aim to promote the best QoL. Treatment decisions should consider:
  - The patient's prognosis and general health
  - Patient's expectations, wishes, and concerns
  - Clinical presentation
  - Potential impact of the chosen management approach on the patient's QoL.

Active treatment
- **Surgical intervention** (if the patient is fit enough), e.g. bypass procedures such as formation of a colostomy or ileostomy, dependent on the confinement of the tumour site. Useful when tumour confined to a single site or low tumour grade.
- **Stenting under radiological guidance:** the stent enables the bowel to remain patent and allows passage of stool through the area affected by the tumour. Less invasive than a surgical bypass. Useful when tumour not confined to one site, shorter prognosis, to facilitate symptom relief.

Medical management

Inoperable bowel obstruction can be managed medically. Treatment will vary, depending on the degree and site of obstruction. The aim is to palliate the symptoms of nausea, vomiting, pain, and constipation.

In advanced cancer, bowel obstruction is unlikely to be a single acute event and more likely to become continuous. For medical management of associated symptoms, see Table 40.5.

Partial obstruction

Proactive management of constipation can help to delay complete bowel obstruction. It may be necessary to stop the stimulant, osmotic, or bulk-forming laxatives, as they could increase peristalsis. This causes abdominal pain and can lead to further complications, such as perforation of the gut, if the bowel is obstructing.

It is preferable to use a faecal softener, e.g. sodium docusate 100–500mg in divided daily doses, to enable the faeces to soften sufficiently to pass through a narrowed bowel.

For complete or partial bowel obstruction, secondary symptom management is important to maintain the patient's QoL. Table 40.6 summarizes the management of secondary symptoms that may be experienced in complete or partial bowel obstruction.

Table 40.5 Management of symptoms associated with bowel obstruction

Management approach	Indications
Dexamethasone 8–16mg daily SC before midday	• To increase water and salt absorption
	• To reduce oedema around tumour (limited evidence of its effectiveness)
	• Adverse effects: prolonged use may lead to problematic symptoms from steroid use, e.g. diabetes mellitus, agitation, depression, oedema, and Cushing's syndrome
NG tube	• Patient experiencing uncontrollable faecal vomiting
	• Large-volume vomits
	• Adverse effects: impact on patient's perception of body image, may reduce fluid absorption
Octreotide Starting dose 250–500 micrograms daily Maximum dose 750 micrograms daily	• For reduction of, and to encourage reabsorption of, gut secretions through:
	• Direct anti-cancer effect on solid tumours of the GI tract
	• Decreasing gut motility
	• Increasing water and electrolyte absorption
	• Decreasing carbohydrate absorption
	• Decreasing nausea and vomiting
	• Adverse effects: insulinoma, dry mouth, flatulence, anorexia, nausea, vomiting, bloating, abdominal pain, diarrhoea, steatorrhoea

Further information on drug management of bowel obstruction and contraindications can be found in the *British National Formulary* (available at: ◌ http://www.bnf.org

Table 40.6 Management of secondary symptoms associated with bowel obstruction

Symptom	Management
Nausea and vomiting (⊖ see Chapter 44, Nausea and vomiting)	• First line: cyclizine 100–150mg SC in 24 hours • Second line: haloperidol 3–5mg SC in 24 hours (this can be either with or without cyclizine) • Third line: levomepromazine 6.25–25mg in 24 hours. Low doses (6.25mg) are effective in the majority of individuals and should not cause sedation.
Abdominal cramp	• Hyoscine butylbromide 40–100mg SC in 24 hours • It may also be necessary to consider centrally acting analgesic drugs if pain persists, e.g. morphine
Loss of appetite	• Control of associated symptoms that reduce appetite, i.e. nausea and vomiting • Small and frequent meals
Constipation (partial obstruction only)	• Stop stimulant, osmotic, or bulk-forming laxatives to avoid pain from peristalsis • Consider faecal softener e.g. sodium docusate 100–500mg in divided doses • Consider rectal laxatives, i.e. arachis oil enema, to soften faeces in the rectum
Diarrhoea	• Codeine 30–60mg orally four times daily • Loperamide 2–4mg orally 4-hourly • This should be considered with caution if there is any chance of the obstruction being reversible, as it could make constipation and secondary symptoms of obstruction (i.e. pain) worse

Further reading

Dalal KM, Gollub MJ, Miner TJ, et al. Management of patients with malignant bowel obstruction and stage IV colorectal cancer. *J Palliat Med* 2011;14:822.

Tuca A, Guell E, Martinez-Losada E, Codorniu N. Malignant bowel obstruction in advanced cancer patients: epidemiology, management, and factors influencing spontaneous resolution. *Cancer Manage Res* 2012;4:159–69.

Cancer-related breathlessness

Causes, diagnosis, and assessment

Breathlessness is the experience of shortness of breath, of difficult or un-comfortable breathing. It is a very unpleasant and frightening experience, often associated with anxiety and distress and a sensation of suffocating. It can cause profound disability, limiting the patient's function and drastically reducing the QoL, for the family as well as the patient. Breathlessness is a complex, multidimensional problem, with physiological and psychological components. It can be associated with a range of malignancies but is most common in patients with primary lung cancer.

There is a role for specialist lung cancer nurses, social workers, and occupational and physiotherapists in the management of breathlessness. Patients being managed at home will need to have the full support of the primary care team to enable them to remain as independent as possible.

Causes

A central feature of the management of breathlessness is dealing with underlying processes, so it is important to establish the cause of the breathlessness.

Breathlessness as a direct consequence of malignancy
- Intrinsic or extrinsic airway constriction or obstruction with associated lung infection or collapse.
- Lymphangitis carcinomatosis or mediastinal lymphadenopathy.
- Involvement of the pleura.
- Pericardial involvement.
- Vessel involvement.
- Chest wall involvement.
- Phrenic nerve paralysis and diaphragmatic involvement.

Breathlessness as an indirect consequence of malignancy
- Embolism, e.g. PE.
- Pneumonia.
- Pneumothorax.
- Symptomatic anaemia.
- Chronic cancer folic acid and vitamin B12 deficiency.
- Respiratory muscle weakness (severe).
- Cachexia–anorexia syndrome.
- Drug-induced (corticosteroids, benzodiazepines).
- Electrolyte imbalances/abnormalities.
- Paraneoplastic syndrome of malignancy.

Breathlessness as a consequence of treatment
- Surgery, e.g. pneumonectomy, lobectomy.
- Radiation-induced pneumonitis or fibrosis, pericarditis.
- Chemotherapy-induced pulmonary and cardiac toxicity,
- Myelosuppression.

Diagnosis

Physical signs, such as nasal flaring, hyperpnoea (↑ rate and depth of breathing), use of accessory muscles, and tachypnoea (rapid breathing), are all associated with the subjective experience of shortness of breath.

Concurrent respiratory and general symptoms associated with breathlessness are important diagnostic features, e.g. cough, sputum, haemoptysis, fatigue, insomnia, pain, loss of appetite, anxiety, and depression.

Accurate diagnosis is dependent on a thorough history, clinical assessment, examination, and targeted investigations. For patients with advanced disease, CXR, routine blood tests, and pulse oximetry are the most useful investigations.

Assessment

Nurses have a considerable contribution to make to a comprehensive patient-centred approach to the assessment of breathlessness. To be effective, an assessment must be individualized. The essential areas an assessment should cover are:

- When did the breathlessness first become a problem?
- How did it start, and was it acute or gradual?
- What does being breathless feel like? Ask the person to think about its emotional and physical characteristics.
- How frequently does breathlessness occur? Is it continuous, occurring even at rest, or does it vary?
- Are there any precipitating or exacerbating factors—activity, wind, temperature, laughing, or eating, for example?
- Has the person experienced any attacks of breathlessness, and if so, how long does it take to recover after an attack?
- Does the breathlessness—or the fear of it—stop the individual from doing things? What does the breathlessness mean to the individual and their family?
- A simple scale of 0–10 (where 0 is not being breathless and 10 is the worst breathlessness you can imagine) can be a quick assessment tool.

Management

Cancer-directed therapies and interventions

Chemotherapy, radiotherapy, and hormonal therapy can provide some symptomatic relief for patients with treatment-sensitive primary and metastatic disease. Breathlessness associated with responsive anaemia, malignant pleural effusions, airway obstruction, ascites, and SVCO is often best managed by treating the underlying cause.

Outside of this, however, breathlessness can be hard to manage, but improvements can be made through a number of approaches, either concurrently or sequentially. Non-pharmacological approaches should be considered in the first instance.

Non-pharmacological approaches

Fan therapy

Orofacial cooling with a fan, especially to the area of the face supplied by the trigeminal nerve, reduces the sensation of breathlessness. This should be explained to patients who should be encouraged to try this, as it can offer some immediate benefit. Handheld fans are cheap, easily available, portable, and safe. Additionally, it acts as a tool over which the patient has a sense of control.

Relaxation techniques

Relaxation strategies can offer some simple steps to help 'undo' established reactions to breathlessness. This can increase a patient's sense of control in recovering their breath (➜ see Progressive muscle relaxation, p. 588).

Positioning

Leaning forward from the hips, when sitting with the forearms resting above the knees, can increase abdominal pressure and promote improved respiratory muscle function. Directing a person to relax with a slow out-breath, as they let their shoulders 'drop and flop' into a relaxed position, can help achieve greater relaxation of the shoulders, upper back, and neck. If accessory muscles are required for breathing, resting a hand on the upper back or moving it slowly in a downward movement can encourage slower breathing.

Controlled breathing techniques

Breathing retraining or controlled breathing techniques involve sitting upright, breathing in through the nose and out through the mouth, and focusing on using the diaphragm. Pursed lip breathing (PLB) helps slow breathing down by prolonging exhalation. These techniques help develop a slower, relaxed, and more efficient breathing pattern.

Activity pacing and planning

Helping the patient and family learn to plan and pace activities is central to promoting self-care and well-being. Finding ways of integrating controlled breathing techniques, relaxation, and new techniques for washing, dressing, and climbing stairs into a person's daily life requires sensitive, skilled, and knowledgeable caring.

Pharmacological approaches

Opioids, benzodiazepines, corticosteroids, bronchodilators, and oxygen (O_2) are the main pharmacological treatments used for relief of breathlessness. The primary aim in the management of breathlessness is to reverse any condition that may result in, or exacerbate existing, shortness of breath. For example, if shortness of breath is caused by sepsis or fluid overload, antibiotics or diuretics may be prescribed. If breathlessness is caused by SVCO, radiotherapy may treat the obstructive effects of the tumour and corticosteroids reduce oedema (➔ see Superior vena cava obstruction, pp. 645–6).

Oxygen

O_2 therapy is commonly used as the first-line intervention for symptomatic relief of an acute exacerbation of breathlessness. However, most breathless patients will not benefit from O_2, unless their O_2 saturations are below the normal range (SaO_2 <90%). Where O_2 is required, administration via nasal cannulae, rather than a face mask, can reduce oral dryness and inhibition of social interaction.

If a patient's O_2 saturations are within the normal range (SaO_2 >90%), the patient and family can be reassured that O_2 is not required and that other non-pharmacological interventions (as described previously) may be more beneficial.

Opioids

Opioids are commonly used for breathlessness management within cancer palliation. In patients who have not taken opioids before (opioid-naïve), doses should start at 2.5–5mg of oral morphine, either 4-hourly or as needed, to bring about therapeutic benefit. In patients already taking morphine, a dose increment may be indicated, although evidence to support this is equivocal. Morphine seems to alter the sensation of breathlessness for some patients by decreasing the ventilatory drive, and thus decreasing the level of distress experienced from breathlessness. There is no evidence to support the use of nebulized morphine.

Benzodiazepines

Benzodiazepines, such as lorazepam, can be used to ease the psychological aspects of breathlessness. Where this is associated with acute feelings of panic, midazolam may be used. Benzodiazepines with opioids may be used to provide a sedative effect for terminal breathlessness during the final hours or days of life.

Other pharmacological interventions

Commonly used methods to relieve breathlessness include: corticosteroids for inflammatory aetiology, bronchodilators for airway obstruction, antibiotics, anticholinergics, nebulized saline, anticoagulants, and diuretics.

Further reading

Barnes H, McDonald J, Smallwood N, Manser R. Opioids for the palliation of refractory breathlessness in adults with advanced disease and terminal illness. *Cochrane Database Syst Rev* 2016;3:CD011008.

Booth S, Burkin J, Moffat C, Spathis A. *Managing Breathlessness in Clinical Practice*. London: Springer-Verlag; 2014.

Bredin M, Corner J, Krishnasamy M, Plant H, Bailey C, A'hern R. Multicentre randomized controlled trial of nursing intervention for breathlessness in patients with lung cancer. *BMJ* 1999;**318**:901–4.

Cancer-related fatigue

Nature and assessment of cancer-related fatigue

Fatigue is one of the most common and distressing symptoms experienced by people with cancer, occurring in up to 80% of people having treatment. Cancer-related fatigue (CRF) is characterized by a subjective feeling of tiredness, weakness, or lack of energy. It is different from the usual tiredness experienced after exertion, as it is not relieved by rest. It tends to be pervasive and affect both mental processes, like concentration and attention, and physical processes, restricting activities and potentially leading to social isolation.

> 'I couldn't overcome it. I couldn't force myself... the fatigue was overwhelming ... there would be times when you might be tired but you can make yourself do it anyway. I couldn't make myself do things anyway during certain phases of it. So it was just overwhelming.'[1]

All patients should be informed of the likelihood of CRF and given advice on self-care, so that they have the means to manage it and not be overwhelmed by it. CRF can occur at any stage of cancer, becoming more common with advancing disease, and it may persist for long periods after treatment. It is associated with all forms of cancer treatments, including surgery, radiotherapy, chemotherapy, and biological therapies. In spite of this, the underlying processes and pathophysiology of CRF are not fully understood. Causes of fatigue are complex and multifactorial.

CRF is associated with the following problems:[2]

- Psychological: depression, anxiety, frustration, irritability, loss of enjoyment of life
- Functional: inactivity, disruption of usual activities, weakness, deconditioning, loss of appetite
- Cognitive: poor concentration and attention, poor problem-solving and decision-making
- Social and occupational: social withdrawal, inability to perform usual roles, at home and at work, inability to work, and loss of income.

CRF can have a profound impact on the person, their sense of self, and their roles in the family:

> ' ... I constantly feel that if I'm not producing something—either a clean house or a beautiful garden or, you know, making something—that there's something, I should be doing something.'[3]

It also commonly occurs with:

- Poor sleep
- Pain
- Anaemia
- Nutritional deficiency
- 'Secondary fatigue': lack of activity, leading to muscular and cardiorespiratory deconditioning.

Assessment of cancer-related fatigue

In practice, if time is limited, the patient may be asked the three following questions to ascertain the presence, severity, and effects of fatigue:[4]

- Are you experiencing any fatigue?
- If yes, how severe has it been, on average, during the past week, using a scale of 0–10 scale?
- How is the fatigue interfering with your ability to function?

Screening for fatigue can be made by asking the patient to rate their fatigue on a scale of 0–10. On this scale, 0–3 can be judged as mild, 4–6 as moderate, and 7–10 as severe. Alternatively, if they find this scale difficult, the patient can be asked to evaluate their fatigue as mild, moderate, or severe. Patients experiencing mild fatigue may be given further information on fatigue and management strategies. Those reporting moderate to severe fatigue should receive a more detailed fatigue assessment. This should comprise the following factors.

- Focused history of the fatigue:
  - Disease and treatment status; is this associated with disease recurrence?
  - Onset and duration of fatigue
  - Nature and effects on lifestyle
  - Factors that make it better or worse
  - Restrictions on function, activity, and daily living
  - Availability of support and carers.
- Assessment of treatable factors:
  - Pain
  - Emotional factors, including depression and anxiety
  - Sleep disturbance
  - Anaemia
  - Dyspnoea
  - Nutritional deficiency and loss of appetite
  - Prescribed medication and side effects
  - Use of alcohol and non-prescribed drugs
  - Comorbidities.

Note that treating contributing factors will not necessarily reduce the fatigue but will improve the overall QoL. Clinical assessment tools for fatigue are also available.[5]

Referencesc

1 Wu H-S, McSweeney M. Cancer-related fatigue: 'It's so much more than just being tired'. *Eur J Oncol Nurs* 2007;**11**:117–25.
2 Given B. Cancer-related fatigue: a brief overview of current nursing: perspectives and experiences. *Clin J Oncol Nurs* 2008;**12**(5 Suppl):7–9.
3 Oktay JS, Bellin MH, Scarvalone S, Appling S, Helzlsouer KJ. Managing the impact of posttreatment fatigue on the family: breast cancer survivors share their experiences. *Fam Syst Health* 2011;**29**:127–37.
4 Portenoy RK, Itri L. Cancer-related fatigue: guidelines for evaluation and management. *Oncologist* 1999;**4**:1–10.
5 Stone PC, Minton O. Cancer-related fatigue. *Eur J Cancer* 2008;**44**:1097–104.

Management of cancer-related fatigue

Many of the fatigue management strategies are psychosocial or behavioural, so education and counselling are central to the effective management of fatigue. Patients on treatment may believe that fatigue is a sign of disease progression and may be cautious about discussing it. It is important to work with the patient's current understanding of the nature and effects of fatigue, to build on this, and to include any positive strategies the patient already has for alleviating the fatigue.

The patient's clinical status, including treatment, comorbidities, and stage of disease, will influence management and treatment strategies. Approaches to managing CRF should address any factors contributing to its onset or maintenance. This includes treating any identified causes or associated symptoms, e.g. pain, depression, anaemia.

Psychosocial interventions for cancer-related fatigue

A number of psychosocial interventions are available to help patients to live and cope with fatigue. It is important to coordinate these interventions with other MDT members, including occupational therapists and physiotherapists. They include:

- **Education**: education or **psychoeducational interventions** will include information about the nature of fatigue and recommendations for self-management, including guidance on activity and exercise, energy conservation, sleep hygiene, attention restoration, and how to seek and use social and professional support. Keeping a diary of activities, fatigue severity, feelings, symptoms, and self-management strategies is one straightforward educational intervention. Psychoeducational interventions are often given in group formats and aim to foster self-efficacy and a sense of personal control.
- **Exercise and activity**: promotes ↑ functional capacity and psychological well-being, and it has a good evidence base. It can include, for example, resistive exercises, stretching, walking, swimming, or cycling. It is advisable to build up the level of activity over time, taking care not to overdo it, but to achieve a degree of balance and consistency. It often helps to have a friend or family member support the patient or, where possible, a professional such as an occupational therapist or a physiotherapist. Activity may be a preferable term if exercise sounds daunting to the patient or if functional capacity is limited. Exercise can also be done in professionally led groups. Caution should be taken if patients have comorbidities like bony metastasis, bone marrow immunosuppression, or other treatment complications.
- **Energy conservation**: is the deliberate planning and management of personal energy resources to avoid exhaustion, balancing activity and rest to enable valued activities to take place. This involves setting priorities and personal goals, pacing activity, and delegating tasks, often based around a structured daily routine and activity scheduling. Rest alone does not improve CRF and may make it worse if it results in deconditioning.

- **Sleep hygiene**: promotes refreshing sleep by establishing a consistent sleep routine, maintaining the bedroom as a place for sleeping and intimacy only, avoiding food and stimulants like coffee just before bedtime, not taking naps, and ensuring enough activity, light, and fresh air during the day.
- **Attention-restoring interventions**: mental fatigue can impair the ability to acquire and retain information, make decisions, or comply with treatment. Attention restoration involves helping the patient to choose activities that help focus concentration and mental energy. These activities should be chosen by the patient and have the following qualities: be interesting and not boring, be a change from routines and concerns, and be enjoyable or pleasing. Activities involving nature are thought to be particularly restful and restorative, so they could include looking at nature, listening to birds, gardening, or involving a favourite hobby like reading or craft work. They should be carried out regularly, e.g. 30 minutes 3–4 times a week.
- **Psychological therapies**:
  - CBT (➔ see Cognitive behavioural therapy, p. 132), including activity scheduling, can be an effective treatment for depression and sleep problems
  - Mindfulness and mindfulness-based stress reduction (MBSR) (➔ see Mindfulness, p. 132) have value in managing depressive mood and stress and improving coping
  - Relaxation techniques, including progressive muscle relaxation (➔ see Relaxation training, p. 588), may reduce tension and feelings of tiredness

Pharmacological approaches to cancer-related fatigue

The most commonly used pharmacological approaches include:
- **Psychostimulants**: commonly used in fatigue management, aiding concentration, and there is evidence to support the use of methylphenidate
- **Treatment of depression**: antidepressants will alleviate mood in depressed patients, though they may not have a significant impact on the fatigue itself
- **Corticosteroids**: such as prednisolone or dexamethasone, are often prescribed for their effects on appetite, mood, and energy levels. However, there is limited evidence for their effectiveness as a treatment for fatigue
- **Treatment of anaemia**: the causes of anaemia need to be properly investigated. Iron or folic acid supplements may help. Red cell transfusions may also be prescribed (➔ see Blood product support, pp. 488–93). Haematopoietic growth factors, including EPO and darbepoetin alfa may improve CRF in anaemic patients; however, there are a number of safety concerns that make them unsuitable for routine practice
- **Progestogens**: such as medroxyprogesterone acetate (MPA) or megestrol acetate (MA), are prescribed to relieve anorexia and cachexia in patients whose fatigue may be related to cachexia.

Websites

Macmillan Cancer Support. *Side Effects and Symptoms: Tiredness (Fatigue)*. Available at: ℘ https://www.macmillan.org.uk/information-and-support/coping/side-effects-and-symptoms/tiredness

National Comprehensive Cancer Network (NCCN). *NCCN Guidelines for Supportive Care*. Available at: ℘ http://www.nccn.org/professionals/physician_gls/f_guidelines.asp#supportive

Further reading

Du S, Hu L, Dong J, *et al.* Patient education programs for cancer-related fatigue: a systematic review. *Patient Educ Couns* 2015;98:1308–19.

Meneses-Echávez JF, González-Jiménez E, Ramírez-Vélez R. Effects of supervised exercise on cancer-related fatigue in breast cancer survivors: a systematic review and meta-analysis. *BMC Cancer* 2015;15:77.

Mitchell SA, Hoffman AJ, Clark JC, *et al.* Putting evidence into practice: an update of evidence-based interventions for cancer-related fatigue during and following treatment. *Clin J Oncol Nurs* **18**(Suppl):38–58.

Scott JA, Lasch KE, Barsevick AM, Piault-Louis E. Patients' experiences with cancer-related fatigue: a review and synthesis of qualitative research. *Oncol Nurs Forum* 2011;38:E191–203.

Malignant effusions

Introduction

Malignant effusions are abnormal collections of fluid. They most commonly occur in the peritoneal or pleural space. They are generally a sign of advanced metastatic disease. They can be managed, but the fluid normally reaccumulates, often within a short space of time.

Malignant ascites

Malignant ascites is accumulation of fluid in the peritoneal cavity. It occurs when the volume of naturally occurring fluid of the peritoneal lining (situated between the parietal and visceral peritoneal membranes) is too great to drain away through the diaphragmatic lymphatic vessels, or when the drainage pathways become blocked. It is most commonly associated with ovarian, colon, breast, and pancreatic cancers and adenocarcinoma of unknown origin.[1]

Aetiology

Malignant ascites may result from:
- Tumour compression of the hepatobiliary blood vessels
- ↑ permeability of the peritoneal lining and cavity (particularly the omentum), or the tumour itself may produce fluid
- Obstruction of diaphragmatic lymphatic vessels
- Hypoproteinaemia (low level of circulating protein), leading to movement of fluid from the circulation into central oedema and ascites.

Most commonly, ascitic fluid is an exudate, which is high in protein. More rarely, where a cancer causes hepatic failure or portal hypertension, ascites can be a 'transudate', which is more dilute and low in protein.

Presenting symptoms
- Abdominal discomfort (pain).
- Feeling bloated and uncomfortable.
- Nausea and vomiting.
- Inability to sit or bend easily.
- Loss of appetite, indigestion.
- Fatigue, breathlessness.
- Distress associated with altered body image.

Diagnosis
- Drainage and cytological examination of the fluid.
- Disease history.
- Detailed observation and assessment of patient problems.

Treatment

Treatment is suggested when the symptoms of malignant ascites are distressing, particularly abdominal pain and breathlessness.

Evidence is limited about which the best treatment is.[1] The main approaches include:
- **Paracentesis**: drainage of fluid from the peritoneal cavity using a catheter. The catheter may be placed by US guidance.
  - Rate of drainage—practice varies. Some centres allow free drainage for the first 5L. There is little evidence of causing hypovolaemic shock.

However, if the patient is hypotensive, drainage can be stopped temporarily. Other guidelines are more cautious—1L every 2 hours.
- No evidence of benefit from albumin post-drainage.
- Catheters are removed generally once drainage has slowed significantly or after 24 hours. Any longer increases the risk of infection.
- Pain management: insertion and removal of the catheters can be painful, and patients may have abdominal pain/discomfort during fluid removal. Adequate analgesia should be prescribed and administered throughout.
- **Indwelling catheter**: a semi-permanent drainage catheter left *in situ* to enable drainage of fluid at home. This requires either stoma nurse or community nurse involvement. There is some evidence that the rate of infection is higher than that for paracentesis alone, but despite this, the methodology is becoming more common. This is largely because it allows patients with a short prognosis more time at home and fewer visits to hospital for repeated paracentesis.
- **Diuretic therapy**: this has been widely used to manage malignant ascites in the past, but in recent years, its popularity has waned as there is real uncertainty about its efficacy. It may cause dehydration, with limited impact on peritoneal fluid volume.
- **Peritoneovenous shunt**: a shunt is placed in the peritoneal cavity, under local anaesthetic. It tunnels under the skin and enters the vena cava. Fluid shifts along the shunt due to pressure changes during breathing. It can reduce the need for further paracentesis and can relieve symptoms. Limitations include shunts blocking or becoming infected.
- **Palliative chemotherapy**: this may be given to try and shrink the tumour, therefore reducing obstruction and potentially relieving ascites.

Nursing management

Malignant ascites is a distressing and debilitating consequence of cancer. Abdominal discomfort, fatigue (➲ see Chapter 42 Cancer-related fatigue), and alterations in body image (➲ see Body image, p. 607) all require skilled nursing support. Comprehensive nursing assessment of this problem will allow nurses to support patients and their families to live with its demands, which often necessitate frequent hospital or hospice admission as the disease advances. Informational support about the different approaches to management is required, particularly as there is limited evidence about their effectiveness.

References

1 Royal College of Obstetricians and Gynaecologists (2014). *Management of Ascites in Ovarian Cancer Patients*. Scientific Impact Paper No. 45. Available at: ℅ https://www.rcog.org.uk/globalassets/documents/guidelines/scientific-impact-papers/sip45ascites.pdf

Malignant pleural effusion

Pleural effusion is the accumulation of fluid in the pleural space (between the parietal and visceral layers encasing the lungs). It can be caused by malignant and non-malignant triggers such as infection, severe burns, or congestive cardiac failure. Almost half of patients diagnosed with lung or breast cancer will develop an effusion during their illness, and malignant pleural effusions are present in ~50% of patients who die of cancer.

Aetiology

Malignant pleural effusions may occur for several reasons:
- Infiltration of the pleura by the tumour
- Alteration in the integrity of the pleural lymphatic system
- Metastatic spread to the visceral pleural surface or to the parietal pleura
- Confounding comorbid conditions such as renal failure, congestive cardiac failure, or PE.

Presenting symptoms

- Breathlessness, cough, chest pain.
- General flu-like malaise.
- Anorexia and weight loss may also be present.

Diagnosis

- Detailed observation and assessment of the patient's presenting problems.
- On auscultation, ↓ breath sounds, dullness to percussion, and ↓ fremitus (vibration felt by a hand placed on the chest when the patient speaks or coughs).
- Tracheal deviation—if the effusion is large.
- CXR.
- US and CT may be helpful if the effusion is small or the fluid is loculated (in pockets).
- Thoracocentesis—if the effusion is confirmed in the absence of an enlarged heart or if cancer is strongly suspected.
- Other options include thoracoscopy, pleuroscopy, or surgical biopsy.

Treatment

- If a patient is asymptomatic, surveillance alone may be the treatment option of choice.
- If the primary tumour is amenable to treatment, the effusion may resolve once systematic treatment is established.

For symptomatic patients

Thoracocentesis and tube drainage
- Small-bore tube introduced after local anaesthetic under CT or US guidance.
- Position and absence of pneumothorax checked on X-ray.
- Tube aspirated and placed on low suction.
- Generally followed by sclerosis to prevent reaccumulation of the fluid.

Sclerosis (pleurodesis)
- Obliterates the pleural space.
- Sclerotic agent introduced into the pleural space.
- Agents used include tetracycline or its derivatives, bleomycin, and sterile talc.

Tunnelled long-term catheters and drainage
- Can be useful in the community setting, reducing the need for regular hospital admission.
- This technique is becoming more popular and widely used, as there is evidence that it is more effective than thoracocentesis and pleurodesis at reducing discomfort, providing long-term effective drainage and improving patient QoL.[2] In addition, patients can be cared for at home with the catheters *in situ*.

Pleuroperitoneal shunting
- Can be used when pleurodesis is not possible or is unsuccessful.

Nursing management
Thoracocentesis
Patients should be pre-medicated with an opioid analgesic and have regular monitoring of pain post-procedure. Patients also need monitoring of temperature, signs of respiratory distress, or bleeding, which could indicate infection, pneumothorax, or haemothorax.

Pleurodesis
Patients often get severe pleuritic pain with pleurodesis, even with intrapleural local anaesthetic. Sedation and opioids may both be required. Patients need assistance with repositioning post-procedure to enable the sclerosing agent to contact the entire pleural surface.

Indwelling pleuritic drains
The insertion of tunnelled indwelling pleuritic drains requires the input of a skilled radiologist and post-procedure observation and monitoring. Following this, the catheter requires some care, observation, and, of course, drainage of the fluid. The tubes have an integrated one-way valve to prevent air from flowing into the pleural cavity. Patients should be cared for at home and regularly observed for signs of infection, increasing shortness of breath, or haemorrhage.

Overall effective nursing management of patients with malignant pleural effusions requires skill and expert knowledge. Presenting symptoms, such as breathlessness (➔ see Chapter 41, Breathlessness), are frightening, and patients normally have a poor prognosis with advanced disease. The choices of treatment are complex and involve procedures that are sometimes invasive, painful, and frightening.

Further reading
Roberts ME, Neville E, Berrisford RG, Antunes G, Ali NJ. Management of a malignant pleural effusion: British Thoracic Society pleural disease guideline. *Thorax* 2010;65(Suppl 2):ii32eii40. Available at: ℘ http://thorax.bmj.com/content/65/Suppl_2/ii32.full.pdf+html

References
2 Demmy TL et al. Comparison of indwelling catheters and talc pleurodesis in the management of malignant pleural effusions. *Clin Oncol* 2010;28(Suppl):15s (abstr 9031).

Nausea and vomiting

Treatment-related nausea and vomiting

Introduction

Definitions

Nausea is an unpleasant feeling of the need to vomit, often accompanied by autonomic sensations. Vomiting is the forceful expulsion of gastric contents through the mouth. Retching is an attempt to vomit that does not expel any stomach contents. Nausea is generally the most distressing long-term symptom of these, but it is often under-assessed.

Physiology

The physiology of nausea and vomiting is not fully understood. Evidence suggests that both are coordinated by the vomiting centre (VC) and the chemoreceptor trigger zone (CTZ) in the midbrain. Key chemoreceptors involved in the process of relaying messages from various organs to the VC include serotonin (5HT3), dopamine, substance P/neurokinin-1, histamine, and acetylcholine.

Common causes of nausea and vomiting

- Chemotherapy or radiotherapy.
- Infection.
- Drugs, e.g. opioids, antibiotics, NSAIDs, digoxin.
- GI stasis, intestinal obstruction.
- Pain.
- Metabolic, e.g. hypercalcaemia, renal failure.
- Brain metastases (raised ICP).
- Psychosomatic, e.g. fear, anxiety.

Radiotherapy-induced nausea and vomiting (RINV)

The site of radiotherapy treatment will determine the risk of nausea and vomiting. Higher doses of radiation, longer duration of treatment, and a larger treatment field will also increase the risk.

High risk	Intermediate risk
• Total body irradiation	• Abdominal pelvic
• Whole or upper abdominal	• Cranium
• Hemi-body irradiation	• Craniospinal
• Lower thorax	• Mantle

For high-risk radiotherapy, administer a 5HT3 antagonist (such as ondansetron) prior to each treatment. Add in dexamethasone if nausea or vomiting is not controlled. If still unsuccessful, follow the chemotherapy-induced nausea and vomiting (CINV) guidelines (→ see Chemotherapy-induced nausea and vomiting, p. 532).

For intermediate risk, use metoclopramide or domperidone. Swap to a 5HT3 antagonist if it is not controlled.

Chemotherapy-induced nausea and vomiting

Nausea and vomiting are two of the most distressing symptoms of chemotherapy treatment. They impact on QoL, cause a range of other side effects such as malnutrition and oesophageal injury, and can affect treatment compliance.

Up to 70% of patients receiving chemotherapy will experience some nausea and vomiting, although it is highly regimen-dependent, though the introduction of 5HT3 antagonists has dramatically improved the management of CINV in recent years.

CINV generally occurs in three distinct phases

1. **Anticipatory nausea and vomiting**: this occurs prior to a new cycle of chemotherapy.
2. **Acute nausea and vomiting**: this occurs in the first 24-hour period after chemotherapy.
3. **Delayed nausea and vomiting**: this occurs >24 hours and can last for several days post-chemotherapy. May have a more complex mechanisms of action than acute nausea and vomiting. Common in platinum-based regimes and anthracyclines combined with cyclophosphamide.

Management of CINV

Pre-treatment assessment

Prevention is key, as once CINV occurs, it can be difficult to control. Accurate assessment is a crucial part of management. The following must be considered:

- Emetogenic potential of the chemotherapy regimen—consider drugs, dose, and schedule (see Table 44.1)
- Other causes of nausea and vomiting (➔ see Common causes of nausea and vomiting, p. 532)
- Patient risk factors: those that increase the risk of CINV include age (being younger), ♀, history of motion sickness, previous uncontrolled nausea/vomiting after chemotherapy, severe pregnancy-related sickness, and high levels of anxiety.

A history of chronic alcohol ingestion actually reduces the risk of CINV.

Table 44.1 Level of emetogenicity of common cytotoxic agents

High-risk agents (>90%)	Moderate-risk agents (30–90%)	Low-risk agents (<30%)
• Cisplatin >50mg/m^2	• Cyclophosphamide <1g/m^2	• Methotrexate <250g/m^2
• Carmustine >250mg/m^2	• Carmustine <250mg/m^2	• Mitoxantrone
• Cyclophosphamide >1g/m^2	• Cisplatin <50mg/m^2	• Asparaginase
• Lomustine >60mg/m^2	• Anthracyclines	• Cytarabine
• Dacarbazine >500mg/m^2	• Carboplatin	• Docetaxel
	• Irinotecan	• Paclitaxel
	• Melphalan	• 5FU
	• Oxaliplatin	• Gemcitabine
	• Methotrexate >1g/m^2	
	• Cytarabine >1g/m^2	

Note: in combination chemotherapy regimes, the level of emetogenicity is based on the combination of drugs. Therefore, two moderate drugs combined may be classed as high risk. Also most of the novel and targeted therapies generally have a low emetogenic potential.

Note: if a patient has two or more risk factors, consider starting them on a higher level of anti-emetic cover than normal for any specific chemotherapy regimen.

Nurses have a major role in both pre- and post-treatment assessment. A thorough initial assessment will establish any risk factors for nausea and vomiting, beyond the actual chemotherapy regimen.

Drug management
- Anti-emetic drugs are the cornerstone of managing CINV. They usually act by competitively blocking receptors for serotonin, histamine, and dopamine at the CTZ and VC.
- Table 44.2 highlights the main approaches for managing both acute and delayed symptoms. If there is a risk of delayed nausea and vomiting, the anti-emetic course should be continued for 72 hours post-chemotherapy. In the UK, each clinical area should have a protocol for the management of CINV, which should be followed.
- Akynzeo® (combination of netupitant/palonosetron capsules) has recently been shown to be more effective than palonosetron alone and may be considered for use in some highly emetogenic regimens and delayed nausea and vomiting.

Table 44.2 Pharmacological management of CINV

Emetogenic risk	Acute symptoms	Followed by	Delayed symptoms
High (including anthracycline + cyclophosphamide)	(aprepitant, or fosaprepitant) + 5HT3 antagonist + dexamethasone	NK1R antagonist + dexamethasone*	Moderate
5HT3 antagonist + dexamethasone	Dexamethasone	Low	Single agent, e.g. dexamethasone, 5HT3 antagonist, or a dopamine receptor antagonist
No routine prophylactic anti-emetics	Minimal	Nothing	No routine prophylactic anti-emetics

Notes:

* Dexamethasone only if fosaprepitant available and used on day 1.

There are no clinically meaningful differences between the currently available 5HT3 antagonists. Oral and IV regimens are equivalent when correctly dosed.

If there is failure at one level, then move up to the next level, i.e. from low to moderate or moderate to high. If failure occurs at the top level, then add in other class of anti-emetic.

Remember to reassess, and consider other causes of nausea and vomiting in cases of resistant CINV, particularly in patients with advanced disease.

Data sourced from UKONs Acute Oncology Prevention & Management Guidelines: CINV 2013 & MASCC/ESMO guidelines 2013.

Note: these have been developed by joint American and European oncology groups and are updated on a regular basis.

Side effects of anti-emetics

Many anti-emetics themselves carry potentially significant side effects. The side effects of the most common anti-emetics, plus their management, are highlighted in Table 44.3.

Management of anti-emetic failure

Despite the use of anti-emetic regimes and effective assessment, many patients will still experience CINV. Once treatment has started, nurses need to assess any nausea and vomiting, including:

- The number of episodes, their time, and their duration. Ensure that you assess separately for nausea and vomiting (see Table 44.4)
- The effectiveness of any drug/non-drug measures
- The behavioural, emotional, and physical impact of the symptoms (➔ see Nursing management of nausea and vomiting, p. 538).

Additional anti-emetics

If one level of the regimen fails, then move the anti-emetics to a higher level, e.g. from a low emetic regime to a moderate one.

If failure persists at the top level, then consider empirical-based additional anti-emetics, e.g.:

- Can consider adding in cyclizine or prochlorperazine
- If still failure, then consider adding in haloperidol or levomepromazine, which has effects on a wide range of chemotherapy receptors.

Table 44.3 Side effects of common anti-emetics

Drug classification	Side effects	Management
NK1R antagonists Aprepitant, fosaprepitant	Moderate CYP3A4 inhibitor	Steroid doses may need to be reduced
5HT3 antagonists	ECG changes, headache, constipation, fatigue, dry mouth, dizziness	Care with elderly patients and in hypokalaemia and hypomagnesaemia. Analgesics for headache. Administration of laxatives as required or prophylactically for constipation
Phenothiazines, metoclopramide, and butyrophenones	Extrapyramidal reactions (EPRs), particularly for patients under 30 years of age. Phenothiazines can also cause sedation	Close observation for signs of EPRs, e.g. agitation, restlessness, tremor, muscular or facial twitching
Corticosteroids	Agitation, insomnia, ↑ appetite, dyspepsia, fluid retention. Perirectal burning when given IV	Give IV infusions slowly
Benzodiazepines	Sedation	Use cautiously if patients have poor respiratory status

Table 44.4 CINV grading and management

Grade 1	Grade 2	Grade 3	Grade 4
Nausea: loss of appetite but maintains normal eating habits	Nausea: reduced oral intake, but no significant weight loss, dehydration, or malnutrition	Nausea: inadequate oral/fluid intake; IV fluids or tube feeding needed for ≥24 hours	Nausea/ vomiting: life-threatening consequences
Vomiting: one episode in 24 hours	Vomiting: 2–5 episodes in 24 hours	Vomiting: ≥6 episodes in 24 hours	
Assess daily for signs of dehydration, weight loss, and electrolyte imbalance	Assess 12-hourly. May require hospital admission if evidence of dehydration	Admission essential. For assessment and IV fluids or tube feeding needed for ≥24 hours	Admission essential. For assessment and IV fluids or tube feeding needed for ≥24 hours

Anticipatory nausea and vomiting (ANV)

This is best described by the concept of 'Pavlovian' classical conditioning; the patient associates aspects of the treatment, such as the nurse or the hospital environment, with nausea or vomiting. On future occasions, these associations are enough to cause further nausea or vomiting, even before administration of the chemotherapy.

Risk factors
- People who have had moderate to severe nausea or vomiting after their previous course of chemotherapy.
- Being under 50 years of age.
- Susceptibility to motion sickness.
- Being ♀.
- High levels of anxiety.

Screening for these risk factors could influence preventative management, e.g. increasing initial anti-emetic cover.

Due to the psychological aspects of the condition, use of progressive muscle relaxation treatment (➔ see Progressive muscle relaxation, p. 588), support of a psychological specialist (➔ see Psychological support, pp. 130–1), or benzodiazepines, such as sublingual lorazepam, can be effective.

Note: prevention is key, as once established, ANV can be hard to manage. Initial, effective anti-emetic management is crucial.

Further reading

MASCC/ESMO. Antiemetic Guideline 2013. Available at: ℛ http://www.mascc.org/assets/documents/mascc_guidelines_english_2013.pdf

National Institute for Health and Care Excellence (2016). *Prevention of Chemotherapy Induced Nausea and Vomiting in Adults: Netupitant/Palonosetron*. Evidence summary [ESNM69]. Available at: ℛ https://www.nice.org.uk/advice/esnm69/chapter/key-points-from-the-evidence

UK Oncology Nursing Society (2012). *UKONS: Acute Oncology Prevention and Management Guidelines: Chemotherapy-Induced Nausea and Vomiting (CINV)*. Available at: ℛ http://www.ukons.org

Nausea and vomiting in advanced cancer

Nausea and vomiting are often multi-causal, with different chemoreceptors involved, and a combination of anti-emetics may be required to manage it successfully. Regular nursing assessment is crucial, as the causes of nausea and vomiting may change over time.

Management

Identify potential reversible causes, and ensure they are treated appropriately:
- Pain
- Infection—give antibiotics
- Cough—give an antitussive
- Hypercalcaemia—give fluids and bisphosphonates (➔ see Malignancy-induced hypercalcaemia, p. 637)
- Raised ICP—give corticosteroids
- Emetogenic drugs—stop or reduce dose
- Anxiety—give anxiolytics or psychological management (➔ see Anxiety management, pp. 588–9).

Administer anti-emetics most likely to resolve nausea and vomiting.
- Always give anti-emetics regularly, not as required.
- Oral medication can control nausea, but alternative routes will be required for vomiting such as per rectum or SC.

If this is not successful or partially successful, the patient may require an ↑ dose or a different anti-emetic may be tried.
- If the cause is certain, then the first step is to increase the dose. Otherwise, combine anti-emetics that have different actions.
- Levomepromazine acts on several receptor sites and can be a useful broad-spectrum anti-emetic, though it can cause sedation at doses above 6.25mg twice daily.

Note: cyclizine may antagonize the prokinetic effect of metoclopramide, and they should not usually be given together.

Common causes of nausea and vomiting and drug management options are highlighted in Table 44.5.

Table 44.5 Causes of nausea and vomiting and drug management

Cause of vomiting	Choice of anti-emetics
Drug or endogenous toxins	Haloperidol 1.5mg twice daily
	Levomepromazine 6.25mg
Constipation	Metoclopramide
Gastric stasis	Domperidone
Intestinal obstruction	(➔ See Bowel obstruction, pp. 510–12)
Raised ICP	Cyclizine 150mg/24 hours orally or SC
	Dexamethasone 4–16mg

Nursing management of nausea and vomiting

- Nurses have a key role in assessment. Separately assess nausea and vomiting. Identify potential causes, and ensure treatment of any reversible causes.
- Ensure regular, safe administration of anti-emetics, including frequent observations for common side effects such as EPRs, constipation, and sedation.
- Inform patients of early signs of side effects and the need to alert a health-care professional about these, e.g. contacting their GP or their cancer treatment centre if they are vomiting or nauseated at home.
- Assess fluid balance and manage fluid replacement, including IV as required.
- Assess weight gains or losses, and provide additional nutritional intake as required (◆ see Nutritional support, pp. 542–5).
- Provide vomit bowls, privacy, and regular oral care to maintain comfort.
- Support and advise patients in using non-pharmacological measures as appropriate.

Further reading

Faull C, De Caestecker S, Nicholson A, Black F. *Handbook of Palliative Care*, 3rd ed. Hoboken, NJ: John Wiley & Sons; 2012.

Watson M, Lucas C, Hoy A. *Oxford Handbook of Palliative Care*, 2nd ed. Oxford: Oxford University Press; 2009.

Nutritional disorders

Nutritional issues

Malnutrition

Malnutrition is defined as a severe deficiency of protein and inadequate caloric intake. It occurs when there is an imbalance between dietary intake and nutritional requirements, resulting in wasting of muscle and multisystem dysfunction. There are usually clinical complications such as delayed wound healing, risk of infection, and ↑ mortality. Malnutrition is common in cancer patients and can adversely affect the patient's QoL and survival.

Incidence

Cachexia occurs in around a quarter to one-third of patients with tumours, such as testicular and breast, to around three-quarters of patients with pancreatic, upper GI, and H&N tumours. Evidence has shown that nearly half of all patients with cancer lose >20% of their pre-illness weight.

Causes of malnutrition

- Reduced oral intake—due to anorexia, nausea and vomiting, and altered taste and smell.
- Effects of tumour—due to odynophagia (pain on swallowing), dysphagia, and catabolic effects of the tumour (⟶ see Cancer cachexia, p. 541).
- Psychological—due to depression, anxiety, and food aversions.
- Effects of cancer treatments—such as surgery, chemotherapy, and radiotherapy (see Table 45.1).

Table 45.1 Some common nutritional side effects of cancer treatment

Surgery	Chemotherapy	Radiotherapy (depends on site treated)
• Intestinal resection can cause malabsorption • Reduced capacity to take normal food portions • Problems associated with chewing and swallowing if surgery to H&N region • ↓ intake due to preoperative starvation	• Nausea and vomiting • Mucositis • Diarrhoea • Anorexia • Stomatitis • Learnt food aversions • Fatigue	H&N: • Mucositis • Dry mouth • Pain on swallowing Chest: • Oesophagitis • Dysphagia • Nausea and vomiting Abdomen and pelvis: • Diarrhoea • Nausea and vomiting • Radiation enteritis • Malabsorption

Note: effects may be exacerbated by combination therapies, e.g. surgery and radiotherapy or chemo-irradiation.

Cancer cachexia

This is a complex, multifactorial syndrome characterized by:[1]
- Progressive involuntary weight loss
- Anorexia and early satiety
- Skeletal muscle atrophy
- Generalized tissue wasting
- Immune dysfunction
- Metabolic alterations
- Early satiety.

Cachexia is commonly associated with advanced cancer, and the weight loss seen is due not only to the problems caused by the reduction in food intake, but also by the metabolic abnormalities occurring. Metabolic abnormalities and immune system responses lead to:
- ↑ resting energy expenditure
- Competition between the tumour and the host for nutrients
- ↑ fat breakdown
- Immune response: release of cytokines, e.g. interleukins, interferon, which increase metabolism and reduce appetite.

Clinical effects of cancer cachexia/malnutrition
- Poor tolerance of treatment and ↑ number of treatment breaks.
- Reduction in QoL.
- Higher morbidity and mortality rates.
- Progressive weakness.
- Apathy and irritability.
- Skin breakdown.
- Impaired wound healing.
- Depressed immune system functioning.

Obesity and cancer treatment

There is some evidence to suggest that obesity, particularly when linked to sarcopenia (loss of body muscle), is linked to poorer outcomes for patients receiving chemotherapy for breast and bowel cancer.[2] This finding may be complicated by the fact that many oncologists cap doses of chemotherapy, based on the body surface area, if patients are obese, thus resulting in relative underdosing. A further study has suggested that reducing dietary fat, with modest body weight reduction, in women undergoing standard oncological treatments for early breast cancer (surgery, chemotherapy, radiotherapy, and hormonal manipulation) significantly improves relapse-free survival, although no significant differences were found in overall survival.[3]

References

1 Fearon K, Strasser F, Anker SD, et al. Definition and classification of cancer cachexia: an international consensus. Lancet Oncol 2011;12:489–95.
2 Griggs JJ, Sabel MS. Obesity and cancer treatment: weighing the evidence. J Clin Oncol 2008;26:4060–2.
3 Chlebowski RT, et al. Dietary fat reduction and breast cancer outcome: interim efficacy results from the Women's Intervention Nutrition Study. J Natl Cancer Inst 2006;98:1767–76.

Nutritional support

The aim of nutritional support is to maintain or improve nutritional status and weight and to maintain strength and energy. This can lead to reduced side effects, improve tolerability of treatment, enhance mobility and independence, and maintain or improve QoL.

The main components of nutritional support are:

- Nutritional screening
- Dietary advice
- Oral nutritional supplements
- Enteral nutrition
- Parenteral nutrition.

Nutritional screening

Malnutrition can occur at any point during the course of the cancer journey, and screening must be performed at regular intervals. Screening should be carried out on admission to hospital or first attendance at outpatients to identify patients who are malnourished or at risk of malnutrition. A validated screening tool used nationally is the Malnutrition Universal Screening Tool (MUST), and there is also an American nutritional screening tool developed specifically for cancer patients known as the Patient-Generated— Subjective Global Assessment (PG-SGA). The screening tool is usually completed by nursing staff and is performed to identify those patients who need to be referred on to a qualified, registered dietician for a full dietary assessment and individualized and specific dietary advice and support.

Dietary advice

Increasingly, patients are seeking good advice and guidance on their diet, whilst having cancer treatments. In part, this ↑ interest has been driven by press coverage of studies linking various foods (e.g. 'superfoods') to favourable or unfavourable cancer outcomes. In general terms, there is little evidence to suggest that anything outside a good balanced diet will be of benefit in improving survival or improving the efficacy of treatments.

Patients may require advice and encouragement to modify their general dietary habits and regular meal patterns. For example, they may currently be using a lot of low-fat or low-calorie food products, which may not be appropriate during cancer treatment. Other patients may need information on reducing dietary fat levels and improving the nutritional balance of their diet. Referral to a dietician can provide advice that is tailored to meet the individual patient's needs, whilst taking into account individual and personal food preferences. Regular follow-up from the dietician or nursing staff can promote adherence to any nutritional regimens. In addition, good general advice on diet can be obtained from websites such as Macmillan Cancer Support[4] or the American Cancer Society (ACS).[5]

Oral nutrition support

Oral nutrition is the preferred source of support in patients who are able to consume food and fluid. It is important to keep the patient's diet as closely as possible to normal, as this reinforces the normality of their everyday life. This can be supplemented by commercially available supplements where necessary.

Dietary management
- Texture modification, such as adapting meals, e.g. soft, mashed, or puree.
- Food fortification, including the addition of extra butter, cream, milk, and sugar, to increase energy and calorie content.
- Adaptation of mealtimes: encouraging small frequent meals.

Oral nutrition supplements

Oral nutrition supplements are widely available, can be readily prescribed on the advice of a dietician, and are useful when inadequate dietary intake is identified. Their use must be monitored and reviewed regularly (preferably by a registered dietician) to ensure their effective use. However, if patients report taste fatigue, supplements can be incorporated directly within a meal without too much disruption. The benefits of oral nutrition supplements are to:
- Increase calorie and nitrogen intake
- Stimulate appetite.

Types of oral nutrition supplements

Oral sip feeds
- Various types available, e.g. milk, juice, yoghurt.
- High in calories and protein.
- Some nutritionally complete.
- Some contain eicosapentaenoic acid (EPA), which are *n*-3 fatty acids, and antioxidants which are thought to be of benefit to patients with cancer-related weight loss, as they interfere with the mechanisms of cachexia at multiple levels.

Fortified puddings
- Useful in the case of dysphagic patients who have a delayed swallow.
- Provide calories and protein in smaller volume.

Modular supplements
- Concentrated sources of calories/protein/fat, either individually or in combination.
- Carbohydrate-based powders and drinks should only be given to diabetics under strict supervision.
- Can be incorporated into everyday foods.

Enteral nutrition

May also be referred to as 'tube feeding' where a tube is placed directly into either the stomach or the small intestine via the nose or direct percutaneous route. Commonly used tubes are NG, gastrostomy, and jejunostomy.

Enteral feeding can be used for patients who are not able to take sufficient nutrients orally due to a variety of reasons, such as anorexia, dysphagia, or mucositis, and when the patient has a functioning gut. It is **not** appropriate for the following patients:
- Patients with a bowel blockage
- Patients suffering from severe nausea, vomiting, and/or diarrhoea
- Patients whose stomach or intestine are not working properly or have been removed.

The type of tube used will depend on the tumour site, the anticipated duration of feeding, and the patient's overall physical condition.

Benefits of enteral nutrition
- Nutrition can be delivered past obstructed areas, e.g. H&N.
- Nutrition can be delivered at a slow, continuous rate, permitting optimal use of a limited absorptive capacity over a long period of time.
- Prescribed feeds may be tolerated better than oral nutrition products.

Enteral nutrition can be used as the sole source of nutrition or used in combination with oral or parenteral nutrition. The dietician will calculate the patient's daily nutritional requirements and devise a feeding regimen that takes into account:
- Assessed nutrition needs
- The patient's preference/wishes
- The treatment regimen
- The ability to administer the feed
- Mobility
- Prognosis.

The feed can be given continuously via a pump or intermittently as a bolus feed. Feeds are ready to use in a liquid form and contain energy, protein, fluid, and vitamins and minerals. Common complications of NG feeding include tube displacement, whereas for gastrostomy tubes, complications include pneumoperitoneum, infections, leakage, hypergranulation, and erosion of the tube flange into the gastric mucosa (buried bumper syndrome).

Typical feeds
- Standard feed: 1kcal/mL.
- High calorie: 1.2–2kcal/mL.
- Fibre feeds: combination of soluble and insoluble fibre added to the above.
- EPAs added.

Patients do not necessarily have to remain in the hospital whilst receiving enteral nutrition, as it can be undertaken at home. To ensure a safe discharge, good communication between the hospital and community teams is required. There should be agreement on who will provide prescriptions for feed and equipment.

In recent years, there has been research in H&N cancer, which suggests that patients who can maintain normal swallowing for as long as possible during cancer treatment have fewer problems with longer-term dependence on tube feeding and have more straightforward rehabilitation of swallowing.

Parenteral nutrition

This is nutrition that bypasses the normal digestive system, instigated when the patient is unable to tolerate oral or enteral nutrition. Nutrients are administered by the IV route via a dedicated central or peripheral placed line.

The provision of parenteral feeding should be used only when all other forms of nutrition support have been tried or if the GI tract is not accessible. There are a number of complications, including:

- Line infection
- Thrombosis
- Metabolic disturbances.

Indications

- Patients with a non-functioning gut.
- Patients suffering from severe nausea, diarrhoea, or vomiting.
- Patients suffering from severe sores in the mouth or GI tract.
- Patients with a fistula in the stomach or oesophagus.
- Patients who have received surgery to the H&N.
- Patients with upper GI obstruction.

Commencing a patient on parenteral nutrition should be a carefully considered decision, involving the patient and members of the MDT, taking into account the potential benefits and risks. It is an invasive and relatively expensive form of nutrition support.

Complications

Though parenteral nutrition can be offered at home, this requires careful facilitation and planning and may delay discharge plans in some situations.

Websites

British Association for Parenteral and Enteral Nutrition. Available at: ℘ http://www.bapen.org.uk/
National Institute for Health and Care Excellence (2006). *Nutrition Support for Adults: Oral Nutrition Support, Enteral Tube Feeding and Parenteral Nutrition.* Clinical guideline [CG32]. Available at: ℘ https://www.nice.org.uk/guidance/cg32

Further reading

Cooper C, Burden ST, Cheng H, Molassiotis A. Understanding and managing cancer-related weight loss and anorexia: insights from a systematic review of qualitative research. *J Cachexia Sarcopenia Muscle* 2015;6:99–111.
Schoeff SS, Barrett DM, Gress CD, Jameson MJ (2013). Nutritional management for head and neck cancer patients. *Practical Gastroenterology.* Available at: ℘ https://med.virginia.edu/ginutrition/wp-content/uploads/sites/199/2014/06/September_13_Head-Neck-CA-21.pdf

References

4 Macmillan Cancer Support. *Healthy Eating.* Available at: ℘ http://www.macmillan.org.uk/information-and-support/coping/maintaining-a-healthy-lifestyle/healthy-eating
5 American Cancer Society. *Benefits of Good Nutrition During Cancer Treatment.* Available at: ℘ http://www.cancer.org/treatment/survivorshipduringandaftertreatment/nutritionfor peoplewithcancer/nutritionforthepersonwithcancer/nutrition-during-treatment-benefits

Support of specific nutritional complications

Anorexia/weight loss

Loss of appetite or desire to eat is a common symptom in patients. This leads to an energy deficit due to poor dietary intake and results in weight loss.

Causes
Multifactorial and can include:
- Pain
- Cancer treatment
- Medication
- Constipation
- Depression.

Dietary management
- Serve smaller portions of food more frequently.
- Increase nutrient density of food, in particular energy, fat, and protein.
- Encourage participation in shopping and preparation at mealtimes.
- Advise methods for simplified meal preparation to reduce anxiety at mealtimes.
- Encourage a social atmosphere at mealtimes.
- Limit drinks at mealtimes to prevent early satiety, whilst ensuring adequate daily fluid intake.
- Drink liquids between meals such as milkshakes and oral sip feeds.
- Seek medical advice for appropriate appetite stimulants.
- Advise gentle exercise and/or a small glass of alcohol pre-meal to stimulate appetite, if appropriate.

Anorexia can cause a great deal of anxiety and upset between the patient and the carer. The patient has no desire to eat and the carer is concerned and may prepare elaborate meals, encouraging them to eat. Management needs to support both parties with advice and encouragement.

Xerostomia

(⊙ See Oral mucositis and related problems, pp. 617–19.)

Definition
- Abnormal dryness of the mouth due to insufficient secretions.

Causes
- Treatment—radiotherapy can affect the production of saliva from the salivary glands, whilst surgery may remove certain salivary glands.
- Medication, e.g. anti-emetics, diuretics, opioids, some antidepressants.
- Dehydration.

Can cause the sensation of food sticking in the mouth, as well as increasing the risk of dental caries and gum disease due to the reduction in saliva.

Dietary management
- Encourage adequate fluid intake (8–10 glasses a day), timed to ensure optimum food intake.

- Ensure effective oral care.
- Use of artificial saliva, e.g. lozenges, sprays.
- Chewing sugar-free gum or sucking on boiled sweets or ice cubes may help to moisten the mouth.
- Softer foods or foods that can be mashed up may be better tolerated.
- Extra sauces, gravy, or butter can be added to moisten meals.
- Sips of fluids with meal. Be warned that excessive fluid intake may lead to early satiety.
- Try very sweet or tart foods and drinks, as may stimulate saliva.

Dysphagia

Definition
- Difficulty in swallowing food or liquid.

Causes
- Mechanical obstruction—due to site of tumour.
- Extrinsic compression—due to tumour in a lung or bronchus, or from chest wall compressing on the oesophagus.
- Neurological dysfunction—due to surgery or a brain tumour blocking innervation of the swallow reflex.
- Inflammatory—due to side effects of radiotherapy or chemotherapy.
- Oral candidiasis.

Symptoms
- Difficulty in mastication and swallowing.
- Coughing or choking during meals.
- Pain during swallowing.
- Aspiration after swallowing.
- Sensation of food lodged in the throat.

Management
Note: ensure advice is provided by the SALT to establish if the patient has a safe swallow or is at risk of aspiration.

Dietary management
- Soft foods and foods that can be mashed might be better tolerated.
- Some patients may need to liquidize, or even strain, their food through a sieve to remove all lumps.
- Milk, cream, white sauces, and condensed soup can be added to foods when liquidizing, to moisten the food more and add more calories and protein.
- Extra sauces and gravies can be added to meals.
- Strained baby foods should not be used, as their nutritional content is low for adults.
- Fluids can aid with swallowing, to 'flush' the food past the obstruction, but must ensure that this does not affect appetite.
- If required (as advised by the SALT), thickened fluids can help ensure the patient consumes sufficient liquid in their diet. SALT can advise on how to thicken to the prescribed consistency.

Note: management only acts as a guideline. Specialized advice should be provided by a registered dietician, based on the patient's reported symptoms.

Pain management

Introduction to pain management

Pain is not an inevitable symptom of advanced cancer; however, it is a common symptom when caring for people with advanced disease. Pain is defined by the International Association for the Study of Pain (IASP)[1] as: '*an unpleasant sensory and emotional experience associated with actual or potential tissue damage or described in terms of such damage*'. In other well-known definitions, pain is described as being whatever the experiencing person says it is, whenever he/she says it does. There is much debate about the adequacy of these definitions in terms of the complex multidimensional nature of pain and indeed in terms of whether patients experiencing pain will necessarily report it.

The perception of pain is determined by

- The patient's mood.
- The patient's morale.
- The meaning of pain for the individual.

Prevalence of pain in cancer

Cancer pain is common, and its prevalence is related to the stage of the illness. It is present in:

- 33% of patients after curative treatment
- 59% of patients undergoing cancer treatment
- 64% of patients with advanced disease.

The European Pain in Cancer (EPIC)[2] survey of 11 European countries indicated an overall pain prevalence of 71% in a cohort of 5084 patients with all stages of cancer in the community.

- 56% experienced moderate to severe pain several times a month or more [Numerical Rating Scale (NRS) ≥5, using a scale of 0–10).
- 26% experienced severe pain (NRS 7–10).
- The mean pain score was 6.4.

The EPIC survey[2] also revealed that cancer pain management in this cohort of patients was suboptimal. Nearly a quarter of patients with moderate to severe pain were not receiving any analgesic medication.

The causes of cancer pain

Pain in patients with cancer may be from many sources. They may have more than one pain, each with a differing cause. Understanding and establishing the cause/causes of cancer pain will lead to optimal pain management.

A person with cancer can have pain related to the following causes:

- The cancer itself:
  - Direct tumour invasion of local tissues
  - Visceral involvement
  - Bone involvement
  - Nerve compression or destruction
  - Ischaemia, e.g. thromboembolism secondary to cancer
  - Inflammatory pain
  - Raised ICP
  - Obstruction, e.g. bowel obstruction

- Pain related to cancer treatments, e.g.:
  - Chemotherapy-induced peripheral neuropathy
  - Chemotherapy-induced mucositis
  - Radiotherapy skin damage
  - Radionecrosis of tumour
  - Post-surgical pain
- Pain related to the cancer and debility, e.g.:
  - Constipation
  - Muscle tension/spasm
  - Lymphoedema
- A concurrent disorder, unrelated to the cancer, e.g.:
  - Osteoarthritis/degenerative joint pain
  - Peripheral diabetic neuropathy
  - Chronic pain from injuries such as rotator cuff tear or hip fracture.

Approach to cancer pain management

Optimal pain management starts with the diagnosis of the cause of pain through careful clinical assessment and by using available information from recent radiological imaging or by considering if more radiological imaging is required. Because pain is multidimensional, a holistic approach in the assessment is necessary, and this should encompass the physical, psychological, social, and spiritual aspects of pain.

Cancer pain management may involve the removal or minimization of the cancer through disease-directed therapies (e.g. chemotherapy, hormone manipulation therapy, radiotherapy, or surgery). Alongside these disease-directed therapies, there are many pharmacological and non-pharmacological therapies which should be tailored for the individual, depending on the specific clinical situation.

A multiprofessional and MDT approach to the management of cancer pain may provide the best support and outcomes for patients. This may encompass and utilize the skills of different nursing and medical specialties (e.g. oncology, pain, palliative care, and psycho-oncology), as well as different therapists (e.g. physiotherapists, occupational therapists, and complementary therapists).

Barriers to effective pain management

- Patient-related barriers:
  - Knowing when to take and titrate analgesia
  - Concerns about the side effects of drugs, e.g. constipation
  - Fears about drug tolerance and addiction
  - Fatalism about pain, i.e. pain is an inevitable consequence of cancer and nothing can be done to relieve it
  - Reporting pain might distract the doctor from treating the underlying disease
  - 'Good' patients do not complain of pain
  - Some religious and cultural beliefs may also impede effective pain control
- Role of carers:
  - Carers' barriers are often similar in nature to patient barriers
  - Carers' beliefs and values about a person's pain experience

- Health-care professionals:
  - Lack of knowledge on pain management
  - Lack of pain assessment skills
  - Inappropriate prescribing of analgesia, e.g. over- or under-prescribing
  - Lack of follow-up and reassessment
  - Lack of knowledge on management of analgesia side effects.

Further reading

Peacock S, Patel S. Cultural influences on pain. *Br J Pain* 2008;1:6–9.

van den Beuken-van Everdingen MH, de Rijke JM, Kessels AG, Schouten HC, van Kleef M, Patijn J. Prevalence of pain in patients with cancer: a systematic review of the past 40 years. *Ann Oncol* 2007;18:1437–49.

Xue Y, Schulman-Green D, Czaplinski C, Harris D, McCorkle R. Pain attitudes and knowledge among RNs, pharmacists, and physicians on an inpatient oncology service. *Clin J Oncol Nurs* 2007;11:687–95.

References

1 International Association for the Study of Pain (IASP). Available at: ℛ http://www.iasp-pain.org
2 Breivik H, Cherny N, Collett B, *et al*. Cancer-related pain: a pan-European survey of prevalence, treatment, and patient attitudes. *Ann Oncol* 2009;20:1420–33.

Pain assessment

Assessing a person's pain requires a number of skills in communication such as listening, verbal and written reporting skills, relationship building, and observation. Patients in pain may have >1 pain, and each of these needs to be assessed and considered separately. Assessment of pain is an ongoing process that requires systematic updating and re-evaluation of the situation, in other words constant reassessment.

A narrative approach to pain assessment is often helpful; it keeps the focus on the patient and their experience of pain. This approach focuses the assessment on the person's story and key issues for them related to the experience. A key question using a narrative approach might be 'Would you tell me all about your pain?' A question like this incorporated within a conversation will enable clinical decision-making regarding the appropriate interventions to manage the person's pain (➔ see Assessment, pp. 462–3).

There are many methods of taking a pain history. If a structured and systematic approach to pain assessment is required, the following themes and questions may be helpful:

- **Location:** Where is your pain? Is there more than one site? Can you point to the area?
- **Radiation:** Does the pain go anywhere else? Does it move around?
- **Quality/description of pain:** What does it feel like? What words would you use to describe your pain?
- **Severity/intensity:** How bad is the pain? How would you describe it: mild, moderate, or severe? What number would you give your pain on a scale of 0–10 (0 being no pain and 10 being the worst pain)? Are you able to divert your attention away from the pain?
- **Duration:** How long have you had this pain? And how long does it last? Is it constant or does it come and go?
- **Relief:** What relieves or helps your pain?
- **Increase:** Is there anything which increases your pain or makes it worse?
- **The effect of pain on function and activities of daily living:** Does the pain impact on your mobility?
- **The impact on QoL:** Does the pain disrupt your sleep? Does the pain affect your enjoyment in life?
- **The impact on psychological well-being:** How do you cope with the pain? Does the pain affect your mood?
- **Understanding of pain and expectations:** What does the pain mean to you and your family? What do you hope we can do for your pain?
- **Medication—current and previous analgesics:** What medicines have helped with the pain? Are there any medicines that have not helped in the past?
- **Anything else I need to know about your pain?**

Pain assessment tools

Pain assessment tools may be helpful in providing documentary evidence of pain management and to aid communication between the person in pain and health-care professionals. However, assessment tools need to be appropriate to the situation and assess what they purport to assess.

The following are a selection of pain assessment tools.

Pain body map

The pain body map is two diagrams side by side, representing the entire body from the front and from the back. This can be helpful to identify where pain is present, as sometimes patients may not know the medical terms but will be able to show where it hurts.

Visual analogue scale

The visual analogue scale (VAS) is a 10-cm line with the anchors or ends marked with 'no pain' and 'worst pain'. This self-reported tool represents the intensity of a person's pain by marking the point on the line which best represents their pain. Some people may find the idea of a line representing their pain as a difficult concept to understand and may not be able to apply this idea to their pain experience. One criticism of this tool is the difficulty associated with the VAS, as a person rating their pain as 'worst pain', which then further intensifies. Progression of pain experience may be more sensitive and more easily understood if the VAS is used vertically, rather than horizontally. This tool only attempts to assess pain intensity, as opposed to the multidimensional aspects of the pain experience.

No pain...Worst pain

Verbal rating scale

A verbal rating scale (VRS) is a tool which uses a series of descriptive words to represent the intensity of pain, e.g.:

None Or	Mild	Moderate	Severe
No pain	A little pain	A lot of pain	Too much pain

The VRS is a simple and quick tool to use; however, it may have little resonance for some people in pain if the descriptive words do not fit with their experience or if a more comprehensive tool is required.

Numerical rating scale

The Numerical Rating Scale (NRS) is similar to the VAS but has numbers along the 10-cm line to indicate the intensity of pain.

No pain ... 1 ... 2 ... 3 ... 4 ... 5 ... 6 ....7 ... 8 ... 9 ... 10 ... Worst pain

It has some of the same problems as the VAS, in that pain may be rated at 10 and then intensifies further, leaving no place on the scale to acknowledge that increase.

Brief Pain Inventory
More complex tools aim to capture the multidimensional nature of the pain experience. An example of these is the Brief Pain Inventory (BPI) (see Fig. 46.1). This multidimensional tool seeks to assess the pain experience in a more comprehensive way. It attempts to use words to describe the pain, a body map to locate the pain, and questions which seek to include the social impact and the physical activity of the person.

Abbey Pain Scale
The Abbey Pain Scale is a tool designed to assist in the assessment of pain in patients who are unable to clearly articulate their needs (e.g. secondary to cognitive impairment or reduced levels of consciousness). It can also be used as a movement-based assessment. The tool depends on the observation skills of the health-care professional to record six separate items, whilst closely observing the patient (e.g. vocalization, facial expression, change in body language, and behavioural changes). The scale does not differentiate between distress and pain, so a comprehensive assessment of the patient should always be considered. To measure for the effectiveness of pain-relieving interventions, it is recommended to make a second assessment 1 hour after any intervention taken in response to the first assessment.

Pain diaries
Asking a person in pain to keep a diary of their experiences can be a helpful way to gain an understanding of how the experience has had an impact on their life and what interventions have been helpful. Some people will find this activity positive, as it enables them to take a more active role in managing their pain.

Pain may be assessed differently, according to the setting. For example, in the acute hospital setting, there may already be a tool in use and practitioners may be expected to utilize the same tool. Tools need to take account of the time available for assessment, resources, staff experience, reliability and validity, and how acceptable they are to the person in pain.

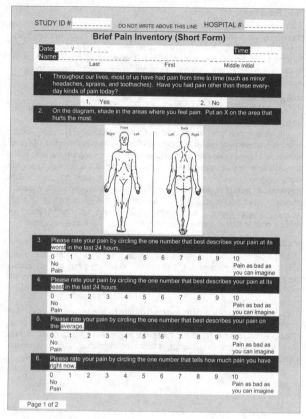

Fig. 46.1 Brief Pain Inventory.

Copyright 1991 Charles S. Cleeland, PhD Pain Research Group All rights reserved. Reproduced with permission.

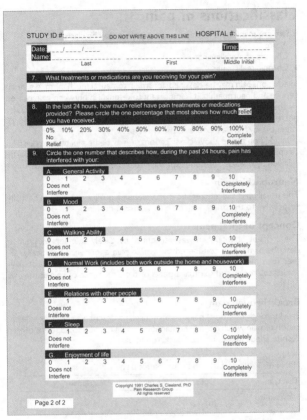

STUDY ID #:_____ DO NOT WRITE ABOVE THIS LINE HOSPITAL #:_____

Date:____/____/____   Time:_____
Name:_____
     Last   First   Middle Initial

7. What treatments or medications are you receiving for your pain?

8. In the last 24 hours, how much relief have pain treatments or medications provided? Please circle the one percentage that most shows how much relief you have received.

0%	10%	20%	30%	40%	50%	60%	70%	80%	90%	100%
No Relief										Complete Relief

9. Circle the one number that describes how, during the past 24 hours, pain has interfered with your:

A. General Activity

0	1	2	3	4	5	6	7	8	9	10
Does not Interfere										Completely Interferes

B. Mood

0	1	2	3	4	5	6	7	8	9	10
Does not Interfere										Completely Interferes

C. Walking Ability

0	1	2	3	4	5	6	7	8	9	10
Does not Interfere										Completely Interferes

D. Normal Work (includes both work outside the home and housework)

0	1	2	3	4	5	6	7	8	9	10
Does not Interfere										Completely Interferes

E. Relations with other people

0	1	2	3	4	5	6	7	8	9	10
Does not Interfere										Completely Interferes

F. Sleep

0	1	2	3	4	5	6	7	8	9	10
Does not Interfere										Completely Interferes

G. Enjoyment of life

0	1	2	3	4	5	6	7	8	9	10
Does not Interfere										Completely Interferes

Copyright 1991 Charles S. Cleeland, PhD
Pain Research Group
All rights reserved

Page 2 of 2

Fig. 46.1 (*Contd.*)

Classifications of pain

There are many ways to classify pain, e.g. pain may be classified as:
- Acute
- Chronic non-malignant
- Chronic malignant.

In addition, pain may be classified according to neural mechanism, e.g. nociceptive and neuropathic. It is important to distinguish between pain caused by the stimulation of nerve endings (nociceptive pain) and pain caused by nerve dysfunction or compression (neuropathic pain) (see Table 46.1). Patients may have a mixture of the two types.

In addition to the above classifications, it may be helpful to consider pain as opioid-responsive (pain relieved by opioids), semi-responsive (pain partly relieved by opioids), or non-responsive (pain not relieved by opioids).

Neuropathic pain

This usually has a characteristic sharp, stabbing quality and is often partially responsive to treatment with opioids such as morphine.

Concept of total pain

The concept of total pain was introduced by Cicely Saunders in 1964 to describe pain which considered the whole pain experience holistically, rather than merely the physical. Total pain encompasses the physical, psychological, social, and spiritual aspects of the experience of pain at the end of life.

Breakthrough pain

Breakthrough (episodic) pain is a term used to describe a transient exacerbation of pain which occurs spontaneously or in relation to a specific trigger despite adequately controlled background pain.[3]

Table 46.1 Nociceptive and neuropathic pain

Pain type	Example	Description
Nociceptive		
Visceral	Liver capsule pain	Sharp
Somatic	Bone pain	Deep aching/gnawing
Muscle spasm	Cramp	Cramp/spasm
Neuropathic		
Peripheral	Neuroma	Burning/stabbing
Central	Spinal cord compression	Numbness/weakness
Mixed	Post-herpetic neuralgia	Cutting/stabbing/shooting/burning

References

3 Davies AN, Dickman A, Reid C, Stevens AM, Zeppetella G. The management of cancer-related breakthrough pain: recommendations of a task group of the Science Committee of the Association for Palliative Medicine of GB and Ireland. *Eur J Pain* 2009;13:331–8.

Principles of analgesic use

Analgesic drugs should be given:
- **Orally**, whenever possible
- **Regularly**, in order to prevent pain in advance, rather than trying to alleviate it once it becomes established
- **Systematically**, according to the 3-step WHO analgesic ladder.[4] If optimizing the dose of analgesic drugs does not give adequate relief, move up the ladder
- **For the individual**, the correct dose of treatment is the one which relieves the pain
- **With adjuvants**, in specific situations to relieve pain and when appropriate to use.

World Health Organization's 3-step analgesic ladder

(See Fig. 46.2.)[4]
- Step 1 is the use of simple analgesics—paracetamol (acetaminophen) or NSAIDs. When regular treatment is no longer adequate to manage the pain or it increases, a 'weak' opioid, such as codeine or tramadol, should be added.
- Step 2: opioids are commonly used for mild to moderate cancer pain. If the pain persists or increases when the maximum therapeutic dose of the 'weak' opioid has been reached, switch treatment to a 'strong' opioid such as morphine, oxycodone, or fentanyl.
- Step 3: opioids are commonly used for moderate to severe cancer pain.
- Adjuvant analgesics can be used at any step in specific situations to enhance the analgesic effect.

European Association for Palliative Care (EAPC) recommendations

- The EAPC produces guidelines on the use of opioids for the treatment of cancer pain.[5]

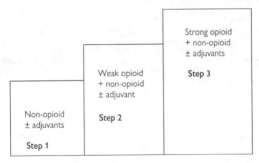

Fig. 46.2 WHO pain relief ladder.
Reproduced from WHO's cancer pain ladder for adults (🔗 http://www.who.int/cancer/pallia-tive/painladder/en/) with permission from WHO.

- Low doses of morphine or oxycodone can be used in opioid-naïve cancer patients with mild to moderate pain (i.e. step 2).
- Oral morphine when used at low doses (e.g. ≤30mg per day) is a step 2 opioid.
- Oral oxycodone when used at low doses (e.g. ≤20mg per day) is a step 2 opioid.
- Morphine has traditionally been used as a first-line 'strong' opioid due to familiarity, availability, and cost. It is acceptable that either morphine or oxycodone can be used as first line.

Adjuvant analgesics

Adjuvant analgesics are defined as drugs with a primary indication other than pain that have analgesic properties in some painful conditions. However, some adjuvant analgesics, e.g. duloxetine, gabapentin, and pregabalin, are now licensed for the relief of various neuropathic pains.

The group includes numerous drugs in diverse classes:
- Corticosteroids (e.g. dexamethasone for spinal cord/nerve root compression or metastatic bone pain)
- Antidepressants (e.g. amitriptyline or duloxetine for neuropathic pain)
- Anti-epileptics (e.g. gabapentin or pregabalin for neuropathic pain)
- Smooth muscle relaxants (e.g. Buscopan®/hyoscine butylbromide or glycopyrronium to relieve visceral distension pain and colic)
- Skeletal muscle relaxants (e.g. baclofen or diazepam for painful muscle spasm)
- Bisphosphonates (e.g pamidronate or zoledronic acid for metastatic bone pain).

Further reading

Lussier D, Huskey AG, Portenoy RK. Adjuvant analgesics in cancer pain management. *Oncologist* 2004;9:571–91.

Twycross R, Wilcock A, Stark Toller C. *Symptom Management in Advanced Cancer*, 4th ed. Nottingham: Palliativedrugs.com Ltd; 2009.

References

4 World Health Organization. *WHO's Cancer Pain Ladder for Adults*. Available at: ℜ http://www. who.int/cancer/palliative/painladder/en/

5 Caraceni A, Hanks G, Kaasa S, *et al.*; European Palliative Care Research Collaborative (EPCRC); European Association for Palliative Care (EAPC). Use of opioid analgesics in the treatment of cancer pain: evidence-based recommendations from the EAPC. *Lancet Oncol* 2012;13:e58–68.

Use of weak opioid drugs

Codeine and tramadol are classed as WHO step 2 opioids and are recommended for mild to moderate cancer pain. [6,7]

Codeine

- Codeine has little or no analgesic effect until it is metabolized by the liver to morphine.
- There is wide inter-individual variation in the production of morphine because of genetic polymorphisms. Some individuals may produce little or no morphine, due to slow metabolism, obtaining little pain relief from codeine. Slow metabolizers may account for 5–10% of the Caucasian population in Europe. Conversely, about 1–7% of this population may be fast metabolizers, producing greater-than-usual amounts of morphine, with enhanced effects seen. [8]
- Codeine is about one-tenth as potent as morphine. Therefore, codeine 60mg is approximately equivalent to morphine 6mg.
- Dose for adults: by mouth, 15–60mg every 4 hours when necessary. Maximum 240mg daily.
- Codeine is often given in a combination product with paracetamol (e.g. co-codamol). Note these combination products come in various strengths of codeine content.
  - Cautions: avoid codeine use in patients with severe renal impairment due to risk of accumulation of morphine.
  - Undesirable effects: similar to morphine (➔ see Use of strong opioid drugs, p. 562).

Tramadol

- Tramadol is a synthetic centrally acting analgesic with both non-opioid and opioid properties.
- Similar to codeine and due to the same genetic polymorphisms, there is wide inter-individual variation in the analgesic effects of tramadol.
- Tramadol is about one-tenth as potent as morphine. Therefore, tramadol 100mg is approximately equivalent to morphine 10mg.
- Dose for adults: by mouth, 50–100mg every 4 hours when necessary or 100–200mg modified-release. Maximum 400mg daily.
  - Cautions: tramadol dose and frequency must be reduced in patients with severe renal or liver impairment to 50mg 12-hourly.
  - Undesirable effects: similar to morphine (➔ see Use of strong opioid drugs, p. 562).

References

6 World Health Organization. *WHO's Cancer Pain Ladder for Adults.* Available at: ◊ http://www. who.int/cancer/palliative/painladder/en/

7 Caraceni A, Hanks G, Kaasa S, *et al.*; European Palliative Care Research Collaborative (EPCRC); European Association for Palliative Care (EAPC). Use of opioid analgesics in the treatment of cancer pain: evidence-based recommendations from the EAPC. *Lancet Oncol* 2012;13:e58–68.

8 Twycross R, Wilcock A. *PCF4: Palliative Care Formulary*, 4th ed. Nottingham: Palliativedrugs.com Ltd; 2011.

Use of strong opioid drugs

Morphine and oxycodone are classed as WHO step 3 opioids and are recommended for moderate to severe cancer pain.[9,10] Morphine has similar efficacy to oxycodone and should be used as first-line opioid in view of familiarity, availability, and cost.

Communication

- When starting a patient on strong opioids, ask them about concerns such as:
  - Addiction
  - Tolerance
  - Side effects
  - Fears that treatment implies the final stages of life.
- Provide verbal and written information on strong opioid treatment to patients and carers, including the following:
  - When and why strong opioids are used to treat pain
  - How effective they are likely to be
  - Taking strong opioids for background and breakthrough pain, addressing:
    — How, when, and how often to take strong opioids
    — How long pain relief should last
  - Side effects and signs of toxicity
  - Safe storage
  - Follow-up and further prescribing
  - Information on who to contact out of hours, particularly during initiation of treatment.
- Offer patients access to frequent review of pain control and side effects.

Common undesirable effects of opioids

- Nausea and vomiting.
- Dry mouth, gastroparesis, constipation.
- Cognitive symptoms, including reduced concentration, drowsiness, and confusion.
- Itching and sweating.

Starting on morphine

- Offer patients regular oral sustained-release or oral immediate-release morphine (depending on patient preference).[11]
- For patients with no renal or hepatic comorbidities, offer a typical total daily starting dose schedule of 20–30mg of oral morphine. For example, 10–15mg of oral sustained-release morphine twice daily, plus 5mg of oral immediate-release morphine for rescue doses (use as required) during the titration phase.
- If the patient is already taking a weak opioid regularly, then switch to oral morphine and convert the weak opioid to approximate the morphine equivalent dose. For example, 240mg of codeine in 24 hours is approximately equivalent to 24mg of oral morphine.
- For elderly or frail patients, a lower dose may be necessary on initiating morphine (e.g. 2.5–5mg 4-hourly).

- Laxatives should be prescribed routinely for the management or prophylaxis of opioid-induced constipation.
- Offer patients frequent review during the initiation phase.
  - Cautions: reduce the dose of morphine for patients with moderate renal or hepatic impairment. Avoid prescribing morphine in severe renal [glomerular filtration rate (GFR) <30mL/min) or hepatic impairment. The opioid of first choice should be fentanyl or buprenorphine.

Titrating the dose of morphine

- Adjust the dose until a good balance exists between acceptable pain control and side effects. Seek specialist advice if balance is not achieved after a few dose adjustments.
- If taking immediate-release oral morphine: increase the regular dose until there is adequate relief throughout each 4-hour period, taking prn into account.
- If taking sustained-release oral morphine: increase the dose every 2–3 days until there is adequate relief of pain throughout each 12-h period and be guided by the as-required use.

Breakthrough dose of morphine

- The breakthrough dose of morphine is usually one-sixth of the total morphine dose in 24 hours. For example, if a patient is taking sustained-release oral morphine 60mg twice daily, then the breakthrough dose is 20mg.

Management of constipation

- It is important to inform patients that constipation affects nearly all patients receiving strong opioid treatment.
- Prescribe laxative treatment (to be taken regularly and at an effective dose) for all patients initiating strong opioids.
- Prescribe a laxative treatment preferred by the patient to enhance adherence and optimize the dose accordingly.
- Ensure adequate hydration.

Management of nausea

- Nausea may occur when starting strong opioid treatment or at dose increase, but this is likely to be transient.
- Prescribing an anti-emetic to take as required may be helpful when initiating strong opioids.
- Prokinetic anti-emetics (metoclopramide and domperidone) are commonly prescribed and lessen the effects of gastroparesis.
- Haloperidol 1.5mg nocte or as required is an alternative anti-emetic.

Management of drowsiness

- Mild drowsiness or impaired concentration may occur when starting strong opioid treatment or at dose increase, but this is often transient.
- Warn patients that impaired concentration may affect their ability to drive and undertake other manual tasks.
- If drowsiness persists, consider dose reduction if pain is controlled, or consider switching opioids if pain is not controlled.
- Seek specialist advice if symptoms remain uncontrolled.

Morphine preparations

Morphine is available in several immediate- and slow-release preparations.

- Immediate-release: Oramorph®/Sevredol® 10mg/5mL, 20mg/mL liquid or tablets (4-hourly).
- Slow-release:
  - 12-hourly: MST and Zomorph® 5, 10, 15, 30, 60, 100, 200mg tablets or capsules
  - 24-hourly: MXL 30, 60, 90, 120, 150, 200mg capsules.
- Rectal morphine, 10, 15, 20, 30mg suppositories.
- Morphine sulfate injection 10, 30, 100mg in 5-mL vials.

Opioid transdermal patches

- Indications: transdermal patches are useful for patients who do not tolerate, or comply poorly with, oral medication.
- They are more suitable for patients whose pain is stable and who do not require rapid changes in dosage.
- A transdermal fentanyl 12-microgram patch equates to ~30mg of oral morphine daily.
- A transdermal buprenorphine 20-microgram patch equates to ~48mg of oral morphine daily.

Diamorphine

Diamorphine is commonly used as an injectable strong opioid in a syringe driver. Its advantage over morphine is that it is more soluble in water.

Typically, the 24-hour dose is divided by 3 to give the 24-hour SC dose. For example, 10mg 4-hourly of morphine is 60mg of morphine in 24 hours, divided by 3, is 20mg of diamorphine in a continuous SC infusion over 24 hours.

Use of other opioids

There are several other strong opioids that are sometimes used in the palliative care, including:

- Hydromorphone
- Methadone
- Buprenorphine
- Alfentanyl
- Fentanyl
- Oxycodone.

Further reading

National Institute for Health and Care Excellence. *Opioids in Palliative Care Overview.* Available at: ℘ http://pathways.nice.org.uk/pathways/opioids-in-palliative-care

References

9 World Health Organization. *WHO's Cancer Pain Ladder for Adults.* Available at: ℘ http://www.who.int/cancer/palliative/painladder/en/

10 Caraceni A, Hanks G, Kaasa S, *et al.*; European Palliative Care Research Collaborative (EPCRC); European Association for Palliative Care (EAPC). Use of opioid analgesics in the treatment of cancer pain: evidence-based recommendations from the EAPC. *Lancet Oncol* 2012;13:e58–68.

11 Wiffen PJ, Wee B, Moore RA. Oral morphine for cancer pain. *Cochrane Database Syst Rev* 2013;7:CD003868.

Use of syringe drivers in pain control

Syringe drivers are used in palliative care to administer continuous SC medication when a person is unable to take medication orally. Medication may be given via a syringe driver for pain management and for the management of other symptoms such as agitation. Prior to commencing a syringe driver, it is important to discuss its use with the patient and/or family. This may help to allay some of the fear and concern attached to the use of a syringe driver, which may be viewed as a last resort. The advantage of a syringe driver is that it enables the continuous administration of several medications, for multiple symptoms, avoiding the peaks and troughs of oral analgesics.

Indications for use include:
• Intractable nausea and/or vomiting
• Difficulty in swallowing (e.g. in the case of H&N tumours)
• Person too weak to take oral medication
• ↓ conscious level.

The use of particular syringe drivers, such as the battery powered MS26 has been discontinued in the NHS due to the danger of opiate overdosing. Nurses should always refer to the local policy when selecting a syringe driver. The analgesic drug of choice for use in syringe drivers is diamorphine because of its solubility; as a result, it can be administered in small volumes of fluid. However, it has been in short supply in some settings, in which case morphine sulfate is used.

The following drugs may be mixed with diamorphine in a syringe driver.

Cyclizine:	anti-emetic
Haloperidol:	anti-emetic/antipsychotic
Metoclopramide:	anti-emetic
Octreotide:	synthetic analogue
Midazolam:	sedative
Hyoscine butylbromide:	anti-muscarinic
Levomepromazine:	anti-emetic/antipsychotic
Ondansetron:	anti-emetic
Glycopyrronium:	anti-muscarinic
Granisetron:	anti-emetic

For more information on drug combinations in syringe drivers, see ஃ http://palliativedrugs.com

The following drugs are not suitable for SC use, as they cause skin irritation or soreness at the injection site:
• Diazepam
• Chlorpromazine
• Prochlorperazine.

It is possible to mix two or more drugs in the same syringe for delivery via a syringe driver, provided they do not react adversely with each other. Care should be taken when mixing diamorphine and cyclizine in higher concentrations, as this can precipitate. The skin site and the driver and tubing need to be checked regularly. Diluting diamorphine as much as possible before adding cyclizine can reduce the risk of this happening.

The infusion is given SC at any suitable site via a 'butterfly needle'. Sites commonly used are the upper arms and the abdomen. The site should be changed if it becomes red, sore, or indurated.

Luer lock connections between the tubing and the syringe provide a safer system. Local guidance relating to the use of syringe drivers are now available in most cancer networks and should be followed, including the procedure for labelling the syringe driver and recommended dilutant.

Further reading

Dickman A, Schneider J. *The Syringe Driver: Continuous Subcutaneous Infusions in Palliative Care*, 2nd ed. Oxford: Oxford University Press; 2005.

Non-pharmacological interventions for pain management

The following measures are helpful in the management of pain, instead of, or in addition to, pharmacological drugs. They provide an opportunity for nurses in particular to utilize their skills to help and support people in pain.

Transcutanous electrical nerve stimulation

TENS is a non-invasive method of pain relief, consisting of a small electrical pulse generator, which connects to two or four electrodes on the skin. The electrical impulse, which is battery-powered, can be adjusted to deliver a variety of strength, duration, and frequency of impulse. One of the positive aspects of this method is that the person in pain controls the impulse.

TENS is effective in some people; however, not everyone will gain relief from this method. Some settings do not endorse nurse administration of TENS and suggest physiotherapists have a key role in the use of this method.

Massage

May be helpful for some people experiencing pain; it is thought to work in a similar way to TENS. Gentle stroking movements of, for example, the hands, feet, or back can be relaxing and provide the comfort of touch and an additional analgesic effect. Massage may be particularly effective when there is muscle tension contributing to the pain experience.

Distraction

Distraction therapy, e.g. television, radio, reading, music, company, talking, puzzles, etc., is commonly used as a method of pain relief. It enables the person in pain to focus on something other than the pain and is commonly used by people with persistent pain. Often people will have their own ways of managing persistent pain developed over time and may include differing strategies for night- and daytime. It is important to try to continue these if the person is admitted to hospital.

Relaxation

Relaxation exercises can be taught. One way is to teach the person in pain to systematically tense and then relax all muscles throughout the body, starting from the toes, until the muscles of the face are reached. Some people find that relaxation audiotapes are of help and are a guide to this process. Others may find music a source of relaxation and distraction. Visualization provides an opportunity to go outside of one's self to another place, as a means of escaping the pain, and can be taught as a non-invasive approach to pain management (➲ see Progressive muscle relaxation, p. 588).

Breathing exercises

These are a helpful strategy to teach a person in pain, particularly whilst waiting for analgesia to take effect. These may be simply helping a person to slow down their breathing rate by breathing with you or by encouraging the person to extend their exhaled breath by breathing slowly through their mouth. Some people find assistance with breathing exercises useful initially but are then able to utilize this as a strategy themselves.

Comfort measures

Comfort measures, e.g. positioning, splinting, heat, and cold, are all part of a skilled nurse's repertoire in caring for people in pain. Other useful strategies that contribute to general comfort are:

• Finding a comfortable position in bed or in a chair
• Using pillows for support
• The use of pressure-relieving mattresses or aids
• Fresh bedding, a pleasant outlook in the room or from the window
• The use of personal effects like family photographs.

Presence—being with the person in pain

Being present with, and hearing about, the person's experience and story can be helpful in itself. If the person alongside the patient is confident and sensitive to the experience of pain and is willing and able to be there, even when it is distressing to watch, this is usually helpful to the person in pain. Being sensitive to the experience means knowing when to talk or be silent, knowing when to use touch, and knowing how to 'be' with the person in pain.

Effective communication

Communication with people who are in pain is particularly important. Having information about the pain experiences, e.g. the cause, potential treatments, drug measures, and side effects, is usually helpful to people. Having a dialogue with a patient about their experience of pain and understanding their perspective, including the impact of the pain on their QoL, is part of effective communication. However, for some people, being able to verbalize their pain is not easy or is impossible. People with dementia may be unable to verbally report or describe their pain, in which case the nurse has to rely on getting to know the person and being alert to changes in behaviour and body language, which may indicate pain.

Radiotherapy

Radiotherapy has a role in managing pain, particularly bone pain associated with metastatic disease (⊖ see Metastatic bone disease, p. 587) and chest pain in lung cancer (⊖ see Management of non-small cell lung cancer, pp. 436–7).

Further reading

International Association for the Study of Pain. Classification of chronic pain. Descriptions of chronic pain syndromes and definitions of *pain* terms *Pain* 1986;3:S1–226.
Watson M, Lucas C, Hoy A, Back I. *Oxford Handbook of Palliative Care*. Oxford: Oxford University Press; 2005.

Symptom management at the end of life

Introduction to symptom management at the end of life

Common symptoms at the end of life include:
- Respiratory secretions ('death rattle')
- Pain
- Restlessness
- Agitation
- Confusion
- Breathlessness
- Weakness
- Nausea and vomiting.

When managing symptoms at the end of life, investigations should only be undertaken if they will influence the choice of treatment offered, e.g. to exclude reversible causes.

When it becomes clear that the person is dying, it is important to review the appropriateness of all medication, and any that does not contribute directly to the comfort of the patient may be stopped. Those required, such as analgesia, anti-emetics, anticonvulsants, and anxiolytics, may be continued via a syringe driver or an alternative route, if the person is unable to take them orally.

A key aspect of end-of-life care, particularly in the community, is the anticipation of needs and forward planning, having the medication and resources available to respond rapidly as needed, as far as the circumstances allow. Coordinated care will be enhanced by ensuring that patient details have been entered onto the locality palliative care register to ensure all service providers are aware of the patient 24 hours a day, ensuring pre-emptive medications—'just in case' boxes—are in the home or prescribed on the ward and ensuring families have all relevant telephone contact numbers.

Although every effort must be taken to relieve symptoms, complete control is not always possible. For this reason, effective communication with the patient and family is essential, to manage expectations and ensure they understand what is being done and why. Care should always be planned in accordance with local and national guidelines in best practice in palliative and end-of-life care (➔ see End-of-life care, pp. 151–3).

Anticipatory prescribing

The pre-emptive or anticipatory prescribing of as-required (PRN) medication for symptoms can avoid great distress. The cost is negligible, and it saves time on the part of both families and out-of-hours health professionals. The doses needed by individuals vary widely; it is more important to assess the effectiveness of each PRN medication before repeating or increasing doses—if a PRN medication is ineffective, then try a different approach or seek advice (see Box 47.1).

> ### Box 47.1 Anticipatory end-of-life prescribing
> A typical anticipatory or PRN regimen for patients approaching the end of life might include:
> - Morphine sulfate 2.5–5mg 1- to 4-hourly PRN SC (or a dose based on prior regular opioid usage) for pain, cough, or breathlessness
> - Midazolam 2.5–5mg 2- to 4-hourly PRN SC for anxiety or breathlessness
> - An antipsychotic for nausea or agitation. Either:
>   - Haloperidol 0.5–1.5mg 2- to 4-hourly PRN SC, or
>   - Levomepromazine 6.25–25mg 2- to 4-hourly PRN SC (use lower end of range for nausea; higher initial doses for agitation)
> - Hyoscine butylbromide 20mg 2- to 4-hourly PRN SC for respiratory secretions
> - Water for injections—10mL (diluent for syringe pump).

Further reading

Twycross R, Wilcock A. *PCF4: Palliative Care Formulary*, 4th ed. Nottingham: Palliativedrugs.com Ltd; 2011.

Respiratory secretions: 'death rattle'

Respiratory secretions can cause noisy, rattling breathing that occurs when the dying person is unconscious and close to death and is unable to cough or clear secretions. It is caused by the collection of secretions in the upper airway and difficulty in clearing them. Although death rattle can be distressing to family members, it does not need to be, if there is adequate explanation, and management should be tailored to the needs of the patient and family.

Nursing management

It is important to observe the patient for signs of a build-up of secretions and assess, where possible, the level of distress experienced by the patient. Families need to know the reason for the noisy breathing and options for treatment, and to be involved in decision-making. The following measures have a role in prevention and management of death rattle:

- Repositioning on the patient's side to aid drainage of secretions
- Frequent mouth care (if the patient is able to tolerate it) is required as any anti-muscarinic drugs will dry the mouth
- If IV fluids are in progress and the volume of secretions is excessive or causing distress, fluids may be reduced or discontinued to maintain patient comfort (➔ see Artificial hydration and nutrition, p. 166)
- There are several options for drug management of death rattle. Anti-muscarinic drugs may be started at the first sign of noisy breathing or if the patient is showing signs of distress
- The following three drugs are commonly used in palliative care centres to treat respiratory secretions at the end of life. There is a lack of evidence regarding the efficacy of one drug over another, and attention should be paid to local protocols:
  - Hyoscine butylbromide (Buscopan®)
  - Hyoscine hydrobromide
  - Glycopyrronium.
- Suction can be distressing for the patient and is rarely necessary. It can damage the mucosa, may increase the amount of secretions being produced, and create a dry mouth. Suction can be used if the above methods do not work or if the patient is distressed by them.

Further reading

Bennett M, Lucas V, Brennan M, et al. Using anti-muscarinic drugs in the management of death rattle: evidence-based guidelines for palliative care. *Palliat Med* 2002;16:369–74.

Wee BL, Coleman PG, Hillier R, et al. The sound of death rattle 1: are relatives distressed by hearing this sound? *Palliat Med* 2006;20:171–5.

Terminal agitation

Terminal agitation is a state of agitation and distress found at the end of life. It can be a very difficult condition for both the patient and their family, and can make the experience of dying a very traumatic event.

There are similarities with acute confusional states (➔ see Acute confusional state or delirium, pp. 594–5), but terminal agitation is associated with the experience of dying and is not clearly caused by reversible factors (though the causes may be multifactorial). The subjective experience of spiritual pain or anguish may be a feature.

It is most important that any reversible causes of agitation at the end of life are identified and treated, e.g. anxiety, pain, breathlessness, dehydration, full bladder or rectum, organic brain disease, or the effects of prescribed drugs.

It is also very important in assessment to differentiate between pain and agitation.

Nursing management

As the patient will usually be acutely distressed by the condition, it is most important to communicate effectively with them and their family, to identify their wishes, and to respond as fully as possible under the circumstances.

The following are key aspects of management:
- Safety of the patient, family, and practitioners
- Maintaining dignity and privacy
- Communicating effectively
- Presence of a nurse or family member may reassure the patient
- Maintaining an environment that is free of disruption and distraction.

(➔ See also Acute confusional state or delirium, pp. 594–5.)

Sedation

Care needs to be taken giving sedation at the end of life. The expressed needs of the patient and family must be taken into account, as well as the need to maintain the comfort and dignity of the patient (➔ see End-of-life care issues, pp. 164–71). The following are options for managing terminal agitation:
- Midazolam 5–10mg stat and 30–60mg/24 hours SC infusion in a syringe driver
- Levomepromazine 25mg stat and 50–100mg/24 hour SC infusion in a syringe driver.

If a syringe driver is not available, other benzodiazepine or phenothiazine drugs may also be used, via sublingual or rectal routes.

Further reading

Maluso–Bolton MN. Terminal agitation. *J Hospice Palliat Nurs* 2000;2:920.

Psychological reactions to cancer

Introduction to psychological reactions to cancer

Having cancer is distressing. Feelings of distress can be expressed in a number of ways, e.g. crying, seeking reassurance, anger, or hostility. People at any stage of cancer can find it hard to concentrate, make decisions, or take in information. Reactions are very individual, and we should avoid making assumptions about how any individual will react or how they will show their distress. People tend to develop characteristic ways of reacting to painful or stressful events in their lives. This will depend on both personal and social factors.

Personal factors

Some people characteristically react by sharing their feelings with friends or family. Others will keep things to themselves and 'bottle things up'. Some people aim to distract themselves by keeping busy, and others avoid problems by using drugs or alcohol, for example. We should be careful not to make assumptions about what is 'normal'. People will react in ways that are 'normal' for them.

Social and cultural factors

Reactions will also be determined by factors in the social or cultural environment. This can include what is expected of gender roles, for example, that men do not cry. Also, roles within families can influence reactions, e.g. some individuals may feel that they have to be 'strong' for other family members.

Distress and mood

There is overlap between the terms **distress** and **mood**. Mood (or **affect**) is a term used to describe someone's emotional state and has a very specific meaning in relation to mental illness, i.e. disorders of mood, including anxiety and depression.

Stress and coping

The concepts of stress and coping are frequently used to understand the reactions of people who are diagnosed with cancer. Stress describes the demands made by the cancer on the individual, and coping describes their efforts to manage these demands. Coping is modified by the appraisal that the individual makes of the stress, i.e. how they appraise their ability to deal with it, and also by the meaning that the stressful event or situation has for them.

Poor coping

Certain factors in the patient's history or environment have been identified as significant in limiting their ability to cope, including:
• Lack of social support or social isolation
• Previous psychiatric history
• Alcohol or drug misuse
• History of recent losses.

These factors are useful in identifying those at risk of poor coping, enabling support to be targeted at those in greatest need.

Adjustment and transition

Another way of understanding people's response to cancer is that of adjustment or transition. This is not about response to an episode of stress, but response to a difficult ongoing and dynamic situation. Rather than being uniformly stressful, a diagnosis of cancer may bring both positive and negative effects. Alongside the losses experienced by people with cancer, many find an enhanced sense of meaning in their lives, closer relationships, and a deepened sense of spirituality. There is the potential for both positive and negative effects of cancer, and the period of adjustment has been described as a 'psychosocial transition'.

Resilience

Resilience is another way of understanding people's ability to recover from adversity and is identified as a personal quality in the individual that buffers against stress. Nurses can support resilience in cancer patients and their families by looking for opportunities to promote control and self-efficacy.

Stress and trauma reactions

Everyone diagnosed with cancer will go through a period of adjustment to the new realities of their situation. In most cases, they will make positive adjustments, with the support of their family, friends, and routine professional care. However, as many as 20% of people with cancer will experience a mental disorder, and up to 30% will experience some form of emotional crisis that is severe enough to disrupt their lives for at least a brief period. This can include:

• Rapid mood changes (fear, anger, despair, elation)
• Distress and tearfulness
• Anxiety and agitation
• Intrusive thoughts that are beyond conscious control, e.g. thoughts of death, pain, loss of loved ones
• Disturbed sleep or nightmares
• Numbness, disorientation, depersonalization (loss of sense of self), or derealization (feeling like you are not really there).

These are most likely to be experienced in the initial phases of diagnosis and treatment but can occur at other traumatic periods of the illness, e.g. recurrence or other significant bad news.

Stress reactions and disorder

When these features are acute and disabling but last only a brief period, such as a few hours or a few days, they are called an **acute stress reaction**. They usually resolve spontaneously, but if they persist for between 2 days to a month, then it is an **acute stress disorder** and may require treatment. This could involve specific psychological intervention or short-term use of anxiolytics such as benzodiazepines. If these features persist beyond 4 weeks, then the patient may be experiencing **post-traumatic stress disorder** (PTSD), a very disabling and distressing condition that can be long-lasting if untreated. PTSD requires referral for specialist psychological treatment (➔ see Psychological support, pp. 130–1).

Post-traumatic growth

It is possible to find positive change, following the diagnosis and treatment of cancer. Post-traumatic growth has emerged as a way of understanding how, in the midst of distress and trauma, people can find positive change in their lives. This can take the form of a reappraisal of priorities in life, enhanced relationships, a stronger sense of personal identity, and greater meaning in life. Nurses can aid this process by supporting the patient in:

• Finding relevant information
• Doing meaningful activities
• Making positive changes to lifestyle
• Sharing their experience and helping others.

Further reading

Brennan J. *Cancer in Context: A Practical Guide to Supportive Care*. Oxford: Oxford University Press; 2004.

Connerty TJ, Knott V. Promoting positive change in the face of adversity: experiences of cancer and post-traumatic growth. *Eur J Cancer Care* 2013;22:334–44.

Supporting the person with cancer

The contact a nurse has with a cancer patient will vary considerably. In brief contacts, e.g. in an outpatient department, support may focus on identifying those who are clearly distressed or need urgent support. In longer-term working relationships, there will be more opportunities to provide support and discuss coping strategies with the patient and their family. Support involves being available to the patient and listening.

Support existing coping strategies

It is important to establish how a patient normally copes with stressful or demanding situations. This gives the best indication of how they will cope with the demands of the cancer. Ask the patient directly how they normally cope by saying, 'What do you normally do to deal with stress?' Identify whether usual coping strategies are working. For example, someone who normally copes by working hard will find it more difficult to cope if they are unable to work.

Review alternatives

If usual coping strategies are not working, discuss alternatives. These would need to fit with the individual's current level of functioning, energy, and capabilities. It is best if these are discussed, rather than suggested, to enable the patient to review what is possible or desirable for them. Below are some commonly used coping strategies:

- Distraction: listening to music, reading
- Doing purposeful and meaningful activity: handiwork, planning trips or holidays
- Physical activity: walking, gardening
- Being in company, talking, sharing experiences
- Relaxation, mindfulness, meditation.

Social support structures

Most people derive great benefit from social support, from a sense that they are valued and loved and are part of a supportive community. These supports are usually there, even when professional support is not. Those with limited social support will need greater professional input. Offering professional support to carers is sometimes the most effective support to the person with cancer.

Provide information and offer choices

Give the patient and their carers information on support available locally and nationally. This may include health and social services and voluntary and charitable organizations. People are more likely to use a service if they make the choice themselves and they feel it will meet their needs.

Intervene and refer when necessary

If the patient does not appear to be coping, then it may be necessary to intervene, to positively offer support or make a referral to a specialist service, e.g. social work, psycho-oncology, or local support group.

Psychological assessment

All health and social care professionals have a role in psychological assessment. However, many aspects of assessment are specialized, particularly where this involves mental health problems. The NICE *Guidance on Supportive and Palliative Care for Adults with Cancer*[1] has provided a four-level model (see Table 48.1), giving guidance on the appropriate level of assessment for different professional groups (compare with levels of support in ➔ Psychological support, pp. 130–1).

Psychological assessment: level 1

All health professionals should have the ability to recognize psychological distress and identify the patient's and family's concerns. This requires an awareness of the problems that patients and their families are likely to experience, as outlined in ➔ Supporting the person with cancer, p. 579, and an ability to elicit concerns.

Psychological assessment: level 2

More experienced and specialized nurses, e.g. site-specific cancer nurses, can be expected to assess the impact of cancer on a patient's daily life, mood, work, and family relationships (including sexual relationships). Some will use specific assessment tools, e.g. the Hospital Anxiety and Depression Scale (HADS) to screen for symptoms of anxiety and depression (➔ see Depression, pp. 581–2).

Psychological assessment: level 3

Some cancer specialists may have special training in counselling or psychotherapy models, e.g. CBT, and be able to undertake assessment of some psychopathology, e.g. anxiety, depression, psychosexual problems. However, practitioners at this level are more likely to be mental health professionals with specialist education and qualifications, e.g. mental health nurses, psychologists.

Psychological assessment: level 4

This level of psychological assessment can only be undertaken by suitably trained mental health professionals, e.g. psychiatrists, psychologists.

Table 48.1 Levels of psychological assessment

Level	Group	Assessment
1	All health-care professionals	Recognition of psychological needs
2	Professionals with additional expertise	Screening for psychological distress
3	Trained and accredited professionals	Assessing for distress and some psychopathology
4	Mental health specialists	Diagnosis of psychopathology

Data sourced from NICE (2004). *Guidance on Supportive and Palliative Care for Adults with Cancer* ℜ https://www.nice.org.uk/guidance/csg4

References

1 National Institute for Health and Care Excellence (2004). *Improving Supportive and Palliative Care for Adults with Cancer*. Cancer service guideline [CSG4]. Available at: ℜ https://www.nice.org.uk/guidance/csg4

Depression

Depression is a persistent and unvarying low mood. It is often experienced as a lack of feeling, an emptiness, or loss of meaning in life.

Depression differs from sadness in both quality and degree (see Table 48.2). The sad person may be cheered up, but the depressed person's mood does not react. Depression is common in people with cancer, with prevalence as high as 20%.

Features of depression

Depression has psychological, physical, and social features or symptoms. These include:

- Psychological: low mood, poor concentration, loss of interest and pleasure in things, guilt, remorse and pessimism (depressive cognitions), suicidal ideas
- Physical: loss of energy, fatigue, slowing up, poor sleep and appetite, tension and agitation
- Social: reduced social interaction, withdrawal or social avoidance.

Assessment of depression

The diagnosis of depression is a specialist mental health activity. However, all health and social care professionals can undertake screening for depression. Some features of depression are also common in people who are physically ill and cannot therefore be relied on for diagnostic purposes. These include fatigue and sleep and appetite disturbance. Other factors that affect psychological assessment include:

- Weakness and exhaustion
- Nutritional deficiency
- Cognitive impairment
- Pain
- Drugs such as opiates, corticosteroids, and benzodiazepines.

Table 48.2 Depression and sadness: differences

Depression	Sadness
Feels outcast and alone	Can feel intimately connected with others
The mood has a feeling of permanence	A feeling that someday this will end
Rumination on past mistakes	Able to enjoy happy memories
Extreme self-loathing	Has a sense of self-worth
Mood is constant and unremitting	Sadness comes in waves
No hope, no interest in the future	Looks forward to things
Enjoys few activities	Retains capacity for pleasure
Suicidal thoughts, suicidal behaviour	Has the will to live

Adapted from Rayner L, Higginson IJ, Price A, Hotopf M. *The Management of Depression in Palliative Care: European Clinical Guidelines*. London: Department of Palliative Care, Policy & Rehabilitation (ℜ www.kcl.ac.uk/schools/medicine/depts/palliative)/European Palliative Care Research Collaborative (ℜ http://www.eapcnet.eu/); 2010.

It is therefore important to identify treatable causes of distress and focus the assessment on psychological and social features that suggest depression.

Key diagnostic features of depression

The primary diagnostic feature of depression is persistent, unvarying mood of at least 2 weeks duration.

In addition, the following features confirm the diagnosis:

- Fearful, depressed, or worried appearance
- Reduced interest and enjoyment of life, social withdrawal
- Depressive thoughts or cognitions, e.g. guilt, remorse, pessimism.

Assessment strategies

The best way to assess for depression is to engage the patient directly in conversation. In this way, the nurse can both observe the patient's behaviour and gain direct information about how the patient is feeling. In observing the patient, note the following signs of depression:

- Avoidance of eye contact
- A lack of rapport or emotional warmth
- Speech lacks spontaneity and is monotonous or monosyllabic.

The most useful single question to ask is 'Do you feel depressed?' If the answer is yes, then it is useful to identify whether any of the other features of depression are also present.

Carers are a very good source of information. They can say whether the patient's current mood and behaviour are normal for them or unusual.

Hospital Anxiety and Depression Scale

The HADS[2] has been developed specifically to detect depression and anxiety in the physically ill, focusing on the psychological and social manifestations of depression and anxiety. It is quick and easy to use, and it can provide a useful score to underpin a verbal assessment. It gives a score for both anxiety and depression on a scale of 0–21. Scores of 11–21 are clinically significant.

References

2 Zigmond AS, Snaith RP. The hospital anxiety and depression scale. *Acta Psychiatr Scand* 1983;67:361–70.

Suicide and suicidal ideas

Suicidal ideas are common in people with depression, and they also occur in people who have been diagnosed with cancer. This may take the form of considering suicide as a future option if life becomes unbearable because of pain or lack of dignity. This can be greatly helped by giving the patient and carers information about palliative care options in advanced disease (➔ see Euthanasia and physician-assisted suicide (assisted dying), pp. 167–8).

People with cancer can also have passive suicidal ideas, i.e. wishing to be dead, but not actively doing anything about it. This can occur at difficult stages of illness and treatment, and is usually transitory. These are different from active suicidal ideas where the person is seriously considering suicide and may be making definite plans.

Suicide itself is not a common event. ~3000 people commit suicide in the UK every year. However, suicidal ideas should always be taken seriously. Most people who have suicidal ideas are willing to talk about them. Although suicidal ideas are not themselves treatable, people experiencing them can be offered support to reduce the risk of acting on them. Suicidal ideas are associated with depression, and depression is treatable.

It is also important to recognize those at ↑ risk of suicide. The following factors increase the risk of suicide in the general population:
- ♂ gender
- Older age
- Mental illness (e.g. depression, schizophrenia)
- Alcohol or drug dependence
- History of previous self-harm
- Physical illness—especially with chronic pain
- Socially isolated

In people with cancer, the risk is higher where there is impaired physical functioning, poor prognosis, or advanced disease.

Nursing management of depression

If patients express suicidal ideas, they should always be taken seriously. It is wrong to believe that someone telling you about suicidal ideas means that they are less likely to do it. Most people who do commit suicide have confided their intentions to someone. Let the patient know that you take their feelings seriously. It is important to make a distinction between passive suicidal ideas (see earlier paragraph) and active suicidal ideas, i.e. when the patient has active intention or plans to kill themselves.
- Spend time with the patient, establishing what their current intentions are.
- Alert your colleagues to what you know of the patient's suicidal ideas, and discuss this as a team.
- Inform senior colleagues who have clinical and managerial responsibility, e.g. senior medical and nursing staff.
- If there is any suspicion that the patient has active suicidal ideas on which they are likely to act, then make a psychiatric referral urgently.
- It may be necessary to observe the patient closely until the psychiatrist or other mental health specialist arrives.

Treatment of depression

It is very important to treat depression. Depression involves considerable suffering for both the patient and their carers. It is also associated with an ↑ risk of suicide. Depressed patients are less likely to cooperate with, and make progress in, their treatment.

Drug treatments for depression

Most episodes of depression will respond to the use of antidepressant medication. Types of antidepressants in common use include:

- **Selective serotonin reuptake inhibitors (SSRIs)** are commonly used with the physically ill, as they have fewer side effects than some alternatives. Examples are citalopram and paroxetine. Potential side effects of SSRIs include nausea, vomiting, and headaches. There is a discontinuation syndrome associated with SSRIs that causes insomnia, fatigue, and agitation. It is advisable to reduce the dose gradually, giving it on alternate days, to prevent this. SSRIs should be used with caution or avoided in any patients with hepatic or renal impairment or who are taking anticoagulants or NSAIDs.
- **Serotonin-noradrenaline reuptake inhibitors (SNRIs)**, including venlafaxine, are a similar group to SSRIs and are also used to treat depression.
- **Tricyclic antidepressants**, including amitriptyline and imipramine, although effective treatments for depression are less commonly recommended for physically ill people, as they can have a range of side effects, including dry mouth, blurred vision, and constipation. They are also very dangerous in overdose.

Psychological treatments for depression

Some depressive episodes can be helped by psychological means alone, and many depressive episodes will be helped by a combination of medication and psychological treatment.

Cognitive behavioural therapy

This is the preferred psychological treatment for depression. CBT focuses on patients' thoughts, feelings, and behaviours and how they interact. There is evidence that negative thought patterns perpetuate a depressed person's pessimistic view of the world, and that helping them to change these patterns overcomes their depressive world-view. CBT is best carried out by a specialist mental health professional trained in its use. Other cognitive behavioural techniques, including **problem-solving treatment** and **activity scheduling**, can be used by cancer care professionals with additional training. There is now very strong evidence that cancer nurses with specialist training can effectively treat depression with problem-solving.

Mindfulness

Mindfulness is another important therapy that can help patients to overcome depression and many other problems. The practice of mindfulness, through techniques like focused breathing and meditation, teaches patients to pay attention to the present moment in a non-judgemental way. This, in turn, helps them to be more aware of, and manage, their thoughts and feelings associated with cancer and its treatment, rather than being overwhelmed by them.

Support of the depressed patient

Alongside specific treatments for depression, effective nursing care can help the patient to make a full recovery. Depression can generate cycles of pessimism and hopelessness, which the nurse can help to counteract. Effective support of the depressed patients involves the following.

- Respect the patient and acknowledge how they feel, but demonstrate confidence that things can get better.
- Actively engage the patient. This shows them that they are worth getting to know and counters any loss of self-esteem. Depressed patients will often withdraw from social contact, and the depression may be missed if efforts are not made to engage with them.
- Be aware of the danger of suicide or self-harming activity. Depression is a high risk factor for suicide.
- Be aware of the danger of self-neglect. Help the patient to maintain adequate standards of hygiene and appearance, as deterioration undermines self-confidence and morale.
- Get to know the social situation. Support family and friends who will find the situation hard to deal with. Identify factors that will perpetuate or prolong the depression, e.g. relationship or financial problems.
- Encourage physical activity which promotes physical well-being and prevents further deterioration.
- Encourage a return to normal activities as soon as possible.
- Refer on for mental health assessment and treatment when necessary.

Further reading

Moorey S, Greer S. *Cognitive Behaviour Therapy for People with Cancer*, 2nd ed. Oxford: Oxford University Press; 2002.

National Institute for Health and Care Excellence (2009). *Depression in Adults With a Chronic Physical Health Problem: Recognition and Management*. Clinical guideline [CG91]. Available at: ℛ https://www.nice.org.uk/guidance/CG91.

Strong, V, Waters, R, Hibberd, C, et al. Management of depression for people with cancer (SMaRT oncology 1): a randomised trial. *Lancet* 2008;372:40–8.

Anxiety

Unlike depression, anxiety is a universal and ever present human experience. Worry, for example, is a common way that people attempt to deal with problems by thinking about them in depth and trying to find solutions. However, anxiety can also become a significant problem in itself if it interferes with coping.

Features of anxiety

The following are common features of anxiety:
- Psychological: fearfulness, apprehension, uncertainty, poor concentration, worrying thoughts, a sense of impending doom
- Physical: tachycardia, hyperventilation, sweating, tremor, frequency of micturition, diarrhoea
- Anxiety is associated with the following behaviour: agitation, seeking reassurance, restlessness, pacing.

Anxiety as a problem

Anxiety disorders, characterized by severe anxiety that disrupts everyday life, include generalized anxiety disorder, phobic disorder, and panic disorder.

Anxiety can have the following effects, which will impair QoL and make treating cancer more difficult:
- Difficulty concentrating
- Loss of patience or irritability
- Difficulty taking in information
- Difficulty making decisions
- Pain may become more difficult to tolerate
- Loss of appetite, nausea
- Sexual dysfunction
- Sleep disturbance
- Fatigue.

Panic attacks

These are intense, acute attacks or episodes of severe anxiety, characterized by:
- Chest pain, palpitations, and shortness of breath
- Intense apprehension or fear, a sense of impending catastrophe
- Fear of losing control or going mad, or that death is imminent.

Anxiety in cancer care

Having a diagnosis of cancer can provoke specific anxieties for patients and their families. As the disease status changes, and the patient progresses through treatment, new situations present new challenges, and there are ongoing uncertainties about the future. Particular situations that can provoke anxiety include:
- Hospital appointments and waiting for the results of investigations. These can have major implications for the patient's future, and many patients report the period leading up to this as a particularly anxious time

- Periods of uncertainty about prognosis or treatment outcome. The period after the end of treatment can be a particularly unsettling time for cancer patients, as they adjust to the challenges of survivorship and deal with fears of cancer recurrence
- Prior to, and during, painful investigative procedures and treatments
- Prior to discharge after a long period of hospitalization
- Social anxiety (fear of being seen in public) associated with changes to physical appearance
- Anxiety associated with breathlessness (➔ see Cancer-related breathlessness pp. 514–15)
- Situations of vulnerability, e.g. being undressed in the presence of staff.

Physical causes of anxiety
- Endocrine disorders, e.g. hyperthyroidism, hypoglycaemia.
- Cardiovascular disorders, e.g. congestive cardiac failure, arrhythmias.
- Respiratory disorders, e.g. COPD.
- Metabolic conditions, e.g. hypoxia, encephalitis.
- Neurological conditions, e.g. delirium.

Drug-related
- Corticosteroids, bronchodilators.
- Drug and alcohol withdrawal.

Anxiety management

Anxiety management is a series of techniques that can be taught to patients as general strategies for coping or for dealing with anxiety and stressful situations during treatment.

General anxiety management strategies

Exercise and rest

Regular exercise, within the limits imposed by the disease, helps to relieve muscular tension and promote a sense of well-being. Good sleep hygiene gives a sense of refreshment and relieves fatigue. Patients who are tense and anxious should avoid or restrict the use of stimulants like coffee, which increase tension and impair sleep.

Time management and goal planning

Using time purposefully enhances the feeling of being in control and reduces opportunities for dwelling on problems. Achieving modest goals can help during periods of adjustment by giving a sense of satisfaction and enhancing self-esteem. Setting unrealistic targets has the opposite effect. You can encourage patients to work with their carers to plan targets to be achieved each day.

Relaxation training

Progressive muscle relaxation (PMR) teaches us to recognize the different feelings of relaxed and tense muscles. PMR usually involves lying or sitting in a calm, comfortable setting and progressively tightening and relaxing groups of muscles, from the head down or the feet up. PMR can be taught to individuals or groups, and there are numerous tapes with which patients can practise at home.

Progressive muscle relaxation

This can be taught to people who are experiencing anxiety or going through a stressful time, as a preventative measure for dealing with anxiety. It can be practised by the person on their own or with others. Twenty minutes a day is a good routine. Audiotapes and CDs are available that take people through the exercises.

- Find a quiet place and make yourself comfortable, removing shoes and loosening clothing, sitting, or lying down.
- Focus on the breathing, breathing in through the nose and out through the mouth. Imagine tension leaving the body with the outbreath.
- Focus on a muscle group, first breathing in and tensing them, holding for a few seconds, then relaxing the muscles and breathing out. Relax before the next stage.
- Go through the following muscle groups: hands, arms, neck and shoulders, face and forehead, chest and back, abdominal muscles, buttocks, legs, and feet. At each stage, tense the muscles as tightly as possible, then release. Focus on the muscle group alone; try to keep the rest of the body relaxed.
- Progress to visualization, or stay relaxed and get up slowly.

Anxiety first-aid

Managing hyperventilation

Hyperventilation (over-breathing or rapid shallow breathing) is a common effect of anxiety, which worsens and extends the episode of anxiety. Managing hyperventilation involves breathing slowly and deeply, by focusing on the breathing. A hand can be placed on the stomach, to observe the rise and fall of the diaphragm. It is helpful to demonstrate this to the anxious person.

Managing panic attacks

Panic attacks are often precipitated by a thought or feeling. Panic then re-inforces whatever fear precipitated the attack. The combination of chest pain, shortness of breath, and tachycardia, with the psychological experience of fear and impending doom, can be very distressing. The following steps can be taught:

• Slow deep breathing
• Identify any precipitants
• Understand the process of panic, and plan how to manage it if it happens again.

Distraction

It can help for the patient to distract themselves from anxious thoughts by finding an external focus for their attention, e.g. by talking to someone, listening to music, or reading a book.

Visualization

This can be developed during relaxation training, visualizing a peaceful or relaxing place that the patient associates with well-being and contentment.

Pharmacological treatment of anxiety

Pharmacological treatment of anxiety should be approached with caution. There are three main reasons for this:

- The most commonly used drugs can develop dependency
- Reliance on drugs can reduce the patient's sense of personal control
- All drugs have side effects which may cause additional problems for the patient.

For these reasons, anxiety management techniques are recommended in the first place for treating anxiety. However, anxiolytic drugs do have a place in the short-term management of anxiety, particularly during acutely distressing or unpleasant medical procedures and in end-of-life care. Benzodiazepines are the main group of anxiolytic drugs in use, e.g. diazepam, lorazepam. Midazolam can be used in situations where rapid sedation is necessary. Problems associated with this group are excessive drowsiness and respiratory depression. Because they can also lead to disinhibition, they should not be given to people who have suicidal ideas.

The other group of anxiolytic drugs in common use are the β-blockers, e.g. propranolol, which are particularly useful for controlling palpitations. Antidepressants, such as SSRIs, e.g. citalopram, can be used for longer-term management of anxiety, particularly if associated with depression.

Assessment and support of the anxious patient

Assessment of anxiety should involve the following:
- How severe and incapacitating is the anxiety, and how long does it last?
- What effect does the anxiety have on the patient's health and QoL?
- Is there a trigger to the anxiety? Identifying what starts off or triggers anxiety will help the patient find alternative ways of responding to their concerns.
- What physical effects is the patient experiencing? This will help the patient distinguish the effects of anxiety from other effects of illness and treatment.
- Are there background factors which maintain the anxiety? This could include any ongoing worries or questions the patient needs to be answered.
- How does the patient normally deal with anxiety? This provides an opportunity for the patient to review the effectiveness of their anxiety management and consider alternatives.

In addition to anxiety management and treatment strategies, the way that care is delivered can minimize anxiety for the patient and aid their coping. Anxiety can be minimized by:
- Helping the patient feel in control
- Involving the patient and their carers in decision-making and offering choices, in a manner and at a pace that is acceptable to the patient
- Providing clear information, based on the patient's view of their information needs.

It is also important to provide reassurance by dealing effectively with treatable causes of anxiety and by demonstrating a professional understanding of anxiety and its management. An important element in the management of anxiety is **containment**, i.e. demonstrating calmness and confidence in managing the anxiety in the face of the patient's uncertainty and apprehension.

Further reading

Butow P, Price M, Shaw J, et al. Clinical pathway for the screening, assessment and management of anxiety and depression in adult cancer patients: Australian guidelines. *Psychooncology* 2015;24:987–1001.

Other psychological problems encountered in people with cancer

Acute confusional state or delirium

Acute confusion or delirium is an acute brain syndrome, characterized by problems with the level of consciousness, attention, and memory. Acute confusion may be transient and reversible. Key features are clouding of consciousness and difficulty registering or making sense of new information. Clouding of consciousness ranges from reduced awareness of the environment or drowsiness to stupor and coma.

Presentation of acute confusional state

It is more common in terminal illness and in older people, particularly when they have been removed from a familiar environment. 'Sundown syndrome' describes a worsening of symptoms towards the evening. The following are common:

• Clouding of consciousness—reduced awareness of the environment
• Impaired attention and memory—especially of recent events
• Disorientation in time, place, or person
• Impaired comprehension and abstract thinking
• Perceptual distortions—illusions or hallucinations
• Transient delusions—usually paranoid
• Disturbed cycle of sleeping and waking, nightmares
• Emotional disturbance—depression, anxiety, fear, irritability, euphoria, apathy, perplexity
• Psychomotor disturbance—agitation, restless, or underactivity.

Patients commonly appear perplexed or apathetic, and sometimes distressed, anxious, or fearful. Misunderstandings, related to poor orientation, or different interpretations of external events may lead to fear and suspicion or paranoid behaviour.

The presentation is similar to that of chronic confusional state or dementia, but unlike acute confusion, these conditions are not associated with clouding of consciousness and are irreversible.

Causes of acute confusional state

There are a number of physical or physiological causes of confusion:

• Prescribed drugs—opioids, corticosteroids, psychotropic drugs
• Drug withdrawal—e.g. benzodiazepines or opioids, alcohol
• Infection—respiratory or urinary infection, septicaemia, encephalitis or meningitis
• Brain pathology—primary or secondary tumour
• Metabolic—dehydration, electrolyte disturbance, hypoxia, hypercalcaemia, organ failure
• Endocrine disorders—hypoglycaemia, myxoedema, thyrotoxicosis
• Trauma—head injury, subdural haematoma
• Severe pain
• Hearing and sight defects.

Nursing management of acute confusion

Assessment

Identify and treat the cause and any contributory factors (e.g. sensory deprivation). Many of the psychological symptoms associated with confusional state are caused by difficulties in processing new information. Assessment may involve using the following tools:
• Mini-Mental State Examination (MMSE)
• Confusion Assessment Method (CAM).

Manage confused thoughts

Aim to keep all communication clear, brief, and to the point. Avoid overtaxing the patient's short attention span. Ask only one question at a time.

Encourage correct orientation

Aid orientation by the use of cues such as mealtimes or visiting times. Make the environment as familiar as possible, using the patient's own possessions. Ensure that the patient's hearing aid or glasses are being worn.

Prevent and respond to distress

Listen to the patient's worries or concerns, which may be expressed indirectly. Use touch to calm the patient, if this proves helpful. Reduce all invasive or painful interventions to a minimum.

Respond to hallucinations and delusions

Try to offer explanations, rather than reassurance. Acknowledge distress and concern when faced with delusional ideas.

Safety issues

Individual nursing care, on a one-to-one basis, will usually keep the confused patient safe. Avoid the use of physical restraint, which undermines the nurse–patient relationship.

Medication

This may be helpful in ensuring a good night's sleep or in calming an extremely distressed patient. The choice of medication will relate to the specific problem, e.g. analgesics for pain, benzodiazepines for anxiety, haloperidol for delirium. Any medication should be kept to the minimum effective dose. Sedating the patient may further impair their consciousness and worsen their confusional state.

Further reading

Folstein M, Folstein S, McHugh P. Mini Mental State: a practical method for grading the cognitive state of patients for the clinician. *J Psychiatr Res* 1975;12:189–98.

Inouye S, van Dyck C, Alessi C, Balkin S, Siegal A, Horwitz R. Clarifying confusion: the Confusion Assessment Method. *Ann Intern Med* 1990;113:941–8.

Schuurmans M, Duursma S, Shortridge-Baggett L. Early recognition of delirium: review of the literature. *J Clin Nurs* 2001;10:721–9.

Psychoses and their management

Psychoses are disorders of thought, feeling, and perception that lead to difficulties relating to both the internal world of self, other people, and the world at large. Psychotic states may be mild and transient, in response to a clear precipitant, or enduring and disabling, e.g. schizophrenia.

The presentation of acute psychosis can be similar to that of acute confusional state, but disturbance in the level of consciousness is rare. Psychotic disorders differ from confusional states in that there is no clear physical cause.

Psychotic episodes are rarely encountered in the cancer care setting, but they are distressing and difficult to manage when they are. There are two main ways in which they will be encountered:

- People with existing psychotic illness who develop cancer
- Acute psychotic reactions in someone with cancer.

Presentation of psychoses

- The person's attention and concentration may be impaired.
- Thought disorders: the person may believe that their thoughts are being controlled, inserted, or removed by others.
- Hallucinations: auditory hallucinations are the most common, but visual, olfactory, and tactile hallucinations are also possible.
- Delusions: incongruous beliefs that are frequently persecutory.
- Mood: may be blunted or inappropriate to the situation.
- Behaviour: may be paranoid or suspicious, impulsive, or unpredictable.
- Appearance: clothing may appear bizarre, or the individual may neglect their appearance.

Nursing management of psychoses

Get expert mental health advice and support

The management of psychosis can be very complex and unpredictable. If the patient is already known to a mental health team, it may be possible to arrange support from professionals, such as mental health nurses, who already know the patient.

Establish a relationship

The experience of psychosis is usually very distressing to patients, relatives, and staff alike. Some nurses may withdraw from, rather than engage with, the patient, but this is likely to alienate the patient and their family. Openness, consistency, and genuine concern on the nurse's part will promote therapeutic rapport.

Maintain safety

Some patients may be at ↑ risk of suicide and self-harm when psychotic. Safety measures should include nursing individuals in observation areas, preferably on the ground floor. Agitation and threatening behaviour are possible (➲ see Violence and aggression, pp. 598–9).

Care of people with long-term psychotic illness

People who have long-term severe mental illness may have a number of physical health problems, in addition to mental illness. This is partly due to the effects of the illness and resulting lifestyle, e.g. poor diet, apathy, and lack of exercise, also of the use of drugs like alcohol and tobacco and the side effects of antipsychotic medication. They are also likely to have secondary social problems as a result of long-term illness that have effects on their health, e.g. social exclusion, poor housing, and limited resources.

Medication

Medication is important in controlling the distressing and disabling symptoms of psychosis. Antipsychotic medication includes the **typical** drugs chlorpromazine, flupentixol, and haloperidol, and the more recently introduced **atypical** drugs such as clozapine, olanzapine, and risperidone. All antipsychotic drugs have difficult side effects, and these should be monitored. **Antidopaminergic side effects** include dystonia, painful muscle spasms, akathisia, a distressing feeling of restless, and Parkinsonian symptoms— tremor, muscle stiffness, and shuffling gait. Tardive dyskinesia, involuntary muscular movements, is associated with longer-term antipsychotic use. **Anticholinergic side effects** include dry mouth, blurred vision, and constipation.

Further reading

Pack S. Poor physical health and mortality in patients with schizophrenia. *Nurs Stand* 2009;23:41–5.

Violence and aggression

Incidents of violence and aggression have been increasingly reported in health-care situations. These are not especially associated with the cancer care setting, but they may occur. There are a number of reasons why people may become aggressive or violent:

- Anger or frustration
- Fear or confusion
- Delusional misinterpretation or intoxication
- Loss of control or disinhibition
- Previous history of violence
- Limited ability to interpret the environment, e.g. learning disabilities.

Assessment

An assessment should establish whether the violent or aggressive behaviour is the result of real and understandable factors in the environment, such as anger or frustration, which are amenable to reason. If the behaviour is the result of an altered mental state, e.g. delirium, psychosis, drugs, or alcohol, they may respond to treatment.

Principles of anger management

- Respond to the person, not the behaviour, as far as possible.
- Maintain your professional composure and priorities.
- Put limits on unacceptable behaviour.
- Ensure a safe environment.
- Defuse the situation by acting calmly and showing concern.
- Acknowledge how the person feels.
- Seek reasons for the behaviour.
- Problem-solve—help the person identify their problems and find solutions.

Principles of dealing with violence

- It is always better to prevent or defuse potentially violent situations than to deal with actual violence.
- Familiarize yourself with the local policy for violent incidents, and know who to call on for assistance.
- Maintain communication, and be clear about the action you are taking.
- Relocate vulnerable people to a safer environment.
- Always act within your own area of confidence.
- Review the incident with the staff concerned, to defuse feelings and learn for the future (debriefing).

Legal and professional framework for action

Most interventions carried out with confused, or potentially violent, patients in hospital are done under common law, i.e. rights and responsibilities that have been established by previous decisions in law courts.

Action is carried out under the following principles

- **Necessity**: staff may need to restrain or treat a patient who is a danger to themselves or others without their consent, in an emergency.
- **Duty of care**: staff have a duty to provide care to those who need it. Failure to do so may result in negligence.

The statutory legal framework for managing people with mental health problems in a hospital in England and Wales includes:

- The Mental Capacity Act 2005, which makes provision for decisions to be made on behalf of patients if they lack capacity, i.e. the ability to make decisions, on the basis of disturbed or impaired mental function. The individual is assumed to have capacity, unless judgement is made that they lack it. **Incapacity** means that a patient is unable to understand, retain, or make effective use of information or is unable to communicate their decision.
- The Mental Health Act 1983 (amended 2007) makes provision for compulsory detention in hospital of an individual, because of the nature or degree of their mental disorder, for assessment or treatment, if they are deemed to be a risk to themselves or others. Section 5(2) can be used in the general hospital to detain a patient for up to 72 hours for assessment of their mental state. Sections 2 and 3 of the Act allow detention for assessment and/or treatment in a psychiatric hospital or general hospital psychiatric unit.

Alcohol misuse

- Alcohol is part of the British and European way of life. Used moderately, it has no harmful effects and may bring positive health benefits, e.g. protection against heart disease.
- Excessive alcohol use is associated with cardiovascular, digestive, neurological, psychological, and social problems, with cancers of the H&N, oesophagus, stomach, pancreas, colon, and breast.
- The incidence of alcohol-related deaths in the UK may be as high as 15,000 per annum, with as many as 25% resulting from accidents.

Alcohol units

Alcohol units are the accepted measurement of alcohol consumption in the UK; 1 unit represents 8g of ethanol. Table 49.1 shows the units in standard measures of alcohol.

Safe drinking

The recommended limits of safe drinking in the UK are:
- 14 units of alcohol per week, or 2–3 units per day
- Spread drinking over 3 or more days
- Have several alcohol-free days a week.

Hazardous drinking

This is regular alcohol consumption in excess of the recommended limits, leading to the risk of physical and psychological harm. As much as a quarter of the UK population drinks in a hazardous fashion.

Binge drinking

This is drinking excessive amounts of alcohol, in order to get drunk. It can be defined as drinking more than twice the recommended number of daily alcohol units in one session, i.e. 6 units.

Table 49.1 Alcohal units in standard drink measures

Beer, lager, cider	Average strength 3–4% alcohol by volume	Half pint	1 unit
		Pint	2 units
Strong beer, lager, cider	5% alcohol by volume	Pint	3 units
		Bottle (500mL)	3 units
Wine	Average strength 12% alcohol by volume (wine ranges 8–14%)	Small glass (125mL)	1 unit
		Bottle (750mL)	9 units
Fortified wine, e.g. sherry, port	20% alcohol by volume	Standard pub measure (50mL)	1 unit
		Bottle (750mL)	15 units
Spirits, e.g. whisky, brandy, vodka, gin	40% alcohol by volume	Standard pub measure (35mL)	1.5 units
		Bottle (750mL)	30 units

Harmful drinking

This is defined as a pattern of heavy drinking which results in damage to physical or mental health: 50 units a week in men; 35 units a week in women.

Alcohol dependence

This is physical dependence on alcohol. The person's behaviour changes, as there is an ↑ emphasis on alcohol within the person's life. This can result in financial and work problems, damaged relationships, a range of health problems, and accidents. It may manifest as:

- A strong or overpowering desire to drink alcohol
- Symptoms of withdrawal, including tremor, nausea, vomiting, perspiration, and seizures. These can start within 3–6 hours of the last drink and may last 5–7 days.
- Delirium tremens: this is a very dangerous condition that occurs in ~5% of people withdrawing from alcohol. It often presents with confusion and agitation, hallucinations (often tactile), and paranoia. Its onset is within 24–48 hours of the last drink.

Websites

Alcohol Concern. Available at: ℘ https://www.alcoholconcern.org.uk/

Department of Health. *Alcohol and Drug Misuse Prevention and Treatment Guidance*. Available at: ℘ https://www.alcohollearningcentre.org.uk/

Further reading

National Institute for Health and Care Excellence (2011). *Alcohol-use Disorders: Diagnosis, Assessment and Management of Harmful Drinking and Alcohol Dependence*. Clinical guideline [CG115]. Available at: ℘ https://www.nice.org.uk/guidance/CG115

Nursing management of people who are alcohol-dependent

A patient who is alcohol-dependent may present with a number of problems in the cancer care setting. The person's use of alcohol may cause additional health problems, may interact with medication, or may make it hard for them to cooperate with treatment or to attend appointments. The disruption of relationships and finances can lead to ongoing problems within the family structure. The resulting loss of trust and confidence can also make it very difficult to offer support to the patient and their family. People who are alcohol-dependent are at greater risk of depression, suicide, and attempted suicide.

Assessment

Dependence is likely to be present in men who consistently drink >50 units a week and in women who drink >35 units a week.

According to the International Classification of Diseases, tenth revision (ICD-10) criteria,[1] alcohol dependence is diagnosed if three or more of the following have been present during the previous year:

- A strong desire or compulsion to drink
- Difficulty controlling drinking
- Physical withdrawal state, drinking to relieve withdrawal
- ↑ tolerance of alcohol, drinking more to achieve the same effect
- Neglect of other interests, more time spent drinking, or recovering from its effects
- Persisting with drinking, despite the harmful effects of alcohol.

Principles of intervention

Do an alcohol assessment. Key questions are:

- How much do you drink?
- How often do you drink?

Alcohol assessment should be undertaken prior to surgery in patients where alcohol abuse is suspected. This should be considered in cancers known to be associated with alcohol abuse, e.g. cancers of the H&N. If undetected, complications due to alcohol withdrawal can occur after surgery. Refer to local guidelines where these are available.

Drinkers are not always honest or accurate about their consumption. Get information from the family where possible.

Intervene at any stage of problem drinking. Provide information on the health risks associated with drinking, what constitutes sensible drinking, and how to cut down.

Many well-motivated people can reduce their drinking with information and informal support from their family and from alcohol support groups. Professional support is targeted on the alcohol-dependent.

Detoxification

Detoxification is the planned withdrawal of alcohol from dependent individuals, under professional supervision. It is usually done at the patient's home or via an outpatient clinic. It can be done in hospital with specialist intensive support. The recommended drug for withdrawal is chlordiazepoxide, which dampens withdrawal symptoms, lowers the risk of convulsions, and is less likely to be misused than other benzodiazepines.

References

1 International Classification of Diseases, tenth revision (ICD-10). Available at: ℜ http://apps.who. int/classifications/apps/icd/icd10online2003/fr-icd.htm

Sexuality and cancer

Introduction to sexuality and cancer

Sexuality is unique to each person and is influenced by a variety of factors throughout lifespan. It is defined by WHO as:[1]

> 'A central aspect of being human throughout life and encompasses sex, gender identities and roles, sexual orientation, eroticism, pleasure, intimacy and reproduction. Sexuality is experienced and expressed in thoughts, fantasies, desires, beliefs, attitudes, values, behaviours, practices, roles and relationships. While sexuality can include all of these dimensions, not all of them are always experienced or expressed. Sexuality is influenced by the interaction of biological, psychological, social, economic, political, cultural, ethical, legal, historical, religious and spiritual factors'.

> World Health Organisation (2006) *Defining sexual health: Report of a technical consultation on sexual health 28–31 January 2002*, Geneva. WHO: Geneva.

Our sexuality is a fundamental part of our identity and includes:
• Physical factors that define biological sex
• Psychological factors that contribute towards gender identity
• Social and cultural factors that influence sexual values, beliefs, and behaviour.

Sexual intercourse is only one aspect of sexuality. Sexuality is expressed in a variety of ways:
• Through our sense of our own masculinity or femininity
• Through our body image and self-esteem
• Through sexual behaviour and sexual activity.

Because our sexuality affects many areas of our lives, the effects of cancer on sexuality are far-reaching. Cancer and its treatments can challenge people's taken-for-granted views of themselves and their sexual relationships. Cancer and its treatments can disrupt: body image and self-image, sexual response and sexual behaviour, emotional life and intimate relationships, and the ability to reproduce. This not only affects those in partnered relationships, but also single people worry about their ability to form future relationships.

Sexual identity

Lesbian, gay, bisexual, or transgender (LGBT) people are a significant group of people who are diagnosed with, and have treatment for, cancer. There is evidence to suggest that, on their cancer journey, they are less likely to feel they are treated with dignity and respect than heterosexuals. It is important therefore that nurses are aware that they may have particular needs, based on their sexual identity and lifestyle, and to help them identify suitable sources of support.

References

1 World Health Organization. *Defining Sexual Health: Report of a Technical Consultation on Sexual Health 28–31 January 2002, Geneva*. Geneva: World Health Organization; 2006.

Body image

Cancer causes changes in appearance through amputation, scarring, hair loss, drug side effects, weight loss, and weight gain. Altered appearance challenges people's views about their body image and can affect self-esteem, feelings of attractiveness, and confidence; these can impede intimacy and sexual relationships.

Strategies for adjusting to altered body image

Patients can be prepared in advance for the possible effects of treatment on lifestyle and self-image. This could involve, for example, providing photographs or other images of how appearance may change after treatment (➲ see Breast reconstruction, pp. 305–7).

If changes have taken place, useful strategies for becoming desensitized to an altered physical appearance include:

• Regularly examining the changed body part
• Regularly looking at oneself in the mirror
• Touching the affected part
• Inviting the partner to look at, and touch, the body.

Each individual should decide which of these tasks they are able to perform first. Through a gradual process of familiarization, they will become less distressed by their appearance; when this happens, they will be ready to move on to the next task. Some will choose to involve their partner from the beginning, whereas others prefer to adjust to their altered body before revealing it to their partner. This is influenced by previous expectations within their relationship.

Some individuals feel they are no longer the person they were and doubt their partner's feelings towards them. It can be helpful if they ask themselves:

• What makes me who I am?
• What do I like about myself?
• What do I value about my partner?
• If their body had changed, how would I feel about them?

Telling one's partner how they feel and voicing their worries and concerns can be helpful. However, they also need to be able to listen to, and hear, their partner's perspective.

Support groups, where people can share their concerns and hear how others are adjusting are often helpful. This could include, for example, Look Good Feel Better groups (➲ see Hair loss (alopecia), pp. 614–15), which support patients through cosmetic options available to them after treatment.

A minority of patients experience ongoing serious problems of self-image. They may benefit from referral for specialist mental health intervention (➲ see Psychological support, pp. 130–1).

Sexual expression

Cancer is associated with a number of sexual problems. Some of these are a direct physical result of the cancer or its treatment (see Table 50.1):
- Disfigurement or loss of sexual organs through surgery
- Nerve damage after pelvic surgery or radiotherapy, affecting sexual response and function
- Disfigurement or loss of sensation to other areas of the body such as the tongue, face, or mouth
- Loss of sensation in the hands due to chemotherapy-induced peripheral neuropathy
- Personality changes or loss of inhibition, resulting from brain involvement or surgery
- Vaginal dryness or narrowing due to chemotherapy or radiotherapy
- Infertility or early menopause through surgery or chemotherapy
- Impotence or loss of sexual response as a consequence of surgery, radiotherapy, or other medication (including some antidepressants, antihypertensives, and anti-convulsants).

Table 50.1 Treatment-related sexual problems

Problem	Management options
• Vaginal dryness, thinning, and loss of elasticity	• Use of suitable hydrating creams, lubricant gels, and oestrogen-based pessaries or creams
• Vaginal scarring and narrowing, causing painful intercourse	• Use of vaginal dilators • Finger stimulation—alone or as a couple • Explore alternative positions (e.g. with the woman on top, so able to control the depth and angle of penetration) • Explore alternatives to sexual intercourse (e.g. mutual masturbation and oral sex)
• Irregular or absence of periods	• Periods usually return—caution: pregnancy can occur in the absence of periods
• Signs of early menopause, e.g. hot flushes, irritability	• HRT if the tumour is not hormone-dependent
• Reduced testosterone in men	• Usually recovers, or testosterone replacement therapy as an option
• Infertility	• Sperm banking • Embryo, egg, or ovarian tissue preservation
• Erectile dysfunction in men	• Use of vacuum devices or medications that improve blood flow to the penis [e.g. sildenafil, medicated urethral system for erections (MUSE) urethral pellets, or penile injections]
• Loss of desire, inability to achieve orgasm	• Thorough physical and psychological assessment • Treatment of any physical causes • Referral to psychosexual therapist

Other sexual problems occur as indirect effects of illness or treatment:
- An altered sense of sexual self because of altered body image, or loss of control of bodily functions
- Loss of confidence due to feeling unattractive, or loss of function
- Loss of intimacy caused by pain, disability, breathlessness, or fatigue
- Erectile dysfunction or loss of sexual response due to anxiety or depression.

Strategies for overcoming sexual difficulties for patients and their partners

During treatment, sexual activity may not be a priority for people, as they concentrate on 'getting through'. However, this cannot be assumed, as each person varies. Even when sexual expression is not possible or does not feel a priority, it is still important to share close, intimate moments that are not sexual and maintain intimacy through hugging, kissing, touch, massage, and shared activities. These can:
- Convey love and affection
- Console and comfort
- Boost self-confidence
- Maintain an emotional bond.

Overcoming sexual difficulties is easier if couples are able to:
- Be flexible
- Be curious and willing to experiment
- Recognize that change takes time
- Communicate openly with each other, voicing concerns, fears, and wishes (e.g. which areas are more/less comfortable to be touched and promote/inhibit arousal)
- Laugh together.

Couples who successfully adapt to the sexual difficulties are able to challenge any previously held expectations about what 'good' sex is (e.g. that it must involve sexual intercourse, must occur spontaneously, and must always end in orgasm). Useful strategies include:
- Making time for intimacy, creating a comfortable and relaxed environment
- Agreeing boundaries, discussing what does not feel possible at the moment, and agreeing which activities or areas of the body are 'off limits' until each partner feels more comfortable
- Avoiding the pressure of sex when tired, uncomfortable, or in pain
- Exploring different positions and options for mutual pleasure and sexual satisfaction
- Exploring other ways of being intimate
- Acknowledging differences in sexual desire between partners and try to work with these.

Despite the effects of cancer and its treatment on sexual expression, couples adjust by re-evaluating the place of sexual activity in their lives. Some couples report becoming closer, despite the long-term sexual problems they experience.

Useful resources
- Cancer Research UK has an information sheet *Sex and Cancer if You Are Single* (available at: ℘ https://www.cancerresearchuk.org)
- The Daisy Network provides information and support for women who have experienced premature menopause through cancer (available at: ℘ https://www.daisynetwork.org.uk)
- Macmillan Cancer Support provides information on cancer and sexuality (available at: ℘ https://www.macmillan.org.uk)
- National LGBT Cancer Project provides information and support for cancer survivors who are lesbian, gay, bisexual, and transgender (available at: ℘ http://www.lgbtcancer.com)
- Relate is a national organization providing relationship therapy and psychosexual therapy (available at: ℘ http://www.relate.org.uk)
- Sexual Advice Association provides information on a range of ♂ and ♀ sexual problems and a booklet *Intimacy and Sexuality for Cancer Patients and their Partners* (available at: ℘ http://www.sda.uk.net)
- Sensate Focus is a practical programme for couples to follow at home, which fosters intimacy and open communication. By shifting the focus from sexual intercourse and orgasm to intimacy, it is possible to re-establish a fulfilling sexual relationship (available at: ℘ http://counselling-matters.org.uk/sites/counselling-matters/files/SensateFocus.pdf

Communication and assessment

The Royal College of Nursing[2] describes sexuality as 'an appropriate and legitimate area of nursing activity'. Research consistently shows that patients want nurses to provide information and **initiate** conversations about sexuality. This requires us to challenge any assumptions we may have about age, gender, ethnicity, sexual identity, and what is important to people.

Communication

Communication about sexuality is frequently a problem, either because of embarrassment on the part of the patient or health-care professional or because of assumptions about its importance during treatment.

In order to effectively address sexuality, health-care professionals should:

• Understand the role of sexuality in personal identity and health
• Have a willingness to discuss sexuality with patients and their partners
• Not assume that if patients or their partners have concerns, they would voice them
• Have an understanding of common sexual problems associated with cancer
• Provide relevant information and give patients and their partners opportunities to express their concerns.

Assessment

When assessing the sexuality needs of an individual, or of a couple, be careful not to make assumptions about their needs on the basis of age or any other personal factors. A person's sexuality is unique to them. There are models designed specifically to assess sexuality, including the PLISSIT[3] model and the BETTER[4] model. They follow similar stages that can be summarized as follows.

• Let the patient know it is acceptable to talk about sexuality, and provide a safe environment to do so.
• Talk about sexuality as an element of health and QoL, encompassing physical and emotional intimacy.
• Provide information about the sexual problems associated with cancer and its treatments as part of informed consent.
• Attempt to address any problems that are raised, within the limits of your own knowledge and competence.
• Find sources of additional support, expert advice, or treatment, and refer on as necessary, e.g. to psychosexual counselling.

The Extended PLISSIT model (Ex-PLISSIT)[5] further emphasizes the importance of developing a climate of permission-giving, through questions such as:

> 'Having cancer and going through treatment can have an impact on people's sex lives. Do you have any questions or concerns about this?'

If patients or partners do not have questions or concerns at this time, it is important not to assume that the issue has been addressed. They may have been surprised or embarrassed by the question and unable to formulate their concerns at that time. The Ex-PLISSIT model emphasizes the importance of 'review'—returning to the topic at a later time and giving further permission, e.g.:

> 'When we last spoke, I mentioned the impact that cancer and its treatments can have on a couple's intimate relationship. Is this something it might be helpful to discuss?'

It is necessary to review and evaluate after each intervention, e.g. asking if written literature was useful and if it raised any issues for the patient or their partner. This may lead to further questions or to a more personal level of disclosure by the patient.

References

2 Royal College of Nursing. *Sexuality and Sexual Health in Nursing Practice*. London: Royal College of Nursing; 2000.
3 Annon J. The PLISSIT Model: a proposed conceptual scheme for the behavioural treatment of sexual problems. *J Sex Educ Ther* 1971;2:1–15.
4 Mick JA, Hughes M, Cohen MZ (2004). Using the BETTER model to assess sexuality. *Clin J Oncol Nurs* 2004;8:84–6.
5 Davis S, Taylor B. From PLISSIT to Ex-PLISSIT. In: Davis S (ed). *Rehabilitation: The Use of Theories and Models in Practice*. Oxford: Elsevier; 2006. pp. 101–29.

Skin and mucosal alterations

Hair loss (alopecia)

Hair loss can be a distressing side effect of cancer treatment; it impacts on body image and feelings of attractiveness, creates anxiety, and causes a visual reminder of the disease and treatment. Alopecia is not a major side effect for most people, but a small group of patients will become extremely distressed by it.

Note: many devout Sikh men and women never cut their hair, and men never shave or trim their beards as one of the five symbols of the Sikh religion is Kesh, the uncut hair and beard which symbolizes spirituality.

Causes

Chemotherapy and radiotherapy damage cells that are dividing. Since most scalp follicles are in a state of rapid growth, patients are susceptible to hair loss during treatment. Alopecia can be a localized effect of radiotherapy, with scalp hair the most susceptible. About half of patients who experience scalp alopecia will also lose other body hair, e.g. pubic, facial, or axillary hair. This may well not be total, as many of the body's hair follicles are not in the growth phase at any one time. Many chemotherapy agents can cause alopecia. Drugs that generally cause severe alopecia include cyclophosphamide, ifosfamide, anthracyclines, vinca alkaloids, and taxanes.

Prognosis

Hair loss generally begins 7–10 days after chemotherapy commences. Many patients get scalp sensitivity during hair loss. Hair will regrow about 4–6 weeks after treatment finishes in virtually all cases. New hair often changes colour and texture—it may be coarser, curlier, greyer, or thinner.

Hair lost due to radiotherapy will start to regrow about 8–9 weeks after treatment. Regrowth tends to be slower, and the texture may be finer. If the radiotherapy dose is particularly high, it can be possible for hair not to regrow.

Nursing support

It is important to prepare patients for their hair loss. As prevention of hair loss is often not possible, emphasis should be on psychological support and measures to minimize the impact on the person's appearance (➔ see Body image, p. 607).

Assessing and understanding the person's sense of loss, or the level of importance the individual and their family attach to their hair loss, allow appropriate support to be planned. This support will include listening to, and valuing, the individual's concerns, considering methods to minimize hair loss, informing them about options, such as wigs, hats, and turbans, and offering practical advice on scalp and hair protection.

Those facing hair loss are often more concerned about the reaction of their friends and family than their own actual loss of hair.

Key areas to cover with patients
• Why hair loss occurs.
• When it will begin and end, and the degree of hair loss, including areas other than the scalp.

- How the hair will fall out—quickly or over time—and any changes in the hair afterwards.
- Scalp cooling options—including potential risks and benefits.
- Other symptoms or complaints associated with hair loss—such as scalp sensitivity.
- Potential psychosocial impact.
- How to cope with hair loss—including information on wigs, hats, turbans, etc.
- Scalp care and eye care—if eyelashes are lost.

Minimizing hair loss
- Advice is often given on minimizing hair loss—this includes cutting it short, reducing washing and shampooing, avoiding hair manipulation, dyes, and perms, use of wide-toothed combs or soft hairbrushes.
- These measures may enable individuals to gain some sense of control in managing their hair loss, but there is little evidence to suggest that they actually reduce hair loss.
- Careful shaving of the head, once hair loss is severe, will allow an even regrowth when it returns.

Wigs and other head coverings
- Wigs are available free of charge on the NHS to anyone facing the prospect of treatment-related alopecia. They can also be bought privately.
- Wigs should be professionally fitted and should be selected before the patient has lost their hair, in order to match the colour, style, and hair texture. Otherwise a photo and a snip of hair can be used to choose an appropriate wig. Some patients find wigs feel strange, uncomfortable, or hot; others may not be satisfied with the final look.
- Most cancer centres also offer a range of headscarves and turbans. Hats and caps can also hide alopecia effectively.

Scalp and face protection
- Patients should wear a head covering to protect themselves from the sun, wind, and cold. A high-factor sun cream should also be applied if any sun exposure is expected.
- If eyebrows and eyelashes have been lost, then sunglasses, wide-brimmed hats, and false eyelashes can all protect the eyes from injury.

Look Good ... Feel Better

A number of centres in the UK offer the '*Look Good ... Feel Better*' pro-gramme where women can have a makeover by a professional beautician. They also receive advice on how to look and feel their best throughout cancer treatment (available at: ℅ https://www.lookgoodfeelbetter. co.uk).

Scalp cooling (scalp hypothermia)

- The most common attempt to reduce hair loss has been scalp cooling. This causes vasoconstriction of the scalp and reduction in the uptake of drugs in the hair follicles, therefore reducing hair loss.
- Because scalp cooling has to be maintained throughout the period that cytotoxic drugs are circulating, it is generally only used for regimens of short duration (<2 hours).
- Cooling commences shortly before chemotherapy administration (normally 15–20 minutes) and is generally maintained after treatment for a period of time, based on the drug's plasma half-life.
- Effectiveness of scalp cooling varies, but in general, around 50% of patients on anthracycline- and taxane-based regimens should have a good to excellent response with scalp hypothermia.

Methods of scalp cooling

The two methods are:
- Refrigerated gel-filled caps: these require changing regularly throughout treatment
- Cooling machines: these attach to caps similar to the above and maintain them at a constant temperature throughout treatment. They are less time-consuming for nursing staff.

Caps need to be close-fitting, and in some centres, the hair is wet before treatment to increase cold conductivity.

Side effects include headache, dizziness, nausea and vomiting, a heavy feeling on the head, and transient light-headedness, following cap removal.

Scalp metastases

- Concern has been raised that scalp cooling may increase the risk of scalp metastases. In the case of solid tumours, this risk is extremely low, and there is no strong evidence to suggest that scalp cooling increases this risk. Further studies are required to clarify this issue.
- Scalp cooling should not be given in cases where scalp skin metastases exist or in haematological malignancies where the risk of scalp metastases is highest, e.g. lymphoma or leukaemia.
- Patients receiving continuous chemotherapy are unsuitable due to the time element.
- Nurses should discuss the risk of scalp metastases with individuals having scalp cooling, to enable informed choice.

Further reading

Massey CS. A multicentre study to determine the efficacy and patient acceptability of the Paxman Scalp Cooler to prevent hair loss in patients receiving chemotherapy. *Eur J Oncol Nurs* 2004;8:121–30.

Oral mucositis and related problems

Oral mucositis (OM) is a major problem for patients receiving cancer chemotherapy and radiotherapy. The oral mucosa is made up of rapidly dividing squamous epithelial cells. With a lifespan of ~1 week, they are extremely prone to damage from chemotherapy or radiotherapy. The impact of OM is severe, including pain, infection, altered taste, ↓ nutritional intake, dehydration, diarrhoea, bleeding, and altered body image. In extreme cases, airway obstruction can occur. It can also lead to unplanned dose reductions or treatment interruptions.

Definitions

The terms oral mucositis and stomatitis are often used interchangeably. Strictly speaking, OM is inflammation of the oral mucosa due to chemotherapy or radiotherapy treatments. This process may also occur anywhere in the gut and is covered by the general term 'mucositis'. Stomatitis is any inflammation of the oral and oropharyngeal mucous membrane and includes infections of oral tissue.

Causes and risk factors

- 90% or more of patients having radiotherapy for H&N cancers get OM.
- Radiotherapy causes mucosal atrophy and fibrosis of the salivary glands, causing not only OM, but also xerostomia (reduced saliva). Radiotherapy damage can be long term.
- Chemotherapy causes reduced renewal, atrophy, and ulceration of the oral mucosa. As patients become neutropenic, superimposed infections cause further ulceration, damage, and inflammatory response.
- Up to 40% of patients receiving chemotherapy have mucositis (higher rates in haematological malignancies). Drugs most frequently used are:
  - Anthracycline antibiotics, e.g. doxorubicin
  - Taxanes, e.g. paclitaxel
  - Antimetabolites, e.g. methotrexate, 5FU, raltitrexed.
- A number of targeted therapies cause mucositis, though the clinical significance is uncertain, as in most cases, it is low grade only. Other risk factors for OM include:
  - Previous radiotherapy
  - Poor oral hygiene
  - Dental cavities
  - Improperly fitting denture
  - Gingival disease
  - Nutritional deficiency
  - Smoking and alcohol consumption
  - Oxygen therapy.

Prevention of mucositis

Practices for preventing and treating OM are many and varied. There is little convincing evidence for one particular unified approach.

Oral care protocols

Recent guidelines from the Multinational Association of Supportive Cancer Care (MASCC)[1] and the UK Oral Mucositis in Cancer Group[2] both suggest that there is limited evidence of benefit from pharmacological intervention. Key recommendations include:

• Oral care protocols and education of both staff and patients
• Use of a soft toothbrush
• Radiotherapy-induced OM:
  • Salivary gland-sparing radiotherapy techniques, e.g. IMRT
  • Benzydamine mouthwash (anti-inflammatory and antibacterial properties)
• Chemotherapy-induced OM:
  • 30 minutes of cryotherapy (sucking ice chips) for bolus 5FU
• In high dose and stem cell transplant settings, palfermin (Kepivance®), a keratinocyte growth factor, has been shown to reduce the duration and severity of oral mucositis.
• Oral zinc supplements are recommended as prevention in patients receiving H&N radiotherapy or chemoradiation.

Treatment of oral mucositis

Treatment is really aimed at the management of pain and other symptoms, e.g. bleeding, superimposed infections.

Management of mucositis

The following advice is based on the best currently available evidence.[3] Due to the limits of this evidence, if a specific treatment is not working for a patient, it is important to be flexible in your management approach and to consider some of the many alternative treatments that are available.

Oral care protocol

A systematic oral care protocol should be used to carry out the management of OM. It should include the following elements:

• Assessment and monitoring
• Managing the process and symptoms:
  • Maintaining integrity of the oral mucosa
  • Preventing secondary infections
  • Providing pain relief—maintain comfort
  • Ensuring adequate nutritional intake
• Patient education.

Assessment

Regular assessment is essential. The oral cavity should be assessed daily. A consistent assessment method or tool should be used such as the WHO grading system (see Table 51.1). Equipment required for an effective assessment includes a pen torch and a tongue depressor. Can use a gloved finger or even a soft toothbrush if the mouth is particularly sore.

Routine dental procedures should be carried out prior to treatment, if possible, including treatment of underlying dental problems. This is not always possible due to the risk of infection or haemorrhage; it may need to be delayed until after some or all cancer treatment.

Table 51.1 World Health Organization assessment scale for oral mucositis

Mucositis grade				
Scale	0	1	2	3	4
WHO oral toxicity scale	None	Soreness and erythema	Erythema, ulcers, patient can swallow solid diet	Ulcers, extensive erythema, patient cannot swallow solid diet	Mucositis to extent that alimentation is not possible

References

1 McGuire D, Fulton J, Park J, et al.; Mucositis Study Group of the Multinational Association of Supportive Care in Cancer/International Society of Oral Oncology (MASCC/ISOO). Systematic review of basic oral care for the management of oral mucositis in cancer patients. *Support Care Cancer* 2013;21:3165–77.

2 UK Oral Mucositis in Cancer Group (UKOMiC) (2015). *Mouthcare Guidance and Support in Cancer and Palliative Care*, 2nd ed. Available at: ℘ http://www.ukomic.co.uk/pdf/UK_OM_Guidelines. pdf

3 Rubenstein EB, Peterson DE, Schubert M. Clinical practice guidelines for the prevention and treatment of cancer therapy-induced oral and gastrointestinal mucositis. *Cancer* 2004;100:S2026–46.

Oral mucositis: managing the process and symptoms

Maintain the integrity of the oral mucosa by the following measures.

Oral hygiene

- Maintaining excellent oral hygiene is important in managing mucositis and preventing superimposed infections. Patients should be encouraged to brush with a soft-headed toothbrush and fluoride toothpaste after each meal and before bed.
- Flossing may be contraindicated if thrombocytopenic or if mucositis increases in severity.
- If wearing dentures, they should be removed from the mouth and brushed after meals and before bed. The oral cavity should also be rinsed clean on each occasion.
- The frequency of oral hygiene should be up to 2-hourly, or even hourly, for those with severe mucositis—or at high risk of developing it—and also for those on oxygen therapy.
- If patients are unable to tolerate a soft toothbrush, foam swabs can be used instead.

Dry mouth and lips

- For patients with low saliva production, regular sipping of water, ice chips, nebulized saline, and saliva replacement products can be tried.
- Sucking pineapple chunks can stimulate saliva production but may cause irritation, so generally avoid in H&N radiotherapy.
- Lips should be moisturized with lubricants such as paraffin gel and aqueous cream.
- If there is bleeding in the mouth, full blood counts and clotting checks may be required, and replacement blood products given as necessary. Tranexamic acid, as a mouthwash, can be used.

Mouthwashes

- There is little evidence that one mouthwash is better than another; the main benefit may be from the mechanical impact of swilling. Commercial mouthwashes should not be used, as they contain alcohol and other astringents, causing oral irritation.
- Chlorhexidine-based mouthwashes (e.g. Corsodyl®):
  - Though these can reduce plaque and oral bacteria and have often been recommended for patients with haematological cancers, there is no evidence that they are effective in managing OM.
  - They can cause burning and stinging due to their alcohol content. Some patients find that diluting it in half with water can reduce the irritation.
  - Therefore, **chlorhexidine should not be used** to manage OM outside of the high-dose chemotherapy setting.
- For standard-dose chemotherapy, normal saline or water may be as effective as any mouthwash; these are not irritants, so they provide a safer option.
- Benzydamine (Difflam®) mouthwash is recommended for patients receiving radiotherapy for H&N cancers due to its anti-inflammatory and cleansing properties. It is often used within the chemotherapy setting.

Prevention of secondary infections

Regular assessment is essential. Swab suspected areas, and administer anti-viral/antifungal treatment if indicated (➋ see Candidiasis, p. 623).

Pain relief

A range of preparations can be used to reduce pain and inflammation:

- Benzydamine (Difflam®) mouthwash—a local anaesthetic mouthwash. Use every 1.5–3 hours. Rinse round, and spit out. Can be diluted in half if it stings.
- Protective gels/coating agents—can be used to ease the pain of mouth ulceration, though again the evidence for their effectiveness is limited. Use 1 hour prior to eating. Orabase® is applied directly to mouth lesions and can include a steroid to reduce inflammation (Adcortyl in Orabase®). Gelclair® is mixed with water and used as a mouthwash.
- Many patients will require opioids to manage pain.
  - Regular oral morphine is the first choice; however, a continuous infusion may be required.
  - Patient-controlled analgesia is recommended, as there is evidence that patients use lower overall doses of opioid for similar benefit.

Maintenance of nutrition

- Food should be tender. Moist sauces and soft, bland foods might help. Foods that irritate the mouth or throat should be avoided.
- If unable to tolerate food, nutritional support such as high-calorie drinks and NG feeding may be required (➋ see Nutritional support, pp. 542–5).
- IV fluids will also be required for patients unable to tolerate sufficient fluid orally.

Patient education

Nurses need to be involved in teaching, and subsequently reinforcing, optimal oral hygiene practices, including proper brushing, flossing, and mouth rinsing. Nurses should also educate patients about the risk of infection and the signs and symptoms that they need to report to their GP or clinic.

Patients should be educated about pain relief measures and on avoiding alcohol and tobacco, to minimize oral complications.

Nursing support

- OM can have a major impact on a patient's QoL. It often occurs in combination with other side effects of treatment. Accurate information, effective assessment, and speedy management are all essential to try to reduce the impact of severe mucositis.
- Consider methods to ease communication difficulties when patients are unable to talk. Asking closed questions that require simple 'yes' or 'no' answers may be the most appropriate at times.
- Do not underestimate the severity of pain, and ensure the most effective analgesia is administered. Patients may have anxieties about using opioids and might need support and education about the safety and effectiveness of their use in these circumstances.

Oesophagitis

Patients with treatment-induced mucositis are also at risk of oesophagitis. Presenting symptoms are dysphagia, painful swallowing, and epigastric pain. Continuous pain indicates progressing oesophagitis. Oesophagitis pain can be extremely distressing, causing severe discomfort every time the person swallows.

Particular risk factors include:
- Radiation to the oesophagus
- Oesophageal cancer, high-dose chemotherapy, and total body irradiation
- Concurrent chemo-radiotherapy
- Ulcer disease, alcohol, and tobacco use.

In immunosuppressed patient, an infective cause must be considered. *Candida* is the most common cause, though herpes simplex can also cause oesophagitis.

Management
- Amifostine can be used to reduce oesophagitis induced by combined chemo-irradiation in patients with NSCLC.
- Consider treatment of possible *Candida* with fluconazole.
- Nursing management is symptom relief and supportive care. Humidifying the bedroom air can help, particularly at night.

Pain management
- NSAIDs should be administered, if not contraindicated.
- Sucralfate solution can relieve some discomfort.
- No smoking and avoid irritants.
- For severe pain, opioids should be used (⊃ see Oral mucositis: managing the process and symptoms, p. 620).
- Anaesthetic sprays can help throat discomfort, but there is a risk of reducing the gag reflex, so they should be used with caution.

Nutritional support in oesophagitis
- Advise moist foods, such as sauces and gravies, and cold foods such as jellies and fruit nectars.
- No citrus juices or hot and spicy food.

(⊃ See Nutritional support, pp. 542–5).

Oral care in advanced cancer

- Most problems in advanced cancer are due to reduced saliva production and poor oral hygiene, leading to xerostomia (dry mouth) and candidiasis.
- Other problems include mucositis, altered taste, and hypersalivation (drooling).
- A dry and dirty mouth should be cleaned as usual by oral hygiene.
- Chewing pineapple can also cleanse the mouth and encourages saliva production.

Xerostomia (dry mouth)

This can impact on speech, chewing, and swallowing. Common causes include radiotherapy, oxygen, anxiety, dehydration, candidiasis, antimuscarinics, antidepressants, and opioids.

Management

Ensure reversible causes are treated. Offer regular water, ice chips, nebulized saline, and saliva replacement products, particularly before meals. Saliva stimulants, such as pilocarpine, can also be effective but are better for non-radiation induced xerostomia (➔ see Nutritional support, pp. 542–5).

Candidiasis

Oral thrush is extremely common, both in immunosuppressed patients and in those with advanced cancer. Accurate and regular assessment of the oral cavity is essential to establish diagnosis and early management.

Presenting features

- Dry mouth, loss of taste
- Smooth, red tongue
- White plaques on tongue or mucous membranes
- Soreness
- Dysphagia.

Management

- Take swabs (not usual in palliative care setting).
- Treat with oral fluconazole or ketoconazole. Nystatin suspension 6-hourly can be used topically.

Note: nystatin has reduced activity if combined with chlorhexidine. Do not administer nystatin until at least 30 minutes after chlorhexidine mouthwash.

Hypersalivation

This is not common in the cancer setting. Hyoscine or a range of antimuscarinic drugs can be used to reduce production of saliva.

Further reading

McGuire D, Fulton J, Park J, et al.; Mucositis Study Group of the Multinational Association of Supportive Care in Cancer/International Society of Oral Oncology (MASCC/ISOO). Systematic review of basic oral care for the management of oral mucositis in cancer patients. Support Care Cancer 2013;21:3165–77.

UK Oral Mucositis in Cancer Group (UKOMiC) (2015). Mouthcare Guidance and Support in Cancer and Palliative Care, 2nd ed. Available at: ℜ http://www.ukomic.co.uk/pdf/UK_OM_Guidelines.pdf

Malignant wounds

These are caused by local extension or tumour embolization into the epithelium. They can be extremely distressing, as they are a visual reminder of the disease and can produce odour, discharge, bleeding, pain, and infection. All of these can impact on body image and QoL.

If appropriate, surgical removal, with or without radiotherapy, can reduce pain, drainage, and odour and provide infection control. The aim is complete excision and healing. This may be contraindicated in widespread disease. If healing is not possible and the prognosis is generally poor, then the principle of management is symptom control.

The nurse's role is crucial in the management of malignant wounds. Flexibility, creativity, and patience are all required, since the potential success of any approach may be limited. There is often a need to systematically try a range of approaches to achieve optimum management. Psychological support throughout is essential for what can be an embarrassing and traumatic symptom.

> The overall aim of treatment for malignant wounds is to reduce the impact on QoL and to optimize comfort. Specific management of each of the following is required:
> * Control of odour
> * Pain
> * Bleeding
> * Infection
> * Cosmesis
> * Comfort
> * Wound exudate
> * Psychological impacts.

It is essential to involve the patient and their family in planning care. They need to have realistic expectations of the likely outcomes of any treatment and support.

There are a variety of different products that can be used to dress malignant wounds, e.g. alginates, hydrocolloids, foams, and charcoals (see Table 51.2).

General guidelines

* **Pain**: ensure this is not caused by the dressing or dressing process. Limit the frequency of dressing changes, if possible. Use of quick-acting analgesia or relaxation techniques during the dressing procedure may make it more bearable for the patient. Background wound pain can be managed by a combination of systemic analgesia and topical analgesia combined with dressings.
* **Exudate**: high-absorbency dressings, e.g. alginates, and extra pads can help. Barrier creams should be used to protect surrounding skin.
* **Bleeding**: avoid any dressing that will adhere to the wound, to reduce trauma. Soak in saline before removing dressings or shower/rinse off. Alginates can turn to gel and be removed with limited trauma. Alginate dressings can also be effective in reducing bleeding. Consider adrenaline-soaked gauze (1:1000) or sucralfate paste. Assess clotting factors/platelet levels and manage, if appropriate.

Table 51.2 Wound products

Type	Indications
Alginates	Extremely absorbent. Useful for bleeding wounds and infected wounds with moderate to high levels of exudate
Hydrocolloids	Used with light to moderate exudate
Hydrophilic fibre dressings	Absorb moderate amounts of exudate. Very comfortable
Foams	Useful for superficial exuding wounds, and also for placing in cavities
Charcoal	Excellent absorbent deodorizer. Useful as a secondary dressing if odour is a problem
Ostomy products	Useful with high-volume fistulae. Liaise with enterostomal therapist

Note: contact a wound specialist for advice on the latest products and on any wounds that are particularly difficult to manage.

• **Odour:** topical metronidazole can be helpful. Long-term use can cause an increase in the number of aerobic bacteria. If systemic infection, then both systemic and topical measures are required. Charcoal dressings may help, as can well-sealed dressings and deodorizers. Act sensitively when changing dressings, and consider the environment in which this is carried out, e.g. well-ventilated area, privacy, etc. Other options include regular baths, showering the area clean, and using perfumes. Though antiseptic solutions may reduce healing, their judicious use may be appropriate in reducing bacterial loads in selected patients. Chlorhexidine and povidine iodine can be considered.

Risk of catastrophic bleeding

Depending on the position, malignant wounds can put patients at risk of a catastrophic bleed, e.g. H&N cancer, so care planning needs to consider prophylactic prescribing and the psychological management of living with this risk (➔ see Bleeding, p. 483).

Dressing products

The goals of wound dressing selection are to manage exudate and odour, reduce bacterial levels, reduce bleeding, and limit dressing changes. Dressing changes should also be atraumatic. Finally, dressings should allow patients to maintain function as much as possible, and they should have a good cosmetic appearance. Liaison with wound care specialists is essential due to the wide range of available products.

Further reading

Watson MS, Lucas CF, Hoy AM, Wells J. *Oxford Handbook of Palliative Care*, 2nd ed. Oxford: Oxford University Press; 2009.

Lymphoedema

Lymphoedema is an accumulation of lymphatic fluid within interstitial tissues. Accumulation and stagnation of plasma proteins in the fluid cause local inflammation and fibrotic skin changes. This leads to skinfolds filled with fluid, which distort the limb or other affected area. This can become very severe, making the limb or affected area grossly distorted, increasing in both size and weight. Lymphorrhoea is the leakage of fluid from damaged skin.

It is a progressive, chronic, and extremely distressing condition that is frequently disabling. Most commonly affecting the limbs, it can also affect the trunk and H&N. It is associated with profound disturbance of physical, psychological, and social functioning.

Lymphoedema is a common problem in breast cancer, cancers of the H&N, and advanced pelvic disease, e.g. prostate and bladder cancers.

Causes

In cancer, it is mostly caused by damage to lymph nodes and vessels, either by treatments for cancer or by the disease itself.

- Fibrosis resulting from surgery and radiotherapy are the most common treatment-related causes, e.g. axillary clearance or axillary radiotherapy for breast cancer.
- Up to 40% of patients having axillary surgery, combined with radiotherapy, develop lymphoedema.

Other potential causes include:
- Local malignant disease
- Blockage of lymphatic vessels
- Inflammatory processes
- Trauma
- Infection
- Invasive procedures such as venepuncture.

Common presentations of oedema

- Locally advanced breast cancer causing oedema of the arm and chest wall.
- Advanced pelvic malignancy causing oedema of the legs, genitalia, and lower abdomen.
- Facial oedema in H&N cancer.

Problems associated with oedema

- Altered body image: the dramatic changes in body appearance and function are associated with a high level of body image disturbance.
- Fatigue, exhaustion: these can be caused by the weight of lymphoedematous limbs, lack of exercise, or underlying pathological processes.
- Sexual problems: many people will feel themselves unattractive or lose interest in sex because of tiredness, pain, or discomfort.
- Disability and loss of mobility: limbs may be heavy, as well as distorted, and this can seriously limit activity.

- Social isolation and reduction of pleasurable activities: loss of function, combined with unease at body changes, can lead to social isolation, involving loss of friendships or other supportive activities, in some cases associated with depression.
- Pain and discomfort: lymphoedema itself does not usually cause pain, but underlying infective or inflammatory processes may. It is frequently associated with discomfort and loss of, or altered sensations in, the affected part.
- Infection: this can be a problem in damaged tissue.

Treatments

Treatments are not generally curative but aim to improve drainage, reduce capillary filtration, and prevent complications.

- **Complete/complex decongestive therapy (CDT)**: consists of modalities that work together to fully address lymphoedema.
- **Manual lymphatic drainage (MLD)**: is a gentle, rhythmic form of massage used to promote movement of lymph from affected areas into the lymphatic drainage system. Simple lymphatic drainage is an alternative, simplified version that patients or their carers can perform.
- **Compression**.
- **Bandaging**: this is the most common treatment for lymphoedema. It involves:
  - **Low-stretch bandages**: these are worn 24 hours a day, being replaced regularly
  - **Compression garments**: including stockings and sleeves, usually removed at night.

Compression should not be used in patients with thrombosis or SVCO, or where the area is infected.

- **Skin care infection prevention**: this aims to restore hydration and reduce microbial count.
- **Exercise**: gentle exercise promotes lymphatic drainage. Activity should be tailored to fit with normal activity as far as possible.

In the palliative setting, CDT can be adapted and tailored to the needs of the patient. Realistic goal setting is essential.

Nursing management

In many areas, specialist lymphoedema units have health-care professionals specially trained to deal with this problem. It is also very important to work together with allied health professionals in the multidisciplinary management of lymphoedema. The following are essential elements of the care of lymphoedema:

- Hygiene and skin care: this guards against infection, skin dryness, and cracking.
- Education and information: the condition can be very distressing and frightening, so patients and their families need accurate information on the condition. This is empowering and promotes self-care.

- Avoidance of trauma: damage to the skin must be minimized. Potential trauma includes venepuncture, sunburn, and accidents. Post-mastectomy, women should not have blood tests or chemotherapy drugs administered into the arm on the same side as their surgery.
- Support: professional support should aim to assist with changes to self-image. There are also patient support groups that can be accessed directly (➔ see website references to this chapter).

Websites

International Lymphoedema Framework. Available at: ℘ https://www.lympho.org (excellent resource of materials focused on lymphoedema and malignant would management).

Section 8

Oncological Emergencies

Oncological emergencies

Introduction to oncological emergencies

An oncological emergency may be defined as any acute, potentially life-threatening event that is directly or indirectly related to a patient's cancer, including paraneoplastic syndromes, or its treatment. They require urgent assessment and management and reversal, if at all possible. They require immediate attendance to hospital and may require escalation to intensive care support, when necessary.

One of the challenges faced by health-care professionals in relation to such emergencies is that initial signs and symptoms are often common problems experienced by individuals with cancer, e.g. nausea, pain, headache, and fever.

Anaphylaxis

Anaphylaxis is a severe, life-threatening systemic allergic reaction with multisystem involvement. Onset is normally immediate, but there can be a delay of hours.

It is caused by the immunologically induced release of chemical mediators (histamine, kinins, prostaglandins, and platelet-activating factors) from mast cells and basophils. This leads to smooth muscle contraction, vascular permeability, vasodilatation, cardiovascular stimulation, and gastric acid secretion.

Common causes of anaphylaxis

- Medical products: antibiotics (especially penicillins), blood products, aspirin, NSAIDs, SACT (see Box 52.1), vaccines.
- Non-medical: insect stings, latex, peanuts, shellfish, strawberries.

Allergic reactions in oncology

These guidelines are for the management of acute anaphylaxis. In oncology, many allergic and hypersensitivity reactions are milder in nature and may be treated successfully with IV steroids and antihistamines, without the need to use adrenaline. However, if anaphylaxis is suspected, then adrenaline is the essential drug of choice.

It is essential to diagnose anaphylaxis early, and not to mistake it for other episodes such as vasovagal (fainting), panic attacks, or other reactions to SACT (e.g. laryngeal spasm with oxaliplatin).

Clinical features

- **Respiratory system:** swelling of the lips, tongue, pharynx, and epiglottis may lead to complete upper airway obstruction. Lower airway involvement may develop with dyspnoea, wheeze, stridor, chest tightness, and hypoxia.
- **Skin:** flushing, erythema, pruritus, urticaria. Often the first sign and present in 80% of cases.

Box 52.1 Systemic anti-cancer agents (SACT) with high risk of anaphylaxis

- Paclitaxel
- Asparaginase
- Carboplatin
- Cisplatin
- Liposomal doxorubcin
- Docetaxel
- Etoposide
- Rituximab
- Cetuximab
- Alemtuzumab
- Trastuzumab
- Ramucirumab
- Obinutuzumab
- Ofatumumab

Prevention of anaphylaxis due to SACT

- Monoclonal antibodies: pre-medication of analgesic and antihistamine.
- Taxanes: pre-medication with corticosteroid, antihistamine, and H2-receptor antagonist (major reactions still around 1–3%).

- **Cardiovascular:** tachycardia, hypotension, arrhythmias, ECG changes, ischaemic chest pain.
- **GI tract:** nausea, vomiting, diarrhoea, abdominal cramps.
- Feeling of impending doom.

Assessment

Prevention
- Nurses must be familiar with the likelihood of a particular drug causing an allergic reaction.
- Identify patients at ↑ risk of SACT-induced anaphylaxis, e.g. previous allergic reactions.
- Inform patients of likely signs and the need to report them urgently.
- Ascertain if any pre-treatment prophylaxis has been taken or need to be administered prior to SACT.
- Prior to administration of SACT, nursing/medical staff should be familiar with the likelihood of the drug causing anaphylaxis and have easy access to emergency equipment and drugs.

Suspected anaphylactic reaction

- STOP SACT or related product immediately. Maintain the cannula, if possible, for easy IV access.
- Follow the latest Resuscitation Council (UK) algorithm.

Nursing care
- **Anxiety:** patients and their families may be extremely fearful during and after an episode of anaphylaxis, and will require a lot of emotional support. If an SACT causes anaphylaxis, it could have implications for their future treatment. This will need to be sensitively explored with the patient.
- **Observation:** if anaphylaxis occurs as an outpatient, then ensure the patient is admitted and observed for at least 24 hours (relapses can occur most frequently in first 24-hour period).
- **Drug reactions:** ensure these are properly reported and recorded in the patient's notes.

Note: for prevention of blood product reactions, ➲ see Chapter 38, Blood product support.

Further reading

Guan M, Zhou YP, Sun JL, Chen SC. Adverse events of monoclonal antibodies used for cancer therapy. *BioMed Res Int* 2015;**2015**:428169.

Resuscitation Council UK (2008). *Anaphylaxis Algorithm*. Available at: ⅊ https://www.resus.org.uk

UK Oncology Nursing Society (2013). *Acute Oncology Initial Management Guidelines*, version 1.0. Available at: ⅊ http://www.ukons.org/downloads/FINAL_GUIDELINE_V_1.0_11.pdf

Disseminated intravascular coagulation

DIC is the abnormal generation of thrombin over a sustained period of time, causing generalized intravascular coagulation, leading to consumption of platelets and clotting factors. DIC can be chronic or acute. DIC may arise in patients with sepsis, malignancy, trauma, liver disease, and vascular anomalies. In the cancer setting, the most common causes are sepsis, leukaemias, and adenocarcinomas.

Note: acute pro-myelocytic leukaemia (AML M3) is virtually always associated with some level of DIC at diagnosis.

Presenting signs and symptoms

- Most common is bleeding, which can be widespread.
- Purpura, ecchymosis (purple marks or skin discoloration), and petechiae (red pinprick marks). There are often multiple sites, e.g. skin, gums, nose, lungs, and venepuncture and central line sites.
- Blood in urine and stools.
- Can cause uncontrollable haemorrhage, leading to shock and death.

Important note: chronic DIC may be subclinical, whereas acute DIC develops over a few hours and is a true oncological emergency.

Diagnosis

By clinical presentation and blood tests showing ↓ platelets and fibrinogen plus ↑ clotting times (see Table 52.1). These should be repeated regularly till the condition stabilizes.

Table 52.1 Diagnostic scoring system for DIC

Risk assessment: Does the patient have an underlying disorder known to be associated with overt DIC?

If yes: proceed	If no: do not use this algorithm

Order global coagulation tests
(PT, platelet count, fibrinogen, fibrin-related markers)

Score the test results
- Platelet count (>100 × 10^9/L = 0, <100 × 10^9/L = 1, <50 × 10^9/L = 2)
- Elevated fibrin marker (e.g. D-dimer, fibrin degradation products) (no increase = 0, moderate increase = 2, strong increase = 3)
- Prolonged PT (<3s = 0, >3 but <6s = 1, >6s = 2)
- Fibrinogen level (>1g/L = 0, <1g/L = 1)

Calculate score:
≥5 compatible with overt DIC: repeat score daily
<5 suggestive for non-overt DIC: repeat next 1–2 days

Reproduced from BJH (2009) Guidelines for the diagnosis and management of disseminated intravascular coagulation. *British Journal of Haematology*, **145**, 24–33 with permission from Wiley.

Management

- The cornerstone of management is to treat the underlying cause.
- Support the patient with blood products if bleeding or if the depletion of clotting factors is well established.
- Therapeutic doses of heparin can be used in cases where thrombosis predominates.
- Prophylactic doses of heparin are recommended in critically ill, non-bleeding patients.

Commonly used blood products

Note: use should generally be reserved for patients who are actively bleeding or undergoing invasive procedure.

- FFP: 2–4U if clotting times are prolonged (there is some controversy as to how helpful FFP is).
- Platelets: 10U for platelet counts of $<50 \times 10^9/L$.
- Cryoprecipitate: (if not responding to FFP) fibrinogen $<1g/L$.

Nursing management

- **Assessment for signs and symptoms of bleeding**: this must be from head to toe and extremely thorough; include all pressure areas, back, mouth, vision changes (retinal bleeding), sputum, nosebleeds, line sites, urine, and stool.
- **Regular administration of blood products**: and regular review of blood counts (➔ see Chapter 38, Blood product support).
- **Bleeding**:
  - **Line sites/oozing venepuncture sites**: apply pressure (5–10min minimum), and change dressings regularly
  - **Nosebleeds**: instruct the patient to sit up, and pinch the soft part of the nose for 10–15min. The nurse may have to do this for the patient.
- **Vital sign measurements**: pulse, blood pressure (cuff may cause extensive bruising), respiratory rate. Look for signs of shock (due to blood loss) and respiratory distress (due to pulmonary oedema). Accurate fluid balance and CVP. Chest pain could signal cardiac tamponade, requiring immediate medical intervention.
- **Fear/anxiety**: the symptoms of DIC can be extremely distressing. Careful explanation of the cause, all the treatments, and their goals and side effects is required. Calm and efficient care, despite the potential emergency, can help to reassure the patient (➔ see Anxiety management, pp. 588–9).

Further reading

Levi M, Toh CH, Thachil J, Watson HG. Guidelines for the diagnosis and management of disseminated intravascular coagulation. *Br J Haematol* 2009;145:24–33.

Malignancy-induced hypercalcaemia

- This is the most common oncological emergency associated with cancer. It occurs in possibly >20% of patients with cancer, in most cases with advanced disease.
- It is most commonly seen in breast cancer, multiple myeloma, and lung cancer. Also in H&N cancer, lymphoma, leukaemia, and renal and prostate cancers. It can be seen in any cancer.
- It can occur with or without bone metastases, though in 80% of cases, patients do have skeletal disease.
- Overall prognosis for patients who develop malignancy-induced hypercalcaemia is poor. The median survival is 3–4 months, with 80% mortality in 1 year, reflecting the advanced state of their disease.

Normal calcium homeostasis

- 99% of calcium is in bones (with phosphorus); 1% in serum—half freely ionized, half bound to protein.
- Calcium has a role in bone formation, muscle (cardiac) contractility, clotting, and nerve impulse transmission.
- Normal homeostasis is controlled by parathyroid hormone (PTH), vitamin D, calcitonin, and renal excretion.
- If serum calcium is low, PTH stimulates bone resorption and renal resorption. It also stimulates gut absorption of calcium via vitamin D.
- Calcitonin antagonizes PTH and is released if serum calcium is high. It is only short-acting.

Causes of hypercalcaemia

There are three major mechanisms (not mutually exclusive).

- Local bone metastases directly stimulate osteoclast activity (causing breakdown of bone structure) and release humoral hypercalcaemia factors.
- Some tumours (e.g. renal, H&N, lung, bladder, breast, and haematological) release systemic parathyroid hormone-related protein (PTHrP) and other cytokines, which stimulate osteoclast activity.
- ↑ calcitriol production (primarily in Hodgkin lymphoma and some NHLs).

In the first two cases, ↑ bone resorption releases calcium into the bloodstream. Renal excretion of calcium is also reduced in PTHrP-induced hypercalcaemia.

With ↑ calcitriol, the main abnormality is ↑ intestinal calcium reabsorption and ↑ bone resorption.

Note: PTHrP has the same effect as PTH (see Box 52.2), but without any feedback loop, so it continues to act, regardless of calcium level.

Presenting signs and symptoms

(➔ See also Early detection of hypercalcaemia, p. 638.)

- Mental status: irritability, lethargy, depression, confusion, psychoses.
- Cardiovascular: ECG changes, bradycardia, atrial arrythmias.
- GI: anorexia, nausea and vomiting, constipation, ileus.
- Musculoskeletal: fatigue, weakness, bone pain.
- Renal: thirst, polyuria, dehydration, renal failure.

Box 52.2 Corrected calcium

Since calcium is bound to albumin, ionized calcium levels vary depending on the albumin level, i.e. patients with a low albumin level have higher levels of ionized calcium.

Corrected calcium (mmol/L) = measured calcium + 0.02 × [40 − albumin (g/L)]

Early detection of hypercalcaemia

Hypercalcaemia can easily be overlooked. Early symptoms include thirst, ↓ appetite, nausea, frequent voiding of urine, ↑ fatigue, constipation, lethargy, and personality changes. These symptoms are non-specific and may have many other causes.

It is important to consider who is at risk and to assess individuals for potential signs/symptoms.

Patient/family education

This is important to support a quick response to possible symptoms. Teaching should include:

• Early symptoms
• Maintenance of mobility and adequate hydration
• The need for early assessment and treatment.

Diagnosis

• Blood test for corrected calcium.
• Normal calcium level 2.12–2.65mmol/L. If >3mmol/L, then start to get signs and symptoms. Untreated levels of >4mmol/L can cause death in a few days.

Drug management of hypercalcaemia

Pamidronate and sodium clodronate are effective in about 70–80% of cases. The effects last for about 2–3 weeks. Zoledronic acid is more expensive, but infusion times are shorter and it may be effective for up to 6 weeks.

• Pamidronate: 60–90mg IV (dependent on calcium levels over 2–4 hours
• Zoledronic acid: 4mg IV infusion over 15 minutes
• Sodium clodronate: 1.5g IV infusion over 4 hours
• Ibandronic acid: 2–4 mg IV infusion over 1–2 hours

Bisphosphonates can cause transient fever and bone pains (manage with paracetamol) and also a risk of hypocalcaemia.

Many patients maintain normal calcium levels through monthly treatment with bisphosphonates (➲ see Metastatic bone disease, pp. 287–9).

Oral ibandronic acid is increasingly used in palliative settings as maintenance therapy. Denosumab, a monoclonal antibody receptor activator of nuclear factor-kappa B ligand (RANKL) inhibitor, is currently being trialled in refractory hypercalcaemia.

Steroids are only used in haematological malignancies to reduce osteoclast activity.

Note: caution is needed in renal failure. Renal function monitoring is recommended after use of zoledronic acid in at-risk patients—especially those with pre-existing renal disorders. Slower infusions of bisphosphonates is also recommended

Management

The key principles of management are:

- Treat the malignancy: radiotherapy, SACT, or surgery should be used as appropriate. If the disease is refractory or at an advanced stage, then palliation is the main aim.
- **Lower serum calcium concentration**: if patient symptomatic or at high risk of becoming so, i.e. rapidly increasing serum calcium.
- Remove any exacerbating causes, e.g. drugs such as vitamins A and D, thiazide diuretics. Immobility may require extra analgesia, mobility equipment, physiotherapy, and occupational therapy input.

Note: there is no need to reduce oral dietary calcium, as absorption will already be low.

- **Mild hypercalcaemia**: calcium <3mmol/L and asymptomatic. Treatment is not normally required. Continue to monitor calcium levels, and give advice on early signs and symptoms of hypercalcaemia. Reduce exacerbating factors where possible, e.g. prolonged bedrest, thiazide diuretics, NSAIDs, angiotensin-converting inhibitor (ACEI). Patients should be encouraged to maintain adequate hydration with oral fluids.
- **Moderate hypercalcaemia**: calcium 3–3.5mmol/L, chronic and asymptomatic or mildly symptomatic. May not require immediate therapy. However, if acute rise in calcium levels or increasing symptoms, then treat as for severe hypercalcaemia.
- **Severe hypercalcaemia**: calcium >3.5mmol/L or symptoms of confusion, change in mental status. **Need treatment using a three-pronged approach.**

Rehydration and bisphosphonate therapy

Hydration

Start immediately if the individual is symptomatic. Two to 4L of normal saline per day will reduce calcium levels, but rarely back to normal. Loop diuretics, such as furosemide 20–40mg, can be used to assist in maintaining fluid balance once the patient is rehydrated. Maintain electrolyte monitoring—check for hypokalaemia and hyponatraemia. Check carefully for fluid overload, as many patients may have impaired renal function.

Bisphosphonate infusion

Bisphosphonates inhibit osteoclast activity and reduce bone resorption. They take 48 hours to work effectively. They are given after initial rehydration therapy.

Nursing management of hypercalcaemia

Patients may be extremely dehydrated, drowsy and confused, nauseated, vomiting, and in pain. They can require intensive nursing support in managing their symptoms, maintaining their safety, and monitoring their response to medical treatment.

Nursing assessment

- Manage fluid balance; accurate monitoring of input and output. The patient may not be mobile for weighing.
- Monitor all vital signs (pulse, blood pressure, respiratory rate), including neurological and cardiovascular status, signs and symptoms of fluid

overload, and renal failure. Monitor for response to treatment, i.e. reduced blood calcium levels, improved consciousness levels, and reduction in fatigue, lethargy, and GI symptoms.

Renal and GI
- Assist with fluid input.
- Assess for nausea; anti-emetics; assist with drinking, administration, and management of IV infusion.
- Check for oliguria and anuria.
- Assess for constipation, and manage as appropriate (➔ see Constipation, pp. 506–9).

Neurological
Patient may be confused or have altered consciousness levels. This can be extremely distressing for the patient and their family (➔ see Acute confusional state or delirium, p. 594).
- Assist patient with activities of daily living.
- Assist in orientating to time and place.
- Reassure that as calcium levels improve, confusion and consciousness levels should return to normal.

Musculoskeletal
Mobility can prevent exacerbation of hypercalcaemia. Encourage walking and weight-bearing exercise, unless contraindicated due to a risk of pathological fractures. Analgesia may need assessment and review to enable mobilization. Patient may need nursing assistance with mobility. Equipment, physiotherapy, and occupational therapy can all be helpful in encouraging and maintaining independence.

Hypercalcaemia in the terminal phase

In some cases, a decision not to treat hypercalcaemia may be taken if the patient is close to death. A full assessment needs to be carried out, considering the patient's symptoms and also their recent response to hypercalcaemia treatment. This requires sensitive management; relatives may be expecting continuing treatment of hypercalcaemia if this has happened in the past. Management is aimed at palliation of the other symptoms such as pain and confusion.

Further reading

Barton R, Allanson D. Managing complications of cancer. In: Faull C, De Caestecker S, Nicholson A, Black F (eds). *Handbook of Palliative Care*, 3rd ed. Hoboken, NJ: Wiley-Blackwell; 2012. pp. 184–206.

Watson M, Lucas C, Hoy A. *Oxford Handbook of Palliative care*, 2nd ed. Oxford: Oxford University Press; 2009.

Metastatic spinal cord compression

- Metastatic spinal cord compression (MSCC) occurs in about 5% of cancer patients. Most commonly in breast, lung, and prostate cancers and multiple myeloma.
- 10–15% of patients with spinal metastases develop MSCC.
- Sites of MSCC: 70% thoracic, 20% lumbosacral, 10% cervical.
  - Different sites can produce different motor neurone signs.
  - Multiple points of compression can occur, producing confusing neurological signs.

Pathology

- **Extrinsic**: vertebral body tumour invading the epidural space, vertebral collapse.
- **Intrinsic**: intradural/intramedullary metastases.

Diagnosis

- Medical history—presenting signs and symptoms.
- Neurological examination.
- MRI is the gold standard—assesses soft tissue, as well as bone. Assess for meningeal metastases and multiple areas of compression. MUST be performed within 24 hours of suspicion of MSCC with ANY neurological symptoms.

Diagnostic delay

- Delay in the diagnosis of MSCC can be devastating in terms of QoL, reducing treatment options and leading to a poorer outcome.
- It is very important to have a high index of suspicion in patients with spinal metastases or those with known advanced breast, prostate, or lung cancers.
- Health-care professionals need to educate patients about what MSCC is, what the risks are, and the common signs and symptoms. They need to know why they must inform professionals of signs such as back pain, difficulties in passing urine, or leg weakness.

Management

Depends, in part, on prognostic factors:
- Patient's performance status. Will they cope with surgery or radiotherapy?
- Is there potential to reverse the compression? If there is severe dysfunction, then the chance of improvement is poor.
- Tumour histology. Haematological malignancies tend to respond best.
- Has the patient a very short prognosis?
- Does the patient want emergency treatment?

Nurses have an important role in supporting the patient and their family with these decisions, clarifying the risks and benefits of different treatment strategies.

Presenting symptoms

(See Box 52.3.)

Box 52.3 Presenting symptoms of MSCC
- Back pain: cardinal sign—present in 90% of cases.
- If any of following signs are noted, must discuss urgently with MSCC coordinator:
  - Pain in the middle (thoracic) or upper (cervical) spine
  - Progressive lower (lumbar) spinal pain
  - Severe unremitting lower spinal pain
  - Spinal pain aggravated by straining (e.g. at stool or when coughing or sneezing)
  - Localized spinal tenderness
  - Nocturnal spinal pain preventing sleep.

Emergency presentation
- Neurological symptoms, including radicular pain, any limb weakness, difficulty in walking, sensory loss, or bladder or bowel dysfunction.
- Neurological signs of the spinal cord or cauda equina compression.
- MUST be seen and imaged within 24 hours of presentation.

Late presentation with profound weakness or loss of sphincter control suggests poor prognosis and little chance of reversing the compression, and therefore the symptoms.

Treatment

Steroids

Immediate treatment is given with high-dose dexamethasone (minimum 16mg), particularly if rapidly progressing myelopathy. This is contraindicated if high suspicion of lymphoma diagnosis.

Radiotherapy

This is the standard treatment, unless there is an unstable spine or vertebral collapse. If the patient has severe back pain, radiotherapy can often be effective, even if there is no improvement in neurological status. Opioids and NSAIDs are also used for pain relief. In lymphoma, chemotherapy should be considered.

Surgery

Relatively few patients with MSCC in the UK receive surgery for the condition. Research evidence suggests that early surgery may be more effective than radiotherapy at maintaining mobility in a selected subset of patients. The aim should be to achieve cord decompression and durable spinal stability.

Good performance status patients with a single site of compression may do better with decompressive surgery combined with radiotherapy.

Options are vertebral body resection or laminectomy. The best results are achieved when the tumour is anterior to the spine.

Surgery is also used where the diagnosis is uncertain or there is a single lesion that might be totally removed.

Mortality rates from surgery can be high in patients with metastatic cancer. Careful patient selection is essential.

Prognosis

Early assessment and treatment are essential. ~70% of patients ambulant prior to treatment will regain full function. Around 30% of these will survive for 1 year. Only 5% of those who were paraplegic will regain function. Those who remain paraplegic generally have a life expectancy of only a few weeks.

Nursing management

Assessment and early detection

Pain assessment is crucial. Knowing the early signs of MSCC and educating patients and their families about these can prevent a late diagnosis (see Box 52.3). It is good practice to give information sheets to patients with bone metastases or at high risk of developing them.

Because of poor outcomes associated with MSCC in patients admitted as emergencies, approved pathways have been established in recent years. All cancer networks in England and Wales must now have designated hospitals which can treat MSCC surgically or with radiotherapy.

They must have a 24/7 rota of staff, taking on the role of an MSCC co-ordinator, with a single contact number.

Unstable spine

Until bony and neurological stability is ensured, patients should be nursed flat, with log rolling, slipper pan for toilet, etc. Work closely with physiotherapist guidance to begin gradual sitting, and continue to unsupported sitting, transfers, and mobilization as symptoms allow (stable blood pressure, no increase in pain).

If pain re-occurs, then return them to a more stable position and get reassessment of stability.

If not for definitive treatment, patients should be helped to position themselves and mobilize as symptoms permit, with specialist seating and equipment.

Rehabilitation

For patients with MSCC, nursing care and goals will depend on the degree of neurological deficit. Realistic goals need to be set in collaboration with the patient and family.

These need to include the preferred place of care, so that the involvement of community or hospice services can be arranged early on.

Early involvement of physiotherapists, occupational therapists, and the palliative care team is essential to maximize the patient's rehabilitation and to enable them to maintain as much independence as possible (➔ see Rehabilitation, p.138).

Symptom management

Patients with severe neurological deficits will require full nursing care. Assessment of their skin condition, regular turning, use of low-pressure mattresses, and maintaining adequate nutrition are all essential to prevent skin breakdown and pressure sores. Bowel or bladder programmes will need to be started.

Education for patients and their family is required about physical care, mobility, injury prevention due to sensory deficits, risks of chest and urinary infection, and management of bowel and bladder care.

Facing the last months of life as a paraplegic can have a huge impact on the QoL. Referral to a specialist palliative care team is essential.

Further reading

National Institute for Health and Care Excellence (2008). *Metastatic Spinal Cord Compression in Adults: Risk Assessment, Diagnosis and Management*. Clinical guideline [CG75]. Available at: ℜ https://www.nice.org.uk/guidance/cg75

UK Oncology Nursing Society (2013). *Acute Oncology Initial Management Guidelines*, version 1.0. Available at: ℜ http://www.ukons.org/downloads/FINAL_GUIDELINE_V_1.0_11.pdf

Watson M, Lucas C, Hoy A. *Oxford Handbook of Palliative Care*, 2nd ed. Oxford: Oxford University Press; 2009.

Superior vena cava obstruction

This occurs when the superior vena cava is obstructed by extrinsic compression (in about 80% of cases), tumour invasion, or thrombosis. It results in impaired drainage of the H&N and upper extremities.

Causes

- 97% are caused by cancer, of which 75% are bronchus, particularly SCLC.
- 15% are caused by lymphoma.
- SVCO can also be caused by thrombus formation from a central line.

Clinical features

- Dyspnoea: the most common feature, caused by tracheal or bronchial compression.
- Face, neck, and arm oedema: often worse in the morning and when bending down.
- Cough, headaches, hoarseness, facial erythema, or superficial vein distension of the upper torso.

There is usually a gradual onset (not a true emergency), but rapid onset can cause severe, life-threatening symptoms such as respiratory distress and stridor. The prognosis is generally dependent on the type of cancer and the stage of the disease.

Diagnosis

Unless it is a life-threatening emergency, it is important to establish an accurate diagnosis of SVCO and the cause. Over 50% of cases present without a known diagnosis of malignancy.

- CT scan: ideally with contrast. Establish patency of the superior vena cava and external or internal compression.
- Venogram: if there is no obvious external cause and/or if stent placement or thrombolysis is considered.
- Blood tests: blood gases, full blood count, urea and electrolytes, clotting.
- Tissue samples: for definitive diagnosis (if unknown).

Treatment

Radiotherapy, chemotherapy, and surgical stenting provide the main treatment options for SVCO.

- Stenting: insertion of a metal stent via the femoral vein. This is the first choice in an emergency, as it provides immediate relief (95% success, with 92% long-term patency). It can also be used when radiotherapy or SACT are no longer options or if non-sensitive tumour. It should be considered as part of initial therapy in NSCLC. If a clot is suspected to be exacerbating SVCO, thrombolysis can be combined with stenting.

Note: if a clot from a central line is causing SVCO, then removing the line normally resolves the obstruction.

- **SACT**: used for chemosensitive tumours, such as SCLC (77% success) and lymphoma, as it provides systemic treatment of disease as well. Symptom relief in 7–10 days.
- **Radiotherapy**: used for NSCLC and also when there is poor performance status or relapse post-chemotherapy in SCLC or lymphoma. Similar overall benefit to chemotherapy. Symptom relief in 3–4 days.
- **Steroids**: dexamethasone 16mg orally/IV. There is a lack of evidence for the use of steroids, but they can reduce radiotherapy-induced oedema and they have an anti-tumour effect in lymphoma.

Nursing management

It is important to be aware of those most at risk of developing SVCO, e.g. people with SCLC. Being aware of early signs, such as increasing shortness of breath, dilated veins, or a feeling of tightness or fullness of the neck, arms, and chest, can allow SVCO to be treated before it becomes an emergency.

Management

This involves the assessment and support of respiratory, cardiac, and neurological systems. Emotional and psychosocial support is important where there is breathlessness and a recent diagnosis or poor prognosis (➲ see Management, p. 516).

Observations

- Look for dilated veins over the arms, neck, and anterior chest wall.
- Observe for signs of worsening SVCO such as increasing anxiety, respiratory distress, ↓ oxygen saturation, stridor, or hoarseness.
- Also look for signs of blurred vision and mental status changes—these are signs of cerebral oedema.
- Vital signs monitoring—frequent respiratory, cardiac, and neurological assessment. Venepuncture, blood pressure, and IVs are contraindicated in upper extremities.
- Fluid balance monitoring—overhydration could exacerbate symptoms.

Interventions

- Maintain the patient's airway.
- Support oxygen perfusion. Oxygen therapy can temporarily relieve dyspnoea; restrict activity, assisting with activities of daily living, and maintain the patient in a supported, upright position.
- Anxiety management. Aim to reduce anxiety and feeling of drowning or suffocating (➲ see Anxiety management, pp. 588–9).

Syndrome of inappropriate antidiuretic hormone

This is a paraneoplastic syndrome, caused by unregulated release of ectopic antidiuretic hormone (ADH) by the tumour.

High levels of ADH lead to water being conserved in the kidney and concentrated urine. This causes plasma hypo-osmolarity and hyponatraemia ('water intoxication'). Plasma volume moves into cells in an attempt to equalize the osmotic gradient. This leads to intracellular oedema; cerebral oedema leads to reduced neural function and eventually death.

Physiology

ADH, also known as arginine vasopressin (AVP), is produced by the hypothalamus and has a role in maintaining accurate fluid balance. It conserves the levels of fluid in the body by reducing the output of urine. It is regulated by plasma volume and osmolarity (the concentration of solutes in blood). Dehydration, vomiting, diarrhoea, or bleeding would all decrease the volume of extracellular fluid, increase plasma osmolarity, and stimulate ADH production and release.

Incidence

- Common in SCLC. Rare, but also found in H&N, oesophageal, and haematological cancers.
- Non-ectopic causes include:
  - Infection, COPD
  - SACT agents (vinca alkaloids, cyclophosphamide, ifosfamide, cisplatin, docetaxel)
  - Other drugs: tricyclic antidepressants, carbamazepine, morphine.

Presentation

- Most patients present with slowly developing asymptomatic hyponatraemia. If hyponatraemia develops rapidly, the symptoms are more severe, as the brain does not have time to effect compensatory mechanisms against cerebral oedema.
- At sodium levels below 125mmol/L, common symptoms are nausea, anorexia, fatigue, weakness, and muscle cramps.
- As hyponatraemia worsens, symptoms include confusion, lethargy, and psychotic behaviour, eventually leading to seizures and death.

Diagnosis

Hyponatraemia is common in advanced cancer due to several causes, including cardiac and hepatic failure, diuretics, and hyperglycaemia. To diagnose SIADH:

- There is a need to exclude all non-ectopic causes.
- The following criteria are essential:
  - ↓ plasma osmolarity, normal plasma volume
  - Serum sodium <130mmol/L
  - Concentrated urine and high urinary sodium levels.

Management

The key is successful treatment of the cause, e.g. the malignancy, and stabilization of the patient by correcting hyponatraemia.

Chronic/asymptomatic hyponatraemia

Fluid restriction to 500–1000mL/24h is generally sufficient. It takes several days to correct sodium levels. This does have QoL implications for many patients.

Oral medication

Demeclocycline can be used. It inhibits the action of ADH on the renal tubules. Renal function must be monitored closely due to the risk of acute renal failure.

- Vaptan therapy: recently developed therapy directly aimed at SIADH. They can result in over-rapid correction of sodium levels.
  - Reduces the need for fluid restriction (helpful to QoL)
  - Correction of hyponatraemia occurs quickly
  - Requires initial very close monitoring of serum sodium levels
  - Currently expensive.

Severe/symptomatic hyponatraemia

- This is a true emergency, with a mortality rate of >5%.
- Management involves conservative measures, as for asymptomatic hyponatraemia. If these fail and the patient deteriorates, administration of IV hypertonic saline (3%) may be tried. This requires meticulous monitoring (1- to 2-hourly) of electrolytes, since correcting hyponatraemia too quickly can cause cerebral dehydration and neurological damage. Best carried out in a high-dependency/intensive care setting.

Nursing management

- Meticulous fluid balance monitoring, including fluid balance chart, signs of fluid overload or dryness.
- Weight, lying/standing blood pressure.
- Urine measurement: volume, osmolarity.
- Educate patients on the need for fluid restriction, and support with the impact of this.
- Support with oral care, managing thirst.
- For management of the confused patient, ⮀ see Acute confusional state or delirium, pp. 594–5.

SACT and SIADH

Patients may present with SIADH as part of their initial diagnosis. They may require treatment with chemotherapy regimens that need high levels of hydration, e.g. cisplatin or cyclophosphamide.

- If they have hyponatraemia, treatment should go ahead since treating the cancer will effectively reduce the SIADH. Balancing the hydration needs for SACT and management of hyponatraemia will require meticulous monitoring.

Further reading

Gross P. Clinical management of SIADH. *Ther Adv Endocrinol Metab* 2012;3:61–73.

Tumour lysis syndrome

This is an oncological emergency caused by tumour cell breakdown releasing cellular contents—uric acid, phosphorus and potassium—into the bloodstream.

TLS is most commonly seen during aggressive treatment of large, rapidly dividing tumours, e.g. high-grade lymphoma, acute leukaemia, and CML in blast crisis. It is rare in solid tumours, although it has been recorded in SCLC and metastatic breast cancer.

Risk factors

- High-risk disease type: Burkitt's lymphoma, Burkitt's type ALL, other acute haematological malignancies with high white blood cell count, aggressive bulky solid tumours, and paediatric malignancy.
- Patients at ↑ risk are those with pre-existing renal impairment, high uric acid or electrolyte levels, and dehydration before treatment.

Timing

The syndrome generally starts within 48 hours of treatment commencing but can last 5–7 days.

Presenting signs and symptoms

(See Table 52.2.)

- **Acute renal failure**: due to uric acid blocking the distal tubules.
- **Cardiac arrhythmia**: due to raised potassium and phosphorus levels (which also causes lower blood calcium levels).
- **GI and neurological effects**: due to raised potassium and phosphorus levels.

Management strategy

Education

- Health-care professionals need to educate patients about what TLS is and the common signs and symptoms. Patients need to know why it is essential to immediately report any of the signs or symptoms of TLS.
- Explain the importance of maintaining a good fluid intake (>3L) and output of urine.

Table 52.2 Common clinical manifestations of tumour lysis syndrome

Renal effects	Cardiovascular effects	GI effects	Neuromuscular effects
• ↓ urine output	• Hypertension	• Nausea and vomiting	• Muscle weakness
• ↑ urea and creatinine	• Tachycardia	• Diarrhoea	• Muscle cramps, twitching
• Flank pain	• ECG changes	• Anorexia	• Paraesthesiae
• Acute renal failure	• Ventricular tachycardia	• Intestinal colic	• Tetany
	• Cardiac arrest		• Confusion, delirium

Prevention of renal failure and electrolyte imbalance

TLS can develop rapidly and is difficult to treat once established. It is therefore essential that effective prevention measures are undertaken.

- Nursing assessment and patient monitoring for risk factors and signs of TLS (see Table 52.2).
- Pharmacological treatment.
  - Rasburicase (IV) converts uric acid into allantoin. It decreases uric acid levels far quicker than allopurinol. It can be used for high-risk patients with a haematological malignancy and a high tumour burden at risk of high-volume cell lysis. Do NOT give together with allopurinol, as allopurinol will reduce its effectiveness.
  - Allopurinol: 300mg, ideally at least 24 hours before and then during chemotherapy. This inhibits the enzyme xanthine oxidase and blocks the conversion of nucleic acids into uric acid. It does not affect pre-existing uric acid and therefore takes 1–3 days to start reducing uric acid levels. A small proportion of patients have severe allergic reactions.
- Aggressive hydration and diuresis: IV fluids, loop diuretics.
- Electrolyte monitoring: urea, creatinine, and electrolytes.

Treatment of established tumour lysis syndrome

- Vigorous hydration to maintain urine output of >100mL/m^2/hour
- High potassium levels (>5mmol/L)—use calcium gluconate and loop diuretics, e.g. furosemide 40mg twice daily.
- Use rasburicase, as described in ➔ Prevention of renal failure and elecrolyte imbalance, p. 650.
- High phosphate levels (>1.45mmol/L)—use aluminium-containing antacids every 4–6 hours (may need laxatives due to constipating effect).
- High uric acid levels. Consider switching from allopurinol to rasburicase. Continue other preventative methods, as described in ➔ Prevention of renal failure and elecrolyte imbalance, p. 650.
- Some patients require intensive nursing support of any symptoms, e.g. nausea and vomiting, diarrhoea, muscle cramps, flank pain, and confusion.
- If the electrolyte imbalance continues to worsen (e.g. potassium levels >6mmol/L), haemodialysis may be required.
- Only use alkalinization if rasburicase is not available and the patient is severaly acidotic.

Further reading

Coiffier B, Altman A, Pui Ching-Hon, *et al.* Guidelines for the management of pediatric and adult tumor lysis syndrome: an evidence-based review. *J Clin Oncol* 2008;26:2767–78.

Acute Oncology Services

One of the most exciting developments within cancer care in the UK in the last 5 years has been the extending provision of Acute Oncology Services. From no acute oncology specialist nurse posts in 2010, by 2014, there were 154 whole-time equivalent nurses in post. This accounts for 7% of the total specialist cancer nursing workforce. There has been an accompanying increase in the number of oncologists who have acute oncology as one of their named specialties.

Background to Acute Oncology Services

In 2008, the National Confidential Enquiry into Patient Outcomes and Death (NCEPOD) reported on the fragmented and variable nature of care experienced by patients with a cancer diagnosis who were admitted via emergency departments across England.

In 2009, the National Cancer Advisory Group (NCAG 2009) published a report highlighting the rapid increase in chemotherapy treatments in recent years, but also the inconsistency in the care of patients who were admitted with chemotherapy-related problems (such as neutropenic sepsis or chemotherapy-induced diarrhoea). This showed that hospitals frequently failed to care for them effectively when they became unwell. NCAG recommended that each hospital admitting acutely unwell cancer patients should have an Acute Oncology Service, through which patients could be reviewed by a consultant oncologist within 24 hours of referral. Each Acute Oncology Service would be staffed by oncologists and specialist nurses, have a multidisciplinary steering group, and also provide education on the management of acute oncological presentations.

Evidence from pilot studies of Acute Oncology Services suggests that early review by an oncologist can reduce cancer patients' length of stay after emergency admissions.

Considerable variations in both the management and outcome of MSCC were also highlighted, and these could also be addressed, in part, by Acute Oncology Services.

In practice, patients seen by Acute Oncology Services tend to fall into three categories:

- Those on treatment who have severe side effects as a result of SACT, e.g. neutropenic sepsis, chemotherapy-induced nausea and vomiting, radiotherapy skin reactions
- Patients who have extension of an existing cancer or have become unwell as a result of their disease, e.g. MSCC, new brain or bone metastases
- Patients who have been admitted acutely and found to have a new diagnosis of cancer. These patients tend to be older, come from a more socially deprived background, and have poorer prognoses than patients who present in a less chaotic fashion. This is particularly true of patients who present with a CUP (➲ see Chapter 25, Cancer of unknown primary).

Models of delivery

There are currently wide variations and different models used to provide Acute Oncology Services across the UK. These range from nurse-led models, with little input from oncology doctors, to services with full coverage of medical and nursing staff.

Characteristics of effective Acute Oncology Services

- Patients reviewed within 24 hours of referral by a consultant oncologist.
- Automated, or at least very easy, referral mechanisms for patients admitted with cancer-related problems.
- Effective protocols for the management of neutropenic sepsis and other oncological emergencies.
- Good links with palliative care services.
- Can improve the care for patients found to have a CUP by reducing delays in diagnostics.
- Good audit information on key performance indicators, e.g. time to antibiotics in patients with suspected neutropenic sepsis and length of stay for patients referred to the service.
- Access to oncology triage beds, so patients can be assessed within the specialty and discharged where appropriate.
- Equal access to the service, regardless of which environment the patient is admitted into.

24-hour advice service

Another previously problematic area which has fallen under the auspices of 'acute oncology' is that of 24-hour emergency advice for oncology patients receiving SACT. Although all centres and units treating cancer patients have had to have a 24-hour emergency advice line in place for patients for some years, there has been variation in the quality of advice given. Out-of-hours calls overnight or on weekends may be routed through to less experienced nurses on the oncology ward who may not be able to effectively triage patients.

In order to address this, the United Kingdom Oncology Nursing Society (UKONS) developed a triage tool. This leads the telephone triage through a number of questions scored green, amber, or red, depending on the response. One red score will lead to the patient being advised to attend hospital for assessment; two ambers or more are equal to a red score and the same advice is given. A single amber score means the patient will be contacted the next day, or within 24 hours, to make sure all is well.

This simple toolkit has been very effective in providing consistent advice and has now been employed successfully throughout many cancer environments and has been very well evaluated.

The role of the nurse in Acute Oncology Services

Acute Oncology Services offer many opportunities for expanded practice to specialist cancer nurses, with many acute trusts choosing to invest in nurses to coordinate and deliver Acute Oncology Services, rather than medical colleagues. The reasons for this are both financial and logistical, but in many environments, e.g. cancer units, it has proved difficult for visiting oncologists to provide a daily review of patients when they may be covering a wide geographical area.

There are a range of skills, competencies, and nursing experience that are valuable when working in Acute Oncology Services:

- >5 years' experience in oncology nursing
- SACT experience valuable
- Experience of audit work
- Advanced communication qualification
- Non-medical prescribing valuable
- Clinical examination skills.

Nurses employed within Acute Oncology Services tend to be experienced oncology practitioners who are able to work autonomously, whilst assessing patients and monitoring the service. This profile is reflected in the grading of these posts, with 88% of acute oncology nurses in England being employed at band 7 or above (in comparison with breast CNS at 74% and colorectal CNS at 79%).

There are currently very few courses aimed specifically at nurses wishing to develop acute oncology skills. It is hoped that more specialist courses will be developed nationally.

Impact of acute oncology

Despite the specialty being in its infancy, studies that have been carried out seem to indicate that Acute Oncology Services can:

- Improve the care of patients presenting with neutropenic sepsis
- Reduce the length of hospital stay in patients with a cancer diagnosis admitted as an emergency
- Improve the care of patients who present with a CUP
- Improve the quality of patient care in general for oncology patients.

Further reading

Anglia Cancer Network (2013). *Competencies Framework for the Acute Oncology Service (AOS) Clinical Specialist*. Available at: ℘ http://www.angcn.nhs.uk/search/

Macmillan Cancer Support (2014). *Specialist Adult Cancer Nurses in England: A Census of the Specialist Adult Cancer Workforce in the UK*. Available at: ℘ http://www.macmillan.org.uk/documents/aboutus/research/researchandevaluationreports/macmillan-census-report-england.pdf

National Peer Review programme (2011). *Manual for Cancer Services: Acute Oncology - Including Metatastic Spinal Cord Compression Measures*. Available at: ℘ https://www.gov.uk/government/publications/manual-for-cancer-services-acute-oncology-including-metatastic-spinal-cord-compression-measures

Index

Figures, tables and boxes are indicated by an italic *f*, *t* or *b* following the page number.